Questions for the
MRCS vivas

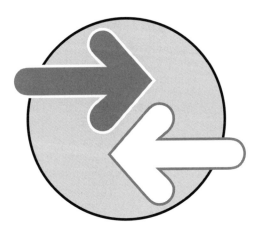

Jeff Garner MRCS (Glasg) MRCS (Ed)
Specialist Registrar in General Surgery in the Defence Medical Services, UK

Peter Goodfellow FRCSI
Specialist Registrar in General Surgery, Sheffield Teaching Hospitals, Sheffield, UK

Hodder Arnold

A MEMBER OF THE HODDER HEADLINE GROUP

A member of the Hodder Headline Group
LONDON

First published in Great Britain in 2004 by
Arnold, a member of the Hodder Headline Group,
338 Euston Road, London NW1 3BH

http://www.hoddereducation.com

Distributed in the United States of America by
Oxford University Press Inc.,
198 Madison Avenue, New York, NY10016
Oxford is a registered trademark of Oxford University Press

Whilst the advice and information in this book are believed to be true and
accurate at the date of going to press, neither the author[s] nor the publisher
can accept any legal responsibility or liability for any errors or omissions
that may be made. In particular (but without limiting the generality of the
preceding disclaimer) every effort has been made to check drug dosages;
however it is still possible that errors have been missed. Furthermore,
dosage schedules are constantly being revised and new side-effects
recognized. For these reasons the reader is strongly urged to consult the
drug companies' printed instructions before administering any of the drugs
recommended in this book.

British Library Cataloguing in Publication Data
A catalogue record for this book is available from the British Library

Library of Congress Cataloging-in-Publication Data
A catalog record for this book is available from the Library of Congress

ISBN-10: 0 340 812923
ISBN-13: 978 0 340 81292 1

2 3 4 5 6 7 8 9 10

Commissioning Editor: Clare Christian
Development Editor: Heather Smith
Project Editor: Zelah Pengilley
Production Controller: Lindsay Smith
Cover Design: Amina Dudhia

Typeset in 10.5/13 Berling Roman by Charon Tec Pvt. Ltd, Chennai, India
Printed and bound in Malta

What do you think about this book? Or any other Arnold title?
Please send your comments to www.hoddereducation.co.uk

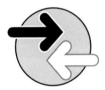

Contents

Foreword

The term 'viva' immediately conjures up the terrifying picture of a confrontational experience facing two examiners across the 'green-baize' table. Indeed, in the past, this was not far from the truth, with pots of ancient specimens swimming in somewhat murky and equally ancient formalin sitting ominously in front of the apprehensive candidate. Fortunately, attitudes have now changed but, even in this so-called enlightened era, the prospect of the MRCS 'viva' can still engender sentiments of fear, concern and apprehension. However, the well-prepared candidate should now find the 'viva' more of an interesting dialogue between two colleagues and, although still an ordeal, it can even be quite enjoyable. The secret of this truth is to be found in the term 'well prepared'. This book is, therefore, a 'godsend' to all MRCS candidates, as it is not only a revision tool, but helps them to formulate their answers and think how they are going to present their knowledge.

The 'vivas' in the MRCS are somewhat arbitrarily divided into:

→ applied surgical anatomy with operative surgery
→ applied physiology and critical care
→ clinical pathology with principles of surgery.

The authors have taken each of these areas of surgery, which inevitably overlap as clinical surgery cannot be so simplistically divided up, and addressed the 'hot' topics as currently being addressed in this examination. They have taken topics that have been asked in recent examinations, phrased them as questions, and then presented the answers in a clear and unambiguous manner. Inevitably, many of the answers have been expanded to allow the reader to use this as a revision book as well as for 'viva' practice. However, there is no doubt that, if candidates knew what is presented in this book, the 'vivas' would hold no threat or fear. Indeed, I can see examiners getting hold of a copy and using it to refresh their own knowledge!

The authors are ideally suited to provide such insight and information having successfully negotiated the hurdle recently and, therefore, have first-hand experience, which they are now imparting to their colleagues. They have done this well and efficiently and, although the book cannot be considered as a surgical textbook, its coverage and contents are far reaching and comprehensive without being exhaustive. It is not pretentious but entirely fulfils its intended objective, and that is to provide MRCS candidates with examples of questions that they may encounter and suggests a way in which each may be answered.

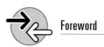

I wish all who read this volume the very best of success as they face the 'vivas' and may they enjoy them.

WEG Thomas BSc FRCS MS

Consultant Surgeon and Clinical Director, Sheffield Teaching Hospitals Trust
Member of Council and Surgical Skills Tutor of the Royal College of Surgeons of England
Past member of the Court of Examiners of the Royal College of Surgeons of England and of the Intercollegiate Board of Examiners in General Surgery

Preface

This book was born out of the frustration of one of the authors at the lack of suitable revision material for preparation for the viva voce section of the MRCS/AFRCS examination. The book itself does not pretend to be a textbook of any type, nor does it try to cover every possible topic; it is purely a revision aid, which demonstrates the types of subjects and questions that are commonly asked at MRCS/AFRCS vivas. It is envisaged that the book will help prospective candidates prepare for the examination and at the same time provide an additional source of information on some topics.

The two authors both qualified from Sheffield University and entered higher surgical training after a wide range of basic training. Jeff Garner is a Specialist Registrar in General Surgery in the Defence Medical Services. He has a wide experience of viva voce examinations, and holds the diploma of Membership from the two Scottish Colleges. Peter Goodfellow is a Specialist Registrar in General Surgery on the North Trent rotation based in Sheffield. He holds the diploma of FRCS. He has taught a local viva revision course twice yearly for FRCS/MRCS/AFRCS for over 5 years, which has a pass rate of over 90 per cent. Both authors maintain an interest in medical education and teach extensively, both undergraduates and junior surgeons preparing for the MRCS/AFRCS examinations.

JPG
PBG
Sheffield 2004

Acknowledgements

We would like to acknowledge the help of our many clinical colleagues who gave help and support during the writing of this book, and for answering our many enquiries to ensure the factual content is correct. We thank all the patients who have consented to allow inclusion of clinical photographs and radiographs. We are grateful to Ian Greaves for his help in the preparatory stages of this book, and his kind assistance in helping us find a publisher, which leads us to Clare Christian and Georgina Bentliff at Hodder Arnold, to whom we are indebted for their help and guidance in negotiating this, our first foray into the world of publishing.

We wish to thank the following for their help obtaining clinical material: Mr K Wembridge, Dr N Morse, Dr C Robb, Dr M Payne, Dr S Cockayne, Miss L Wylde, Mr C Stoddard, Mr S Kohlhardt, Dr M Collins, Mr DJ Gerrard, Mr BSI Montgomery and The Department of Military Surgery, Royal Defence Medical College. Kate Nardoni of Cactus Design also deserves special mention for producing the many splendid illustrations that add so much to this book. Finally, we would like to acknowledge and thank our wives for their unstinting support while we neglected both them and our children to spend our free time working on this book.

JPG
PBG
Sheffield 2004

Abbreviations

AAA	abdominal aortic aneurysm
AC	alternating current
ACE	angiotensin-converting enzyme
ACTH	adrenocorticotrophic hormone
ADH	antidiuretic hormone
ALG	anti-lymphocyte globulin
APACHE	Acute Physiology and Chronic Health Evaluation
APTT	activated partial thromboplastin time
ARDS	adult respiratory distress syndrome
5-ASA	5-aminosalicylic acid
ASG	American Gastroenterology Society
ASIS	anterior superior iliac spine
AST	aspartate aminotransferase
AXR	abdominal x-ray
BCC	basal cell carcinoma
BCG	bacille Calmette–Guérin
BKA	below-knee amputation
BMI	body mass index
BP	blood pressure
BSG	British Society of Gastroenterology
CBF	cerebral blood flow
CHI	Commission for Health Improvement
CIS	carcinoma *in situ*
CMV	continuous mandatory ventilation
COPD	chronic obstructive pulmonary disease
COX	cyclo-oxygenase
CPAP	continuous positive airway pressure
CPD	continuing professional development
CPP	cerebral perfusion pressure
CRC	colorectal cancer
CREST	Calcinosis, Raynaud's phenomenon, oEsophageal motility disorders, Sclerodactyly and Telangectasia
CRH	corticotrophin-releasing hormone
CRP	C-reactive protein
CSF	cerebrospinal fluid
CT	computed tomography
CVP	central venous pressure
CXR	chest x-ray

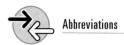

DHS	dynamic hip screw
DIC	disseminated intravascular coagulation
DMSA	dimercaptosuccinic acid
DOPA	dihydroxyphenylalanine
DPG	2,3-diphosphoglycerate
DTPA	diethylenetriamine penta-acetic acid
DVT	deep vein thrombosis
ECF	extracellular fluid
ECG	electrocardiogram
EMD	electromechanical dissociation
EMLA	eutectic mixture of local anaesthetics
ER	oestrogen receptor
ERCP	endoscopic retrograde cholangiopancreatography
FAP	familial adenomatous polyposis
FBC	full blood count
FFP	fresh-frozen plasma
FiO_2	concentration of inspired oxygen
FNAC	fine-needle aspiration cytology
FRC	functional residual capacity
FSH	follicle-stimulating hormone
GCS	Glasgow Coma Scale
GFR	glomerular filtration rate
GH	growth hormone
HAFOE	high air flow oxygen entrainment
Hb	haemoglobin
HCG	human chorionic gonadotrophin
HDU	high-dependency unit
HIV	human immunodeficiency virus
HRT	hormone replacement therapy
HTR	haemolytic transfusion reaction
HU	Hounsfield unit
ICP	intracranial pressure
IDDM	insulin-dependent diabetes mellitus
IGTN	ingrowing toenail
ILs	interleukins
IM	intramuscular
INR	international normalized ratio
IPPV	intermittent positive pressure ventilation
ITU	intensive treatment unit
IV	intravenous
IVC	inferior vena cava
IVU	intravenous urogram

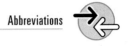

JVP	jugular venous pressure
LATS	long-acting thyroid-stimulating hormone
LDH	lactate dehydrogenase
LFT	liver function tests
LH	luteinizing hormone
LHRH	luteinizing hormone-releasing hormone
LMA	laryngeal mask airway
LSV	long saphenous vein
MALT	mucosa-associated lymphoid tissue
MAP	mean arterial pressure
MCPJ	metacarpophalangeal joint
MEN	multiple endocrine neoplasia
MIBG	^{123}I-metaiodobenzylguanidine
MMA	middle meningeal artery
MODS	multiorgan dysfunction syndrome
MRCP	magnetic resonance cholangiopancreatogram
MRI	magnetic resonance imaging
MSH	melanocyte-stimulating hormone
NBM	nil by mouth
NdYAG	neodymium, yttrium, aluminium, garnet
NICE	National Institute for Clinical Excellence
NIDDM	non-insulin-dependent diabetes mellitus
NPI	Nottingham Prognostic Index
NSAIDs	non-steroidal anti-inflammatory drugs
ODP	Operating Department Practitioner
OGD	oesophagogastro duodenoscopy
OPSI	overwhelming post-splenectomy infection
PAFC	pulmonary artery flotation catheter
PCA	patient-controlled analgesia
PCV	packed cell volume
PDS	polydiaxanone suture
PE	pulmonary embolus
PEEP	positive end expiratory pressure
PEFR	peak expiratory flow rate
PIC	peripherally inserted central (line)
PIPJ	proximal interphalangeal joint
POSSUM	Physiological and Operative Severity Score for the enUmeration of Mortality and morbidity
PR	per rectum
PSV	pressure support ventilation
PTH	parathyroid hormone
RRT	renal replacement therapy

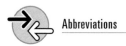

RTA	renal tubular acidosis
SAA	serum amyloid A
SCC	squamous cell carcinoma
SFJ	saphenofemoral junction
SIADH	syndrome of inappropriate anti-diuretic hormone secretion
SIMV	synchronized intermittent mandatory ventilation
SIRS	systemic inflammatory response syndrome
SLE	systemic lupus erythematosus
SSG	split skin graft
SUFE	slipped upper femoral epiphysis
SVC	superior vena cava
SVR	systemic vascular resistance
TCC	transitional cell carcinoma
TENS	transcutaneous electrical nerve stimulation
TIPS	transjugular intrahepatic portosystemic shunting
TPN	total parenteral nutrition
TRAM flap	transverse rectus abdominis myocutaneous flap
TSH	thyroid-stimulating hormone
TURP	transurethral resection of prostrate
U&E	urea and electrolytes
UICC	Union Internationale Contrele Cancer
USS	ultrasound scan
UTI	urinary tract infection
VMA	vanillyl mandelic acid
vWF	von Willebrands factor
WCC	white cell count
WLE	wide local excision

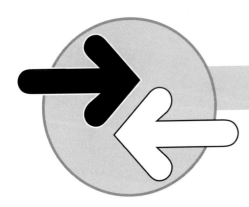

SECTION ONE

INTRODUCTION

This book is designed to help in preparation for the MRCS/AFRCS viva voce examination by providing a series of practice vivas specifically written to reproduce the flowing style a candidate will encounter in the actual examination.

Organization of the book

The book is organized into six sections representing each of the six broad areas defined by the Royal Colleges in the surgical syllabus. The sections are:

→ applied physiology
→ critical care
→ operative surgery
→ surgical anatomy
→ clinical pathology
→ principles of surgery.

Each section covers 25 topics and each is dealt with in a similar manner. An initial question is followed by its answer, then a supplementary question often based on the preceding answer followed by its answer, and so on. This replicates most closely the actual style of the viva examination, where the discussion flows from one point to the next. Clinical material, including photographs, laboratory values and radiographs, has been used to make it as realistic as possible, since this is the practice of many examiners.

The questions have been drawn from feedback from a large number of candidates who have attended the examination at one of the four colleges. All the subjects covered in this book have, at one time or another, been asked in an actual viva examination.

It is hoped that these questions will be both a useful revision aid and a stimulus for further reading. We have not attempted to cover the entire surgical syllabus but have included a representative sample of questions. There are numerous topics that have not been covered, some of which may seem to be surprising omissions, but in a book of this type there simply isn't room to include everything. We have included some historical and biographical notes on eponyms; they are not specifically examined and a candidate cannot be penalized for not knowing such details, but we think they add interest to the toil of revision and may allow a candidate to demonstrate an interest in surgery beyond the scientific.

While making no attempt to be a surgical textbook, each answer contains as much information as possible. Owing to the structured nature of the actual viva examinations, many answers will contain far more information than any single candidate will be expected to reproduce, let alone have sufficient time in which to do so. Although the candidate is likely to be asked only some parts of the whole question as written here, each component of every question could be examined, hence the fullness of each answer. In addition, there is some overlap between topics and chapters, which again replicates the style of the actual vivas. A discussion in the surgical anatomy viva on the femoral canal may easily stray into the surgical approaches and techniques of femoral hernia repair. The answers in this book have copied this style in many areas by including relevant information from more than one section in individual answers. This has allowed presentation of the maximum amount of information in the space available without unnecessary repetition.

It is important to remember that there is often more than one correct answer and more than one correct way of performing an operation; different answers may be acceptable, providing that they are backed by an appropriate justification. In this book we have attempted to provide a generally accepted answer to all the questions and avoid areas of contention, although inevitably some of these answers will be prejudiced by our own experiences, training and personal preferences. Similarly, we have become acutely aware that what we would regard as surgical fact, such as the incidence rates of disease and complications, may vary widely between different surgical reference books. Again, we have tried to avoid controversy and have quoted figures that we believe would be acceptable to the majority of surgeons in practice and examiners.

How to use this book

The topics in this book are set out in a sequential question and answer format, and should be used to identify areas of weakness and potentially act as a source of additional knowledge. This book could easily be used by an individual working through each question and resisting the temptation to look at subsequent answers; alternatively, it could form the basis of practice vivas for use in a revision group. Answering a selection of questions from each chapter at each revision session may sustain interest for longer than doggedly working through the book from start to finish.

Certain key phrases have been highlighted in the text using **bold** type and an arrow logo. Within the context of that particular question, examiners will expect to hear these phrases and their use will demonstrate to them that you understand the crux of the issue under discussion. It should be noted, however, that mere regurgitation of the phrase without understanding is less impressive and may lead to embarrassing silences as your parrot learning is exposed. Every effort should be made to use these key phrases within a well thought out response.

Format of the examination at each college

The format of the viva examination varies slightly between colleges and the following descriptions are only guidelines. Candidates are advised to confirm with their college the dates and requirements of the relevant examinations. In the examination, each viva generally consists of questions on three separate subject areas, asked in a structured manner, to avoid a candidate being unduly penalized on a topic about which they have little knowledge. Questions regarding each topic may proceed for a variable amount of time but seldom more than 5–6 minutes is devoted to any one subject.

Royal College of Surgeons of England

The viva examinations are held twice a year in June and December at the College in London. There are six vivas, each of 10 minutes duration, organized into pairs:

→ applied physiology and critical care
→ clinical pathology and principles of surgery
→ applied surgical anatomy and operative surgery.

There are two examiners for each pair. In the first viva, one examiner will ask the questions, while the other takes notes on the candidate's answers. After 10 minutes, the candidate is asked to withdraw while the examiners confer, after which the candidate returns, usually to a different table, and a second examiner conducts the second half of the viva pairing. In the operative surgery viva, there is a third examiner present to allow scrutiny of the candidate's surgical logbook. In the surgical anatomy viva, the candidate may be taken to prosections or live patients to demonstrate certain features. A large lecture room is allocated for candidates to relax in between the pairs of vivas and candidates may use the college library. The three viva pairs may be spread over the course of the entire day, so there may be a lengthy gap between examinations. At the end of the day, candidates are invited to congregate within the college and the examination numbers of the successful candidates are announced.

Royal College of Surgeons of Edinburgh

The viva examinations are held twice a year, in April and September, in the College in Edinburgh. There are three vivas, each of 20 minutes duration, on the following areas:

→ critical care
→ principles of surgery, including operative surgery and applied anatomy
→ clinical surgery and pathology.

As in London, candidates are examined by a pair of examiners, one examining each 'half' of the viva; the candidate remains at the same station throughout the viva. The candidate may be presented with clinical photographs, radiographs, pathology 'pots' or plastinated specimens. All vivas are completed in one half-day and the list of successful candidates is posted in the College entrance hall the following morning.

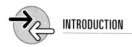
Royal College of Physicians and Surgeons of Glasgow

The viva examinations are held twice a year, in April and September, in Glasgow. There are two half hour vivas:

→ applied anatomy/operative surgery and practice of surgery
→ applied pathology/bacteriology and critical care/surgical physiology.

There are two examiners for each viva. In the applied anatomy section, the candidate may be taken around a series of specimens, radiographs and laboratory reports displayed on a central table within the examination hall. Vivas are completed over the course of the whole day and a list of successful candidates posted in the College entrance hall that evening.

Royal College of Surgeons in Ireland

The viva examinations are held twice a year, in February and October. There are three 20-minute vivas on each of:

→ principles of operative surgery and surgical anatomy
→ critical care, surgical emergencies and applied physiology
→ surgical management and principles of pathology.

Two examiners examine each viva. One of each pair of examiners will be a basic science examiner. At the examination, the operative surgery and surgical anatomy viva will be held in the anatomy department, when both prosections and live patient models may be shown. The other vivas are held consecutively on opposite sides of a large hall. A candidate will sit one viva, and after 20 minutes will immediately swap sides of the hall and sit the remaining viva. The anatomy and operative surgery viva may be before or after the paired vivas. The results will usually be posted in the college foyer the evening of the last vivas or occasionally the following morning in case of a late finish (dependent on the number of candidates). The surgical logbook is not a requirement for this examination.

Presentation of a completed and up-to-date surgical logbook is a requirement of the examination in London, Edinburgh and Glasgow.

Examination technique

As in most areas of surgery, there is no single 'correct' way of succeeding in a viva voce examination but there are several general principles that merit consideration.

→ *Presentation.* Dress smartly in a jacket and tie, or suit if you have one; women should wear an equivalent conservative outfit. Hair should be well kept; men are advised that long hair and designer stubble are generally poorly received. Adopt a neutral body posture; sit up straight with hands folded on your lap or resting on your knees – this also helps to disguise tremors!

→ *Be polite.* Respect the examiners, who by definition are the senior members of our profession and holders of the status to which you aspire.

→ *Do not argue.* If an examiner clearly holds an opposing view to you, do not labour the point and demur gracefully. Under no circumstances should you enter into an argument with the examiner.

→ *Accuracy.* Be sure to answer the question you were asked, rather than either the question you *thought they would ask* or the one you would *want to answer.* Do not mention rarities first. Do not include 'extra' information, which may open a route of enquiry you did not want to get into, unless you are confident that this is to your advantage. You may occasionally be able to 'lead' your examiner into an area in which you are particularly confident by this tactic, but it is a high-risk strategy.

→ *Confidence.* Try to be confident and authoritative when answering, particularly when describing what *you* would do in a given situation. There is nothing wrong with pausing to collect your thoughts before answering: it shows you are rational and not intimidated.

→ *Honesty.* If you have never actually performed the procedure you are describing, it will be evident to the examiner. If you say you haven't done it before, but that you know how it is done and can describe it, then it will be apparent you have revised well. A useful introductory phrase is '… **although I have never seen this operation before, I understand that the principles are …**'. Never guess or lie. You will be found out and examiners take an exceedingly dim view of a candidate who is untrustworthy.

→ *Safety.* The examiners are looking for a safe surgeon, so ensure you do not describe anything that would put a patient at risk. Think clinically and describe what *you* would do in a particular clinical scenario if you were on the ward during the course of your normal 'on-call' duties. Another useful phrase worth remembering is '… **I would call for senior help while proceeding with my initial management …**'.

Revision for the examination

The vivas can be an intimidating experience and it is important that you have a good knowledge base, can think clearly, and can vocalize your thoughts in a clear and logical manner. Practice at viva technique is essential and can make a huge difference to your performance at the critical moment. Some aspects can be practised alone, such as describing how you would perform a particular operation; whereas other facets are best practised in a group, such as discussion of different hernia repair techniques. Whatever their personal preference, candidates should take every opportunity to practise their viva

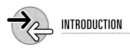

technique, whether in theatre with a senior colleague or in a revision group with their peers.

In many hospitals, small group teaching is available prior to the exam, usually by a few individuals interested in teaching, some of whom may even be examiners. It is well worth joining any such group locally, or even approaching clinicians to try and establish one. There are also likely to be colleagues who have recently taken the exam, and any information they can offer is useful. Find out as much as you can about other people's experiences, since this equips you with a better idea about what it might be like for you, and raises additional topics to think about prior to the exam.

It is also worth reading the current surgical journals to keep up to date with recent advances in surgery – but be selective, as you won't have time to read every journal from cover to cover and continue with your normal revision programme.

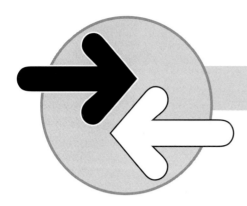

APPLIED PHYSIOLOGY

1. AUTOREGULATION

What is autoregulation and give an example of it at work?

Autoregulation is the ability of an organ to maintain a constant blood flow over a wide range of mean arterial pressures within certain limits. It is seen in the heart and kidney but is best demonstrated by examining cerebral blood flow.

Cerebral perfusion pressure (CPP)
= Mean arterial pressure (MAP)
– [intracranial pressure (ICP) + central venous pressure (CVP)]

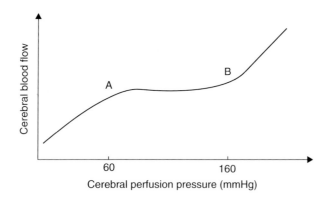

Figure 2.1 The brain autoregulation curve.

This curve (Figure 2.1) shows that, up to a CPP of 60 mmHg (point A), an increase of pressure will increase cerebral blood flow (CBF). Between pressures of 60 and 160 mmHg (A to B), any increase in CPP does not result in alteration of CBF but, with a CPP of over 160 mmHg, the blood flow increases with pressure again.

Draw the brain compliance curve and explain what it means in practical terms

See Figure 2.2. As volume increases, compensation occurs so that almost no rise in intracranial pressure (ICP) follows (A to B on the curve). This works up to a critical point (C), after which even a small increase in volume causes a rapid rise in ICP (C to D).

How do you manage a patient with raised intracranial pressure after closed head injury?

The Munro–Kelly doctrine points out that the cranium is a fixed-volume box, the contents of which – brain, CSF and blood – are not compressible. Rises in

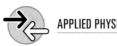

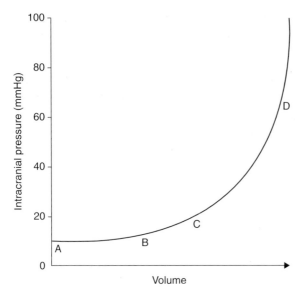

Figure 2.2 The brain compliance curve.

volume cause a rapid rise in ICP at that point on the compliance curve. The brain constitutes 85 per cent of the intracranial volume but is the least amenable to manipulation of its volume. CSF represents 10 per cent and blood, the most accessible, 5 per cent. The following measures all aim to reduce the volume of one or other of the three contents of the box, and thus protect adequate cerebral oxygen delivery:

→ Posture – 15° of head up tilt will reduce venous congestion. The avoidance of venous obstruction also helps, such as keeping the head central without tapes or lines around the neck.
→ Ventilation – protection of the airway and maintenance of good oxygenation are essential. Avoid hypercarbia as CO_2 is a potent vasodilator, which at first seems like a good idea in order to maintain cerebral oxygen delivery, but the increased blood volume actually increases ICP and is counterproductive. Aim for low normal CO_2 levels.
→ Mannitol – an osmotic diuretic. It increases colloid osmotic pressure, and draws water into the vascular space and is a potent free-radical scavenger. It causes a decrease in CSF production and causes a reduction in blood viscosity, allowing increased CBF. Too much mannitol, however, may cause a rebound phenomenon, as the leaky capillaries allow mannitol into the interstitium reversing the colloid gradient.
→ Steroids are only useful when dealing with organized masses, such as tumours and the inflammatory reaction that accompanies them. They are not indicated in closed head injury.

→ CSF drainage – placement of an intraventricular catheter not only allows accurate measurement of ICP, thus allowing calculation of cerebral perfusion pressure, but allows therapeutic drainage.

Whilst these measures are aimed at ensuring adequate O_2 delivery, the patient will also be helped by decreasing O_2 demand. Thus a sedated well-analgesed patient with adequate anti-epileptic prophylaxis will have lower oxygen demands than an awake, anxious, fitting patient. Similarly, surface cooling will reduce the overall metabolic requirements.

2. CATECHOLAMINES

Describe the synthesis and metabolism of catecholamines

Catecholamines are synthesized by chromaffin cells of the adrenal medulla and sympathetic nervous tissue; both are derived from embryonic neural crest. Adrenaline is predominantly produced in the adrenal medulla and noradrenaline in the sympathetic tissue. The pathway begins by hydroxylation of tyrosine to dihydroxyphenylalanine (DOPA) followed by decarboxylation to dopamine. This is further hydroxylated to noradrenaline and then methylated to adrenaline.

They are metabolized in the liver by further methylation and then deamination into vanillyl mandelic acid (VMA), which is excreted in the urine. Urinary VMA and metanephrines may be measured.

How might an excess of catecholamines present clinically?

Catecholamine excess, as in phaeochromocytoma, presents with hypertension as the commonest symptom, which is paroxysmal in 50 per cent of patients. Other symptoms include sweating and flushing, and there is often hyperglycaemia. Phaeochromocytoma is known as the 10 per cent tumour because 10 per cent of all tumours are extra-adrenal, bilateral, malignant, familial or occur in children.

How is the diagnosis confirmed?

The presence of excess circulating catecholamines is confirmed by raised urinary VMA and metanephrines (adrenaline, noradrenaline and dopamine) in a 24-hour urine collection. After the diagnosis is established, the tumour must be localized and magnetic resonance imaging (MRI) scanning is now established as the procedure of choice, since functioning and non-functioning adrenal tumours have different characteristics on MRI, unlike computed tomography (CT). In addition, the need for contrast, which may trigger a hypertensive crisis, is avoided in MRI scanning. If the tumour is not localized by MRI, then MIBG (^{123}I-metaiodobenzylguanidine) scanning is both sensitive and specific for localization of phaeochromocytoma.

What considerations need to be taken into account before embarking on surgery in these instances?

Operating for phaeochromocytoma is not for the occasional surgeon or faint-hearted anaesthetist. Inadvertent handling of the tumour can stimulate an enormous outpouring of catecholamines; even induction of anaesthesia in the unprepared patient can have the same effect. The patient must be fully α and β blocked before surgery. The long-acting α blocker phenoxybenzamine is used, along with a β blocker, such as propranolol. The timing of β blockade is not critical, but the α blockade requires careful optimization. The patient is started on phenoxybenzamine 7–10 days before surgery, and the dose increased until hypertension is controlled and the patient develops orthostatic hypotension. The surgery itself is now routinely performed laparoscopically for tumours less than 6 cm. The approach is most commonly transabdominal but smaller tumours can be removed endoscopically by a posterior retroperitoneal approach. After removal of the tumour, the patient's venous tone may disappear altogether, causing a massive relative hypovolaemia. Thus the anaesthetist should be warned when removal of the tumour is imminent in order to maximize the circulating volume.

Might it be associated with other conditions?

Ten per cent of phaeochromocytomas are familial, associated with the multiple endocrine neoplasia (MEN) syndrome Type II, sometimes referred to as Sipple's syndrome. The other components of MEN II are hyperparathyroidism, which may be due to either parathyroid adenoma or hyperplasia, and thyroid medullary carcinoma. The condition is autosomal dominant with the genetic defect located on chromosome 10. A further variant, MEN IIb, encompasses these same abnormalities, but demonstrates mucosal neuromatosis, marfanoid habitus and musculoskeletal abnormalities in addition.

What is the prognosis for patients with malignant phaeochromocytoma?

Overall, 10 per cent of phaeochromocytomas are malignant, but 50 per cent of all extra-adrenal phaeochromocytomas are malignant. MIBG scanning is useful to assess metastatic spread. Surgery is the mainstay of treatment as the tumours are unresponsive to chemotherapy; radiotherapy to bony metastases will provide local palliation. The 5-year survival is around 40 per cent.

J.H. Sipple (b. 1930): an American physician who described MEN II in his only publication on an endocrine subject.

3. ACID–BASE BALANCE

Interpret the arterial blood gas readings shown in Figure 2.3

Blood gas values	
pH	7.268
pO_2	24.3 kPa
pCO_2	5.05 kPa
Acid – base status	
cBase(Ecf)$_c$	−8.9 mmol/L
cHCO$_3^-$(P,st)$_c$	17.1 mmol/L
Electrolyte values	
cK^+	5.0 mmol/L
cNa^+	137 mmol/L
cCa^{2+}	1.16 mmol/L
cCl^-	115 mmol/L
Metabolite values	
cGlu	9.0 mmol/L
cLac	0.9 mmol/L
Oximetry values	
ctHb	5.3 g/dl
FO_2Hb	97.6 %
FMetHb	0.7 %
FHHb	0.5 %
Hct$_c$	16.8 %
FCOHb	1.2 %

Figure 2.3

- pH is $\log_{10} 1/[H^+]$ and is a measure of hydrogen ion concentration, i.e. acidity or alkalinity. Normal blood pH is 7.35–7.45.
- pO_2/pCO_2 measure the partial pressures of oxygen and carbon dioxide in the blood. They are affected by changes in respiratory function, and the pCO_2 is particularly affected by acidity, since H^+ ions will combine with CO_2 to form bicarbonate and water. Normal ranges are pO_2 10–13.3 kPa, and pCO_2 4.8–6.1 kPa.
- Standard bicarbonate is the amount of HCO_3^- in the sample when equilibrated at 37°C, pO_2 13.3 kPa, and pCO_2 5.3 kPa. Normal values are 22–30 mmol/L. Lower values imply a metabolic acidosis.

→ Base excess is the amount of acid or alkali that needs to be added to the sample at 37°C to achieve a pH of 7.4, with pO_2 13.3 kPa, and pCO_2 5.3 kPa. Positive base excess is an alkalosis and negative base excess is acidosis. Normal values are −2 to +2.

→ Tissues metabolizing glucose with an inadequate oxygen tension produce lactate. Lactate rises with decreased tissue perfusion or with tissue ischaemia. Normal values are less than 1.0 mmol/L.

This patient has a profound acute metabolic acidosis. The pH is low with a low bicarbonate and a significant base deficit. The pO_2 is high (this patient is receiving oxygen therapy) and the pCO_2 is in the normal range. Common potential causes of this picture are shock, renal failure and tissue ischaemia, such as ischaemic bowel.

How does the kidney handle bicarbonate ion?

Bicarbonate is freely filtered at the glomerulus and is resorbed by the renal tubular cells, but these cells are actually impermeable to bicarbonate. The mechanism of bicarbonate resorption is as follows: cellular hydrogen ion is exchanged through an ion transport mechanism with sodium in the filtrate. The H^+ combines with HCO_3^- forming H_2CO_3, which then dissociates into carbon dioxide and water. The carbon dioxide freely diffuses into the renal tubular cell whereupon it reforms H_2CO_3, catalysed by carbonic anhydrase and the sequence starts again. This works in a steady state but, if the kidney is presented with acid to excrete, then it must generate more bicarbonate.

Explain the role of phosphate and ammonium as urinary buffers

These come into play when the kidney has to excrete a hydrogen load. The hydrogen ion transported out of the cell in exchange for sodium combines with the phosphate ion, which is excreted in the urine. The conversion of cellular water and carbon dioxide, again catalysed by carbonic anhydrase, provides the stream of hydrogen ions for excretion and generates one molecule of bicarbonate each time. In the case of ammonium buffering, glutamine in the renal tubular cells splits into glutamate and ammonium ion, which further dissociates into ammonia and H^+. This hydrogen ion is incorporated into 2-oxyglutarate formed from the continued deamination of glutamine to form glucose and the ammonia couples with the free H^+ ion to be excreted as ammonium chloride.

Discuss renal tubular acidosis

Renal tubular acidosis (RTA) may be acquired or inherited, and both types are rare in adults. There are four types described. RTA Type I is a distal tubular defect and is often referred to as classical RTA. The luminal cells are abnormally permeable to H^+ and cannot establish an ion gradient across which the normal cellular mechanisms can excrete hydrogen ion. Type II RTA is a proximal tubular abnormality in which sodium bicarbonate cannot be resorbed proximally. This loss of bicarbonate leads to a systemic acidosis and excretion of bicarbonate in the urine. Type III is a combination of I and II, and is very rare indeed. Type IV is the condition of hyporeninaemic hypoaldosteronism and is commonly caused by non-steroidal anti-inflammatory drugs.

4. CALCIUM HOMEOSTASIS

Describe how calcium homeostasis is maintained

Calcium homeostasis is maintained by the interplay of three factors, namely, parathyroid hormone, calcitonin and activated vitamin D. Parathyroid hormone (PTH) is a single-chain polypeptide of 84 residues that stimulates the increased release of calcium and phosphate from bone. It also increases renal resorption of calcium but decreases resorption of phosphate. Its secretion depends on the free calcium ion concentration and is controlled by a negative feedback loop. The medullary C cells of the thyroid produce calcitonin, the actions of which oppose those of PTH on bone, but it is a relatively weak contributor to calcium homeostasis. Cholecalciferol is formed by the action of ultraviolet light on cholesterol derivatives in the skin. It is 25-hydroxylated in the liver before being further hydroxylated in the kidney. When serum calcium is low, it is 1-hydroxylated to activated 1,25-dihydrocholecalciferol, but when there is calcium excess, it is 24-hydroxylated to the inactive form, 24,25-dihydrocholecalciferol. Its production is stimulated by decreasing plasma phosphate concentrations and increases in PTH, oestrogen concentration, prolactin and growth hormone. It increases intestinal absorption of calcium and acts synergistically with PTH to mobilize calcium from bone.

What effect does an acidosis have on calcium?

Serum calcium is present both bound to albumin and in an unbound form. Hydrogen ions compete with calcium for the ion binding sites on albumin, thus an increase in hydrogen ion concentration – acidosis – will displace calcium, increasing the unbound fraction; in extreme cases, this may cause hypercalcaemia.

How do you 'correct' the serum calcium measurement and why?

As 45 per cent of serum calcium is albumin bound, the albumin concentration directly affects the total calcium concentration measured in plasma and variations in albumin concentration, and, therefore, total plasma calcium, may not accurately reflect the concentration of ionized calcium. It is variations in the plasma calcium ion content that give rise to symptoms, but unfortunately it is difficult to measure free calcium concentrations, so a standard correction is made to the total calcium concentration to account for variations in plasma protein. For each gram per litre the albumin concentration is below 40, the calcium concentration is increased by 0.02 mmol/L. An identical negative adjustment is made for albumin concentrations above 40 g/L.

Outline the causes and clinical presentation of hypercalcaemia

Raised serum calcium may be the result of a wide range of underlying pathologies. Malignancy is the commonest cause followed by increases in the concentration of parathyroid hormone, hyperparathyroidism, and these two causes are responsible for more than 90 per cent of all cases. Malignant neoplasms may elevate the calcium levels by direct osteolysis from secondary deposits or a primary tumour. Myeloma, for example, may mobilize skeletal calcium or may be a focus of ectopic PTH secretion, in common with other tumours, such as small cell lung cancer. Less common causes include thyrotoxicosis, Addison's disease, sarcoidosis, milk-alkali syndrome and familial hypocalcuric hypercalcaemia.

The clinical presentation is the classical student rhyme of 'bones, stones, abdominal groans and psychic moans'. Bone changes range from the florid pepper-pot skull to subtle subperisosteal erosions of the phalanges and commonly present with pain. The urinary tract is susceptible to recurrent stone formation and the patient may display polyuria, haematuria and hypertension from nephrocalcinosis. A variety of gastrointestinal symptoms are attributed to hypercalcaemia; certainly there is a higher incidence of peptic ulceration owing to the gastrin-stimulating action of calcium, and patients become prone to constipation and gallstones. Vague symptoms of lethargy and depression are evident in one-third of these patients.

Classify hyperparathyroidism

Hyperparathyroidism represents an increase in the concentration of circulating parathyroid hormone, and it may be classified as primary, secondary or tertiary.

→ *Primary hyperparathyroidism* occurs with excess PTH production, so PTH and serum calcium are both elevated. A total of 80 per cent of cases are due to a single adenomatous gland; generalized parathyroid hyperplasia accounts for a further 15 per cent of cases, while multiple adenomata are responsible in approximately 5 per cent. Parathyroid carcinoma may also be the cause of primarily elevated PTH but with an incidence of less than 1 in 100 cases.

→ *Secondary hyperparathyroidism* occurs when there is excess calcium loss, usually in renal failure. Calcium is normal or low, but PTH is raised in an attempt to increase calcium mobilization.

→ *Tertiary hyperparathyroidism* occurs in patients who have had their cause of secondary hyperparathyroidism treated, typically individuals whose renal failure was treated by transplantation. Although the stimulus has been removed, the parathyroids remain hyperplastic and secrete excess PTH, i.e. autonomously; both PTH and calcium are elevated.

Hyperparathyroidism may occur as part of the multiple endocrine neoplasia syndromes and, as such, may be familial with an autosomal dominant inheritance. Both parathyroid hyperplasia and adenoma are included in the disease, which is common to MEN types I and II.

How would you treat acute severe hypercalcaemia?

Hypercalcaemia has an enormous range of consequences, including renal tubular damage, peptic ulceration, hypertension, cardiac arrhythmias and bone pain. As an acute severe event the mainstay of therapy is volume repletion, as patients are usually markedly dehydrated. Frusemide will help to increase renal clearance. Biphosphonate infusion binds hydroxyapatite in bone and decreases bone turnover, after which attention must be turned to identifying the cause of the hypercalcaemia.

5. OXYGEN TRANSPORT

Describe the relationship that governs O$_2$ transport in the blood and draw the oxygen–haemoglobin dissociation curve

Ninety-nine per cent of oxygen is carried bound to haemoglobin with only 1 per cent carried in solution in plasma in proportion to the partial pressure. The relationship between partial pressure (oxygen tension) and percentage saturation is given by a sigmoid-shaped curve shown in Figure 2.4.

Point A is known as the p50 point and is the oxygen pressure at which haemoglobin (Hb) is 50 per cent saturated. It is important for two reasons: firstly, it helps to draw the curve and, secondly, it is often used to compare the effects of conditions that shift the curve to either the right or the left. 'B' is the normal mixed venous point and 'C' is the normal arterial point.

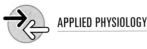

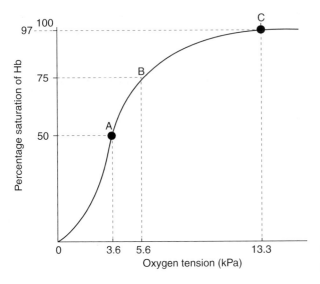

Figure 2.4 The oxyhaemo-globin dissociation curve.

Why is the curve shaped like it is?

It is a sigmoid curve because haemoglobin exhibits peculiar binding character-istics. Binding of one oxygen molecule to one haem molecule makes it easier for further binding to occur, which is represented by the steep mid-portion of the curve. It demonstrates large increases in percentage saturation for minimal increases in partial pressure, i.e. oxygenation of haemoglobin is relatively easy. This facilitation occurs until three out of four binding sites are occupied after which it gets slightly harder again, reflected by the curve flattening out at the higher saturations.

What conditions 'shift' the curve to the right and what is the practical significance of this?

Shifting the curve to the right represents a decrease in affinity in the Hb-O_2 binding, which in practical terms means that haemoglobin will offload oxygen more easily. Conditions that achieve this shift are increasing concentrations of CO_2, 2,3-diphosphoglycerate (DPG), acidity [H^+] and increasing temperature. These four conditions are found in the respiring cell, thus haemoglobin is most effective in offloading oxygen where it is most required.

What are the Bohr and Haldane effects?

The shift in the curve due to changing [H^+] is known as the Bohr effect and is due to binding effects with the imidazole groups of histidine. The Haldane effect describes the effect of the differing buffering capacities of CO_2 for both oxyhaemoglobin and deoxyhaemoglobin. At the cell, deoxyhaemoglobin has a high buffering capacity for CO_2 and accepts it readily. Once returned to the pulmonary circulation, the binding of oxygen converts it to oxyhaemoglobin, which has a low buffering capacity, and thus offloads CO_2 readily.

What do the curves for myoglobin, carbon monoxide and fetal haemoglobin look like?

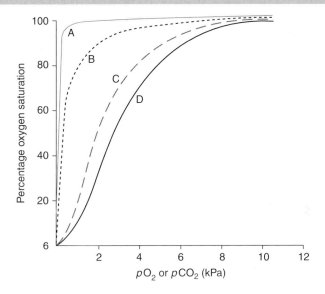

Figure 2.5 Oxygen dissociation curves for myoglobin, carboxyhaemoglobin and fetal haemoglobin. Curves: A, carboxyhaemoglobin (HbCO); B, myoglobin/oxygen (MbO_2); C, fetal oxyhaemoglobin (Hb_fO_2); D, adult oxyhaemoglobin (HbO_2).

See Figure 2.5. The implications are as follows. For myoglobin, it is positioned such that it will release its single molecule of oxygen only at low oxygen tensions, thus is not useful as a transport mechanism. Carbon monoxide has an avid affinity for haemoglobin, some 200 times that of oxygen: the molecule is saturated at even very low tensions of CO and is very difficult to displace. Fetal haemoglobin, which has δ instead of β globin moieties, has a left-shifted curve, increasing its affinity for oxygen at the lower tensions found in the fetus.

6. CARDIAC FUNCTION

What are the differences between the right and left ventricles?

Unsurprisingly, the differences between the two ventricles are a representation of their differing functions and requirements. The right ventricle's thin walls are a reflection of the low afterload, i.e. the low-pressure pulmonary circulation. It is able to cope with large changes in preload, one example being the changes in venous return between lying and standing. It is not, however, very good at coping with an increase in afterload, and rises in pulmonary pressure badly affect right heart function. The left ventricle, on the other hand, is thick walled because of the high afterload and, consequently, it can deal with changes in afterload relatively easily – but it is sensitive to changes in preload, i.e. it needs filling.

This description of the right ventricle explains some of the problems of ventilating asthmatics. To overcome the high airway pressures associated with intermittent positive pressure ventilation of an asthmatic, high pressures are needed. This will compress the pulmonary blood vessels, resulting in an increased right heart afterload. This, in turn, can lead to right heart failure in this group of patients.

What governs cardiac output?

Cardiac output is the product of heart rate and stroke volume, i.e. how much blood does the heart eject at each contraction and how many times a minute does it do it? Cardiac output is also related to the blood pressure (BP) and systemic vascular resistance (SVR) according to the equation:

$$BP = \frac{CO}{SVR}.$$

How can the contractility of the heart be described?

It is the amount of force generated for a given inotropic state. It is described by Starling curves that plot force generated against initial fibre length. A rise in the inotropic state will move the curve into a higher position, indicating greater contractility. It is an intrinsic property of the myocardium.

In the transplanted heart, does Starling's law apply? What is the resting heart rate?

Yes. Starling's law of the heart – 'force generated is proportional to initial fibre length' – is a local mechanosensitive mechanism that is intrinsic to the cardiac muscle fibres. The resting rate is about 80–90 beats per minute, which represents the intrinsic rate of the pacemakers without any vagal slowing.

How well does a cardiac transplant function? What is the rate of developing angina?

Postoperative function is usually good, enabling normal day-to-day activity. Survival rates are 90 per cent at 1 year and 70 per cent at 5 years. There is no angina, because by definition the transplanted heart has been completely disconnected from any nerves and, as such, there is no pain pathway to transmit the sensation of angina; that is not to say that coronary ischaemia does not occur.

What factors affect the working of the transplanted heart?

As stated, Starling's law still holds, as does the Bainbridge reflex (increased venous return causing right atrial distension, and sino-atrial node distension and a reflex increase in heart rate). Although separated from neural autonomic influences, the heart will respond to circulating catecholamines, and may mount a response to stress or exercise.

What is an inotrope? What do they do and give examples?

An inotrope is a substance that alters the inotropic state of the heart, i.e. it affects the myocardial contractility. The phrase is commonly used to refer to those agents that increase contractility, although negative inotropes do exist. Exogenous inotropes are analogues or derivatives of endogenous catecholamines, and act on a variety of receptors including the α, β_1, β_2 adrenergic and dopamine receptors. Adrenaline acts mildly at α receptors, but mainly at β_1 and β_2 receptors to increase heart rate and contractility, and causes vasodilatation because of relaxation of smooth muscle. Noradrenaline acts predominantly at the α receptor causing peripheral vasoconstriction and increase in systemic vascular resistance. Noradrenaline also has some mild β_1 stimulatory properties. Dobutamine is a synthetic derivative of dopamine and causes mainly β_1 effects.

Ernest Henry Starling (1866–1927). British physiologist. In 1892 he described the presence of osmotic pressure due to capillary proteins. He later coined the term 'hormone', and discovered the hormone secretin and elucidated its role in pancreatic secretion. He worked at the Pasteur Institute in Paris and University College, London. His 'Law of the Heart' was described in 1915 when Starling gave his famous Linacre Lecture on the subject. He died aboard ship, while cruising the Caribbean, and was buried in Kingston, Jamaica.

7. GASTRIC FUNCTION

What are the three phases of gastric secretion?

→ *Cephalic phase.* The sight, smell, taste or thought of food stimulates the stomach to secrete hydrochloric acid via vagal cholinergic stimulation. This cholinergic stimulation also stimulates gastrin release from antral G-cells, which in turn increase acid secretion. Low antral pH is a negative feedback stimulus for acid secretion at this stage. This phase accounts for about 10 per cent of secretion.

→ *Gastric phase*. This begins when food enters the stomach, distension and the presence of peptides being the stimuli responsible, and continues throughout the several hours that food remains in the stomach. It is the predominant phase of acid secretion responsible for approximately two-thirds of all secretion, with continuing negative feedback regulation by antral pH. Calcium, alcohol and caffeine all increase acid secretion.

→ *Intestinal phase*. This commences when chyme enters the duodenum. In the early phase, when the pH is greater than 3, there is a continued positive stimulus to acid secretion but, when the pH falls below 3, acid secretion is inhibited. Highly acid solutions in the duodenum stimulate secretin, an inhibitor of gastrin and a potent stimulus to the release of bile from the gallbladder and alkaline pancreatic juice.

What are the functions of the stomach?

The role of the stomach is to provide a reservoir for intermittent large-volume boluses of food, and to perform mixing and rudimentary digestion of proteins and carbohydrates. It is able to deliver smaller, more manageable quantities of material to the duodenum as required and reject potentially harmful substances before absorption. It renders the ingested contents relatively free of bacterial contamination by way of the bactericidal action of hydrochloric acid, and is involved in the facilitation of absorption of certain specific minerals and nutrients such as iron.

What is pernicious anaemia?

The parietal cells of the stomach that secrete HCl also secrete a glycoprotein known as intrinsic factor, which is essential for vitamin B_{12} absorption. Intrinsic factor binds to B_{12} and protects it from acid digestion in the stomach, and aids its absorption by pinocytosis at the intestinal brush border of the terminal ileum. Deficiency of intrinsic factor, either as a result of chronic atrophic gastritis or the generation of autoantibodies to the parietal cell, gives rise to a megaloblastic anaemia known as pernicious anaemia. A similar event occurs after gastric resection and is easily treated by 3-monthly vitamin B_{12} injections. There is a lag period of several years between abolition of intrinsic factor function from whatever cause, and the development of pernicious anaemia as the body's reserves of vitamin B_{12} are considerable.

What factors increase the risk of developing gastric carcinoma?

Certain factors are recognized as risk factors for the development of gastric cancer (see Figure 2.6), not least of which is a geographical distribution of the disease with a high prevalence in the Japanese. Whether this is diet-related or not is unclear. The other notable risk factors are:

→ pernicious anaemia
→ chronic atrophic gastritis
→ gastric polyps
→ family history – a small group of patients have a defect of the E-cadherin gene, which predisposes them to gastric carcinoma at a young age
→ the postgastrectomy/gastrotomy stomach
→ intestinal metaplasia
→ cigarette smoking
→ blood group A
→ gastric ulceration.

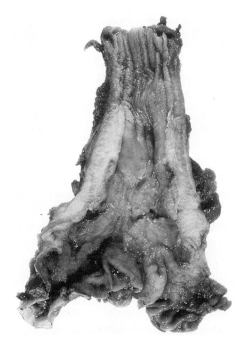

Figure 2.6 Resected specimen of tumour at the gastro-oesophageal junction.

Where in the stomach do most cancers occur?

Two-thirds occur in the pyloric region, one-quarter in the body, with only 6 per cent occurring in the cardia. A further 3 per cent will be the diffuse infiltrating carcinoma known as linitis plastica involving the whole stomach. However, these figures are continuously changing, since the distribution of gastric cancers has been changing over the last decade with a gradual decrease in distal cancers and an increase in proximal cancers.

8. RESPIRATORY ASSESSMENT

Draw a respirometry trace to show the volumes and capacities of the lung

See Figure 2.7.

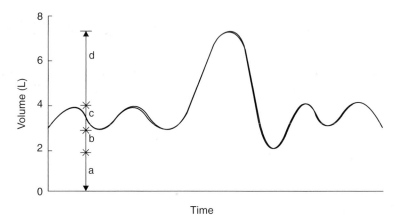

Figure 2.7 The volumes and capacities of the lung: a, residual volume; b, expiratory reserve volume; c, tidal volume; d, inspiratory reserve volume; a + b, functional residual capacity; b + c, expiratory capacity; c + d, inspiratory capacity; b + c + d, vital capacity; a + b + c + d, total lung capacity.

What is the difference between a volume and a capacity?

A capacity represents the sum of two or more volumes.

What is the functional significance of the functional residual capacity?

The functional residual capacity (FRC) is effectively the body's reservoir. It is that volume of gas remaining in the lung after a normal exhalation. It is the volume in which gas exchange actually occurs and, as such, is of the utmost significance. In patients with respiratory failure, attempts are made to increase the FRC, by using continuous positive airway pressure (CPAP) or positive end expiratory pressure (PEEP), in order to recruit more alveoli for gas exchange.

Vitalography is generally a laboratory tool. What other simple measurements may help you assess respiratory function?

A good history will allow you to make an assessment of respiratory function by gauging ability to perform everyday tasks '... do you get out of breath climbing the stairs … or getting dressed?', for instance. Examination of the chest may reveal clubbing, barrel chest, wheeze, or the crackles of fibrosis or failure. A chest x-ray will reveal much in the way of pulmonary pathology, such as emphysema, basal fibrosis and right heart enlargement, and arterial blood gas analysis will give useful information regarding the state of gas exchange in the patient. A non-invasive measure of respiratory capacity can be provided by using a hand-held flow meter to measure peak expiratory flow rate (PEFR).

What would you expect your PEFR to be … and that for an acute severe asthmatic?

An average adult would have a PEFR between 450 and 650 L/min depending on sex, build and degree of fitness. In acute severe asthma, the PEFR falls to between 33 and 50 per cent of normal or best predicted for that patient. If the PEFR falls below 33 per cent of best predicted, then it is termed life-threatening asthma and warrants careful consideration of ITU treatment.

9. RENIN–ANGIOTENSIN

What is the body's primary mineralocorticoid? Describe its synthesis and control of its secretion

Aldosterone is the major mineralocorticoid. It is synthesized in the zona glomerulosa of the adrenal cortex by 18-hydroxylation of a cholesterol skeleton. It is under the control of the renin–angiotensin system and not the hypothalamic–pituitary axis. A decrease in the glomerular filtration rate (GFR) stimulates release of renin from the juxtaglomerular apparatus, which in turn cleaves angiotensinogen to angiotensin I. This is, in turn, acted upon by angiotensin-converting enzyme (ACE) to cleave the decapeptide into an octapeptide, angiotensin II, one of the most potent vasoconstrictors yet isolated. The effect of angiotensin II is to increase peripheral resistance, particularly at the efferent renal arteriole, and to stimulate synthesis of aldosterone. The primary role of aldosterone is regulation of sodium. It increases sodium resorption in the kidney and water will follow by osmosis, thus increasing extracellular volume and hence correcting the decreased GFR. It should be noted that when sodium is resorbed under the control of aldosterone, it exchanges at the cell membrane with either potassium or hydrogen ion; thus aldosterone excess can lead to hypokalaemia. Alternatively, if potassium is already low, the Na^+ will exchange for H^+, which increases bicarbonate production leading to a hypokalaemic alkalosis. Aldosterone is metabolized by hepatic conjugation and urinary excretion.

What is Conn's syndrome and how does it present?

Conn's syndrome is primary hyperaldosteronism. Over half of the cases are due to a single benign adrenal cortex adenoma, 10 per cent are multiple adenomata and one-third due to bilateral hyperplasia. Secretion from a carcinoma is extremely rare. Excess plasma sodium, freed from normal negative feedback control, stimulates increased antidiuretic hormone (ADH) secretion. ADH acts in response to increased extracellular fluid osmolarity by increasing distal tubular permeability and increasing the volume of resorbed water; thus ADH excess leads to water retention and an expanded extracellular fluid volume.

The clinical features of this are hypervolaemic hypertension, hypokalaemic alkalosis, which may be so severe as to lead to tetany owing to the effect on calcium binding. Muscle weakness and even paralysis due to the hypokalaemia, increased plasma bicarbonate, hypernatraemia and low urinary sodium concentration also occur.

What are the causes of secondary hyperaldosteronism?

Secondary hyperaldosteronism occurs when there is a low GFR in spite of normovolaemia. Good examples are damaged renal vessels from either hypertension or renal artery stenosis, reduced colloid osmotic pressure, as in the nephrotic syndrome or cardiac failure, causing poor renal perfusion. In secondary hyperaldosteronism plasma renin is elevated because of the mechanisms described overstimulating the juxtaglomerular apparatus. In the primary condition, aldosterone is elevated, which increases plasma volume and, therefore, results in low levels of plasma renin.

Outline your management of an adrenal lesion identified as an incidental finding on CT scanning

So-called 'incidentalomas' are thought to arise with an incidence of up to 10 per cent. Initial investigation is to determine whether the lesion is functional or not and a combination of biochemical screening tests, such as serum aldosterone and cortisol, urinary catecholamines and cortisol, and a low-dose dexamethasone suppression test should establish this. Neither biochemical markers nor scanning will reliably distinguish benign from malignant tumours in most cases. In most centres, management depends on the size of the lesion and age of the patient. Lesions greater than 4 cm in size in patients under the age of 50 should be surgically removed. Smaller lesions should be monitored closely with serial scanning; the risks of malignancy increase with the size of the lesion and the relative risks for a given size of tumour are higher the younger the patient's age.

Jerome W. Conn (1907–81) graduated from the University of Michigan School of Medicine in 1932. He spent his entire career at the University of Michigan as researcher, physician and professor. In 1954, he presented his extensive clinical investigations of this new syndrome, which he called primary aldosteronism, at the Central Society for Clinical Research.

10. THERMOREGULATION

How do we regulate our body temperature?

Core body temperature is normally maintained fairly rigidly within fine limits. The central control of thermoregulation is the hypothalamic thermostat, which not only contains its own thermosensory cells that are exquisitely sensitive to temperature change, but also receives the input from skin temperature receptors. There are many more 'cold' receptors than 'warm' ones, hence we recognize cooling of our environment much more easily. There are three principal mechanisms for heat loss as follows.

1 *Vasodilatation* of the cutaneous venous plexuses, which are tonically constricted under sympathetic control. Full vasodilatation compared with full constriction has an eightfold increase in heat conductance.
2 *Sweating* allows a significant increase in the amount of evaporative losses. Initially, in a hot environment, this is maximal at about 700 ml of sweat per day with a heavy salt loss but, after 4 weeks of acclimatization, this system will produce up to 2000 ml of low sodium sweat, increasing the efficiency of the evaporative loss system by tenfold. Sweating is under the control of sympathetic cholinergic receptors, although circulating catecholamines can also influence sweating.
3 The final mechanism of heat loss is to *decrease heat production*, and mechanisms such as shivering and chemical thermogenesis are inhibited.

Similarly, there are three mechanisms of heat production. Skin vasoconstriction as mentioned above reduces radiant heat loss from the skin. Piloerection, although somewhat rudimentary in humans, is an attempt to create a larger air pocket around the body, and decrease conductive and convective losses. Increased heat production is established by shivering – under direct hypothalamic control – which increases muscle production of heat. Chemical thermogenesis results in uncoupling of oxidative phosphorylation in the cells regulated by catecholamines to produce an increased rate of cellular metabolism. Brown fat is extremely important in this mechanism owing to the large number of mitochondria in its cells. The final mechanism is a general up-regulation of metabolism by the increased secretion of the thyroid gland, again mediated by the hypothalamus, which increases secretion of thyrotrophin-releasing hormone and is perhaps another form of chemical thermogenesis.

Aside from these inherent physiological systems for controlling body temperature, humans possess an even more potent mechanism – behavioural control. A human adult can increase its temperature by putting on warm clothes, getting out of the cold environment, drinking hot drinks and turning the central heating up. The converse is obviously true for the human in the warm environment.

How does thermoregulation differ in Eskimos and children?

Brown fat plays an important role in chemical thermogenesis. Unfortunately, adult humans possess almost no brown fat; only infants do, in small patches between the scapulae. In children, chemical thermogenesis can increase heat production by 100 per cent, which may be in compensation for the inability of babies to shiver. Eskimos have very high basal metabolic rates mediated by the thyroid gland in an attempt to maintain adequate heat production. Children lack the behavioural control to allow them to modify their environment as circumstances dictate.

Which anatomical sites are commonly used for measuring temperature and are there variations according to site?

The most commonly used sites and their normal readings are oral (37°C), tympanic (37.5°C) and axillary (35–36°C) and these variations should be borne in mind when examining patient charts. More accurate readings of core temperature (37°C) can be obtained by rectal and oesophageal measurements; an oesophageal probe is often used intraoperatively.

How might you manage a grossly hypothermic patient?

Management is by gradual rewarming, whilst correcting any metabolic disturbances and arrhythmias. A temperature rise of 1°C per hour is ideal. The patient should be placed in a warm room with warming blankets. Warmed intravenous fluids can be given. In extreme cases, peritoneal wash out with warmed saline has been used.

11. SPINAL CORD AND REFLEXES

Describe in general terms the internal organization of the spinal cord

See Figure 2.8. The internal architecture of the spinal cord consists of grey and white matter, the grey matter forming proportionally more of the content at the

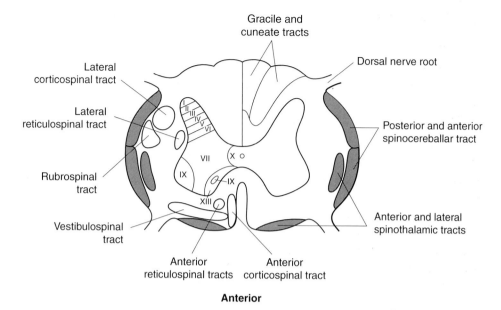

Figure 2.8 Internal organization of the spinal cord. The descending tracts and laminae of the grey matter are shown on the left and the ascending tracts on the right.

cervical and lumbar enlargements. The grey matter is arranged in a 'butterfly' shape centrally and is organized as ten numbered laminae each side, lamina I lying posteriorly. The posterior laminae, I–VI, receive the cutaneous and visceral primary afferent fibres. Laminae VII, VIII and X lie centrally and do not receive peripheral fibres. Lamina IX occupies the anterior horn and contains the α and γ motor neurons. The white matter contains the ascending and descending long tracts. The descending corticospinal, vestibulospinal and reticulospinal tracts lie in the lateral white fibres. The corticospinal tract is the principal descending motor tract and is also known as the pyramidal tract, thus the other two descending tracts constitute the extrapyramidal network and are responsible for controlling tone and posture. Ascending fibres make up the primary afferent posterior columns, and the anteriorly situated spinoreticular and spinothalamic tracts.

Where do motor and sensory pathways decussate?

The descending motor pathways of the corticospinal tract decussate as they exit the medulla and so travel down the cord on 'the opposite side'. Ascending spinothalamic and spinoreticular tracts cross obliquely in the cord before ascending. The obliquity increases the more cranial the segment.

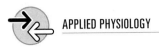
What would happen if you hemisected the cord?

Hemisection of the cord gives rise to the well-described entity of Brown-Séquard syndrome: ipsilateral spastic weakness due to division of corticospinal tracts, and dorsal column division gives loss of joint position sense and vibration sensation. There is a contralateral loss of pain and temperature sensation due to division of the crossed spinothalamic tract – this loss is noted between two and six dermatomes lower than the level of the lesion owing to the obliquity of the crossing fibres.

What is a reflex?

It is defined as a stereotypical response to a sensory input. It must involve, as a minimum, a sensor, an afferent neuron and an efferent neuron. All reflexes except the stretch reflex also include interneurons.

Describe the pathway of a simple reflex

The simplest reflex of all is the stretch reflex, which is monosynaptic. Striking the patellar tendon with a tendon hammer activates muscle spindle endings that are 'stretched'. The stimulus travels by 1a afferent fibres into the posterior horn of the spinal cord, where they synapse with α motor neurons anteriorly that travel to the neuromuscular junction in the quadriceps, which contracts.

What is a crossed reflex?

Before describing the crossed extensor reflex, it is necessary to describe the flexor or withdrawal reflex. Standing on a drawing pin with an unshod right foot sends pain stimuli into the dorsal horn via nociceptive pathways. Here, the stimulus passes into the interneurons, which eventually sends the stimulus to the motor neurons of both the hip, causing iliopsoas flexion, and knee, resulting in hamstring flexion to withdraw the foot. At the same time, inhibitory motor stimuli are sent to the opposing muscle groups to allow the flexion to occur unhindered. This is the withdrawal reflex. In addition, interneurons pass to the contralateral cord at the same segmental levels to stimulate the motor neurons of the left leg to cause extension, thus allowing the right foot to come off the ground, and the drawing pin, whilst the left leg supports the body's weight.

Charles-Edouard Brown-Séquard (1817–94). Born a British subject in Mauritius, he later became a French citizen when he became Professor of Neurology in Paris. In 1858, he lectured at the Royal College of Surgeons in London on hemisection of the spinal cord and thereafter was physician to the National Hospital for Neurology in Queens Square for 5 years before moving on to further posts in America and Paris where he eventually died.

12. SMALL INTESTINE

What is the function of jejunum?

The jejunum has five broad functions, namely: transport of chyme between duodenum and ileum, mixing of this digestive fluid, absorption of various nutrients and electrolytes and water, secretion – both exocrine and endocrine – and a lymphoid function.

A transport function is obvious, as the jejunum provides continuity of the gastrointestinal tract and it is associated with the mixing function, as the repetitive churning is accompanied by contraction of the villi to help pump nutrient-rich lymph away from the brush border. Interspersed with this action are sudden propulsive contractions of the jejunum to propel the bolus of chyme down the gut. The jejunum is the site of absorption for carbohydrate, protein, iron and folic acid, as well as most of the water and electrolytes. In addition, fat and fat-soluble vitamins are absorbed mainly in the jejunum, although more distal absorption does occur. Zinc and copper have been shown to be absorbed mainly in the upper gastrointestinal tract, but the routes of absorption of other trace elements and vitamins are much less clear.

Although a tremendous volume of fluid enters the upper gastrointestinal tract, and is supplemented by the secretions of the gut itself, the overwhelming majority of fluid is resorbed mainly in the jejunum. This part of the gut has been shown to be much more freely permeable to the passage of water than the lower gut and resorption is driven by the osmotic forces generated by nutrient absorption. In the jejunum, a large proportion of the electrolytes (Na^+, Cl^-, HCO_3^-) are resorbed, in part by simple diffusion, in part by active transport mechanisms and partly due to the osmotic pull of nutrient absorption, an effect known as solvent drag. Many hormones have been isolated from the whole length of the small intestine and produce a variety of effects, both truly endocrine and paracrine, such as somatostatin, secretin and motilin, which is implicated in coordinating the intrinsic rhythmicity of the various gut segments.

The entire gut performs an important immune function and is endowed with its own system of lymphoid tissue collectively known as mucosa-associated lymphoid tissue (MALT). It occurs in concentrated areas such as the Peyer's patches, as well as a diffuse distribution of intraepithelial lymphocytes and mucosal mast cells, which help protect the gut from the constant exposure to antigens within the gut lumen.

How would you differentiate jejunum from ileum in a pathology specimen?

The gut wall of jejunum is thinner, but with a thicker more vascular mucosa than the ileum and, overall, the jejunum has a larger circumference; under a microscope, the villi are taller and more numerous in the upper gut. The arterial arcades

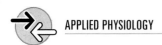

supplying the jejunum are more obviously arborized (tree-like) and plentiful. There is much more fatty infiltration of the ileal mesentery than in the jejunum, where the mesentery is often transparent.

Describe the functions specific to the terminal ileum and the consequences of resection

Effective absorption of bile salts and vitamin B_{12} only occurs in the terminal ileum, since they require specific transport channels that are only situated there. The bile salts are normally returned to the liver and recycled – this is known as the enterohepatic circulation. Resection of the terminal ileum prevents this pathway from functioning and an excessive loss of bile salts occurs. This, in turn, leads to malabsorption of fats and steatorrhoea owing to the diminished bile salt pool.

Vitamin B_{12} is not absorbed when the ileum has been resected, and patients who have undergone resection should have regular blood checks, and receive parenteral B_{12} regularly if needed.

What are the causes and features of 'short bowel syndrome'?

Short bowel syndrome occurs when there is insufficient bowel remaining to support the absorptive function required for normal growth and life. The minimal amount of small bowel needed for normal absorption is approximately 100 cm, although as little as 50 cm may be adequate, if a complete functioning colon is *in situ*. The symptoms are due to the intestinal decompensation from both reduction in absorptive area and a greatly reduced transit time. Absorption of fats and proteins are most severely affected, followed by carbohydrates. The patient is malnourished and underweight, with diarrhoea or steatorrhoea. There are deficiencies of most vitamins and trace elements. With time, the bowel adapts with increased numbers of enterocytes and heightened villi in the remaining bowel, and compensation to some degree can occur. The principal reason for short bowel syndrome is extensive small bowel resection; indications include Crohn's disease, mesenteric infarction, radiation enteritis, mid gut volvulus and small bowel tumours, although loss of bowel length from congenital atresias and loss of functional length due to multiple fistulae may also be responsible.

13. ACTION POTENTIALS

What is an action potential? Draw a representative one for skeletal muscle

It is a rapid change in the membrane potential followed by a rapid return to the resting membrane potential. It is due to voltage-dependent ion channel proteins in the plasma membrane. The size and shape of action potentials differ considerably from one tissue to another. See Figure 2.9.

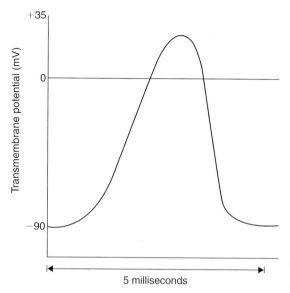

Figure 2.9 A representative action potential for skeletal muscle.

What do the terms 'threshold', 'all or none' and 'summation' mean with reference to the action potential?

The cell membrane has a resting potential across it, with the inside usually ~70 mV negative compared to the outside. Application of a current will decrease this difference – depolarization – up to a point known as the 'threshold' after which an action potential is generated by reversing the membrane polarity, i.e. the inside now becomes positive with regard to the outside. This generates an action potential, which is then propagated, without decrement, down the entire length of the fibre. Depolarization occurs because opening of Na^+ channels allows a large rapid influx of Na^+ into the cell, changing its polarity. Almost as soon as the sodium gate is opened, it begins to close and a potassium gate opens to allow repolarization.

The all or none phenomenon indicates that a larger depolarizing current does not create a larger action potential; similarly, once initiated, an action potential will spread across the whole membrane. If the current is big enough to create an action potential in one small corner of the membrane, it will depolarize the whole membrane; if it is not sufficient, none of the membrane depolarizes, i.e. all or none.

Summation refers to a phenomenon of muscle fibres whereby the addition of individual muscle twitches creates a stronger and more concerted twitch. It occurs by, firstly, increasing the number of motor units contracting simultaneously and, secondly, by increasing the frequency with which they contract.

What is the difference between the action potential of skeletal and cardiac muscle?

In the above description of the phenomenon of depolarization, the ingress of potassium is followed by a refractory period when the system is not susceptible to another depolarizing current and a relative refractory period in which the fibre will respond only to a greater than normal stimulus. In cardiac muscle fibres, the mechanism is different. As well as the opening of fast sodium channels, slow calcium channels open allowing a slow ingress of calcium that gives the action potential a plateau period, making the cardiac muscle fibre contraction many times longer than that of skeletal muscle. It also gives it a longer refractory period to avoid undue cardiac stimulation and allowing the rhythmicity of the heart to remain undisturbed. See Figure 2.10.

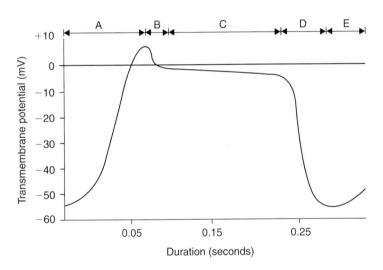

Figure 2.10 Cardiac action potential: A, fast influx of Na^+ – rapid depolarization; B, incomplete early repolarization; C, plateau phase due to slow Ca^{2+} influx; D, rapid K^+ efflux – repolarization; E, refractory period.

14. BREAST

Describe the function of the breast

The only physiological role of the breast is lactation. Thus, it fulfils its role for only a short period of time in less than half the population and, as such, is a physiological oddity.

Which hormones are involved?

At puberty, the female breast develops under the influence of oestrogen and progesterone. Oestrogen is responsible for the growth of ductal epithelium, whilst progesterone mediates the growth of the lobular complex. Many other factors, such as growth hormone, insulin and prolactin, have a complementary effect on oestrogen/progesterone-induced growth but, in the absence of those two sex hormones, will have no effect themselves.

During pregnancy, the breasts enlarge under the influence of oestrogen, progesterone and human chorionic gonadotrophin (HCG) and epithelial proliferation is pronounced. High oestrogen levels inhibit milk production, so it is only after separation of the placenta that milk production is initiated and the consequent low oestrogen levels stimulate prolactin release from the anterior pituitary gland to provide a continued stimulus for milk production.

Suckling is the vital stimulus to the posterior pituitary to release oxytocin, which stimulates the milk to be ejected from the terminal duct lobular system, where it collects under the influence of prolactin, into the large ducts leading to the nipple.

High prolactin levels inhibit gonadatrophin secretion and thus inhibit ovarian follicle maturation, i.e. continued breast-feeding produces relative infertility.

What role do hormones play in breast cancer?

In essence, oestrogen exposure has a small but significant role in breast cancer. Situations that increase the amount of unopposed oestrogen exposure predispose to an increased risk of breast cancer. This may be typified by the woman with early menarche and late menopause. An early age of first pregnancy has been shown to decrease the risk of developing breast cancer, while being nulliparous increases the risk. Breast-feeding will reduce the risk. The oral contraceptive pill and hormone replacement therapy (HRT) are implicated in a small increase in risk. It should be remembered that other factors, such as genetic and family history, and dietary intake of saturated fat, are also implicated in the genesis of breast cancer.

Oestrogen receptor (ER) status of an excised tumour or biopsy is now known to give important prognostic information in breast cancer. ER status is a useful predictor of response to chemo/endocrine therapy after first relapse, with ER-positive women doing better.

What drugs are used for endocrine manipulation in the treatment of breast cancer and how do they work?

The commonest drug in use is tamoxifen, an oestrogen receptor antagonist. It inhibits the growth of oestrogen-dependent breast cancer cells and has been credited with a reduction in the mortality from this disease over the last 15 years. As a result of its anti-oestrogen effect side effects are common, and include hot flushes, pruritus vulvae and vaginal bleeding. There is a small risk of inducing uterine malignancy with tamoxifen use and it is, therefore, only recommended for a maximum of 5 years usage.

Anastrozole and related drugs are newer anti-oestrogens, taken orally, which work by inhibition of the enzyme aromatase, which is responsible for the peripheral aromatization of oestrogen in adipose tissue. Initially licensed for second-line use after relapse on tamoxifen, recent studies have shown improved efficacy over tamoxifen in both adjuvant therapy and treatment of advanced tumours. Older treatments, such as the progesterone megestrol acetate, and aminoglutethimide, a blocker of peripheral conversion of androgen to oestrogen, are less commonly used because of their non-specific nature and subsequent side effects.

15. CORTICOSTEROIDS

Describe the arrangement, function and control of the adrenal cortex

The adrenal cortex consists of three distinct zones: glomerulosa, fasciculata and reticularis. The inner zona reticularis secretes steroid-based sex hormones, such as androsterone, androstenedione and small amounts of oestrogen and progesterone. The outer zona glomerulosa produces aldosterone, a potent mineralocorticoid responsible with the renin–angiotensin system for salt and water homeostasis in the kidney. The middle layer is the zona fasciculata which produces the body's glucocorticoids, primarily cortisol with small amounts of cortisone. Their release is controlled by the pituitary secretion of adrenocorticotrophic hormone (ACTH) via a negative feedback mechanism. ACTH is in turn secreted under the control of hypothalamic corticotrophin-releasing hormone (CRH).

What are the typical manifestations and common causes of hypercortisolism?

The clinical picture of hypercortisolism, commonly referred to as Cushing's syndrome, is one of the most striking of all the endocrine diseases. Glucocorticoid action stimulates appetite and gluconeogenesis, resulting in obesity and fat deposition in particular sites, creating a buffalo hump, moon face and central obesity. In association with muscle wasting owing to the toxic effects of cortisol on muscle, the classical appearance of 'a lemon on toothpicks' occurs. Decreases in collagen synthesis give rise to thin skin, which bruises easily, heals poorly and stretches, causing striae. Diabetes mellitus ensues owing to the glucocorticoid action, and the mineralocorticoid effect of cortisol causes marked salt and water retention giving rise to hypertension. Increased adrenal androgen secretion, if there is increased ACTH, accounts for the acne and hirsutism often seen, and there is often marked osteoporosis and pathological fractures.

The commonest cause is iatrogenic – patients on long-term exogenous steroids for immune suppression or treatment of diseases, such as brittle asthma. Increased autonomous secretion of ACTH from a pituitary micro-adenoma drives the adrenals into bilateral hyperplasia and hypercortisolism with increased androgen secretion as well – this is Cushing's disease. A variety of extra-adrenal tumours produce ACTH-like substances, such as bronchogenic tumours and small carcinoid neoplasms; this gives the 'ectopic ACTH syndrome'. A primary adrenal tumour, either adenomatous or carcinomatous, may produce excess cortisol directly with normal or usually low ACTH.

How would you diagnose Cushing's syndrome?

I would take a thorough history and examination, bearing in mind that none of the above clinical findings are *diagnostic* of Cushing's syndrome. A methodical approach to the diagnosis is needed and, initially, I would aim to confirm the diagnosis of hypercortisolism before attempting identification of the cause. In the first instance, I would perform serial plasma cortisol estimations looking for persistently raised levels, and a loss of diurnal variation as cortisol levels are highest at about 9am and lowest around midnight. I would then perform an overnight dexamethasone suppression test by administering 1 mg dexamethasone at midnight and measuring the morning cortisol levels. Failure to suppress cortisol levels to less than 50 per cent of basal values points towards a diagnosis of Cushing's syndrome.

A high-dose dexamethasone suppression test (2 mg 6 hourly for 48 hours) will suppress ACTH secretion in pituitary Cushing's, resulting in a decrease of at least 50 per cent in plasma cortisol or urinary 17-hydroxy steroids. If this test proves positive, then I would arrange a cranial MRI to examine the pituitary fossa.

If the high-dose dexamethasone test were negative, I would then assay plasma ACTH levels. Very high levels are consistent with ectopic ACTH secreting tumours, whilst low plasma ACTH points to a primary cortisol secreting adrenal tumour. Having differentiated between the two, CT or MRI scanning should be undertaken to image the lesion responsible.

What is Nelson's syndrome and explain its pathogenesis?

It is the combination of hyperpigmentation following bilateral adrenalectomy. In pituitary-dependent hypercortisolism treated by bilateral adrenalectomy, up to 30 per cent of patients develop unrestrained growth of the pituitary tumour with enlargement of the sella turcica and very high levels of plasma ACTH. Residues

1–13 of the ACTH precursor molecule correspond exactly to α-melanocyte-stimulating hormone (α-MSH) and account for the skin pigmentation that is the striking feature of Nelson's syndrome. The syndrome may develop acutely but is more commonly a chronic event with the mean time from adrenalectomy to onset being 3 years. Bilateral adrenalectomy is less commonly performed these days, but anyone who has been treated in this way should be followed up regularly with cranial CT or MRI to look for an expanding sella turcica lesion.

Harvey Cushing (1869–1939) was the father of modern neurosurgery. An American, he published widely on topics such as 'The pituitary body and its disorders' (1912), 'Syndromes of the cerebellar/pontine angle' (1917), and 'Intracranial tumours' (1932) amongst many others. He served with distinction in WWI, later publishing 'From a Surgeon's Journal 1915–18' about his experiences. He won a Pulitzer Prize for his biography 'A life of Sir William Osler'. His greatest contribution though was to reduce the mortality of neurosurgery from 90 per cent to 8 per cent. He died of a myocardial infarction in 1939.

16. BILIARY SYSTEM

What is in bile and what is the difference between hepatic and gallbladder bile?

Bile is manufactured in the liver and transported by the bile ducts to be stored in the gallbladder in preparation for release in response to the stimulus of a meal, mediated by the hormone secretin. Bile contains bile acids, cholesterol, lecithins and phospholipids and bile pigments. The contents of the two sorts of bile are similar, although gallbladder bile is between 5 and 20 times more concentrated because of active resorption of sodium and water.

How much bile is produced per day and what is its function?

Between 250 and 1500 ml of concentrated bile are released per day into the duodenum. Its purpose is to emulsify fats in the duodenum to increase the surface area available for lipolysis and to aid absorption of digested fats at the intestinal brush border. It is also the body's major excretory pathway for cholesterol.

What are the common types of gallstone?

Gallstones may be made of pigment, cholesterol or both. Mixed stones account for 90 per cent, with cholesterol stones adding a further 6 per cent and pigment stones the remainder. Pigment stones occur as a result of excess haemolysis with increased bilirubin formation and the stones are formed of the bile pigments; they are small, hard and dark green in colour. Cholesterol stones precipitate, if the bile becomes supersaturated, owing to an alteration in the balance between cholesterol and the bile salts and lecithin that hold the cholesterol in solution. The stones are usually fewer in number than pigment stones but larger with a pale yellowish cut surface. They may also contain precipitated calcium ions and, therefore, be radio-opaque. The vast majority of gallstones are, however, radiolucent, with only around 10 per cent being visible on x-ray. The mixed stones contain a cholesterol nucleus and an outer pigment shell with variable amounts of calcium bilirubinate, calcium phosphate, calcium carbonate, calcium palmidronate and proteins.

What problems may gallstones cause?

The majority of gallstones are asymptomatic and of those that do cause problems they may do so within the gallbladder itself, within the biliary tree or outside of the biliary system altogether. **The site of the stone determines the** **further management of the patient.** Gallstones are a predisposing factor for carcinoma of the gallbladder.

Within the gallbladder
→ *Biliary colic* – obstruction of the gallbladder neck by a gallstone gives rise to a severe colicky pain, which may, in contrast to most colics, last for several hours.
→ *Cholecystitis* – the stones cause inflammation of the gallbladder wall. Presents as right upper quadrant pain, fever, leucocytosis and systemic upset.
→ *Mucocele* – impaction of a stone in Hartmann's pouch can completely occlude the cystic duct. The gallbladder fills with mucus.
→ *Empyema* – infection of an obstructed gallbladder; it turns into a bag of pus.

Within the biliary tree
→ *Obstructive jaundice* – because of occlusion of the common bile duct by a stone. It tends to be painless as there is no muscle in the common duct wall to produce colic.
→ *Ascending cholangitis* – is produced by infection in the stagnant bile of an obstructed system. The duct fills with pus and the patient is markedly unwell and septic.
→ *Pancreatitis* – due to impaction of a stone at the ampulla.

Outside the gallbladder
→ *Gallstone ileus* – erosion of the stone through into the duodenum and passage through the small bowel may present with small bowel obstruction owing to the blockage of the ileocaecal valve by the gallstone. X-rays reveal the stone in the right lower quadrant and gas in the biliary tree, which is pathognomonic of this condition. See Figure 2.11.

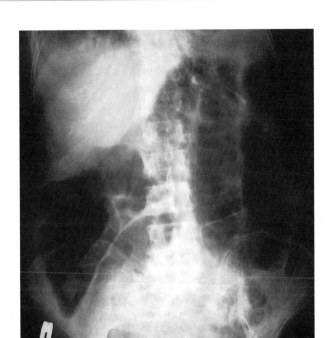

Figure 2.11 Abdominal radiograph showing gallstone ileus with the stone clearly visible.

When is a T-tube used and for how long?

A T-tube is a rubber tube used to drain the common bile duct after surgical exploration. It gives the bile a safe route to the surface, and forms a tract. The tube can be used to perform cholangiograms, and can be removed after 10–14 days, by which time a track will have formed. In the event of bile duct stones remaining, they can sometimes be removed by the use of mechanical graspers down the tract under radiological control.

17. OXYGEN FLUX EQUATION

What is the oxygen flux equation?

This equation represents the amount of oxygen delivered to the tissues per minute

$$DO_2 = [Hb] \times 1.34 \times SaO_2 \times CO \times 10 + (0.025 \times PO_2)$$

where [Hb] = haemoglobin concentration in g/dl;
1.34 = constant representing the amount of O_2 that Hb can carry (ml/g);
SaO_2 = oxygen saturation (per cent);
CO = cardiac output (L/min);
PO_2 = oxygen tension (kPa) multiplied by a constant (ml/dl per kPa) to represent the oxygen in direct solution.

The factor of 10 is included to ensure uniformity of units as haemoglobin is in g/dl but cardiac output is in L/min. In practice, the amount of oxygen in direct solution is minimal (~1 per cent) and is generally ignored in this calculation.

How would you measure the cardiac output?

The cardiac output is the stroke volume of the heart multiplied by the heart rate. The measurement can be made directly using a Swan–Ganz cardiac catheter and a thermodilution technique, which utilizes the Fick principle. This states that the rate of flow, which in this case is the cardiac output, can be measured if an indicator substance is added to a moving flow of liquid at a known rate and the concentration of indicator substance is known both proximal and distal to the point of addition. In common practice, the indicator substance is a bolus of cold saline injected through a side port some distance proximal from the tip of the catheter, where a thermistor records the drop in blood temperature. The change in temperature of the blood allows direct calculation of cardiac output. It can also be calculated using a Doppler measurement of aortic flow in the aortic arch.

What is shock?

Shock can be defined as an acute circulatory disturbance resulting in inadequate tissue perfusion and tissue hypoxia.

What is the relevance of the oxygen flux equation to the management of shock?

The oxygen flux equation tells you how much oxygen is being delivered to the tissues. Shock is by definition an inadequate amount of oxygen delivered to the tissues, thus the management of shock is the maximization of the flux equation in practice. Sequential analysis of the equation and comparison to clinical events will make sense of this.

In order to maximize DO_2, any one of the individual terms could be maximized, hence if the shock is haemorrhagic in nature, there will be a decrease in the haemoglobin concentration and the [Hb] term of the equation will be lower than previously. The solution would be to transfuse blood to restore the haemoglobin concentration, thus increasing the value of DO_2. Similarly, giving the patient supplemental oxygen will serve to increase the SaO_2 phrase of the equation. Cardiac output is defined as heart rate multiplied by stroke volume, thus maximization of these parameters by manipulation of inotropes is another important method of increasing oxygen delivery. Additionally, if cardiac output is considered mathematically as blood pressure over systemic vascular resistance (BP/SVR), then inotropic manipulation of these will also allow manipulation of DO_2. In occasional situations, hyperbaric therapy may be used to increase the final, and normally ignored, part of the flux equation, although this is more likely to be in a case such as carbon monoxide poisoning than hypovolaemic shock.

Discuss the role of 'goal-directed therapy' in the management of the critically ill

'Goal-directed therapy' stems from work by Shoemaker in the early 1980s when he noted that patients in intensive treatment units who achieved a certain level of oxygen delivery according to the flux equation did better than those who did not. This led to patients being aggressively fluid filled and inotropically driven to achieve preset goals of oxygen delivery, and was the vogue in many ITUs for a while. Later work has shown that achievement of these goals in itself does not improve outcome, and the current view is that patients who reach these goals without heavy inotrope support do indeed do better; this is more likely a natural reflection of the fact that they are physiologically able to reach that target. Forcing physiologically incapable patients to meet preset goals by inotropic manipulation has a deleterious effect.

18. ELECTROCARDIOGRAM (ECG)

Draw a diagram to show how cardiac contractions are linked to the ECG trace (see Figure 2.12). Describe the salient points of the ECG waveform

The P wave represents the electrical activity as the atria depolarize. As conduction must spread through the whole chamber before muscle contraction can occur, this must represent the activity immediately before contraction of the atria. Similarly, the QRS complex is the depolarization wave for the ventricles and occurs immediately prior to contraction of the ventricles. The T wave represents the repolarization of the ventricles, which remain contracted until this has happened, so ventricular relaxation happens immediately after the T wave. A small atrial repolarization wave gets hidden in the much larger QRS complex.

What produces the heart sounds?

Simplistically, the closing of the coronary valves produces the heart sounds. To be more precise, after the valves have snapped shut, a backflow of blood against

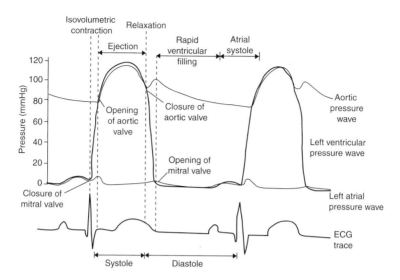

Figure 2.12 Relationship of the ECG trace to atrioventricular contraction.

them causes them to bulge taut into the adjacent chambers and then rebound, forcing blood back into the chamber in turbulent flow. It is the rebound of the taut valve cusps and turbulent flow that causes the heart sounds.

The first sound is caused by the closure of the atrioventricular valves, namely the tricuspid and mitral valves, and the second heart sound by the closure of the semilunar (aortic and pulmonary) valves. Rarely, third and even fourth heart sounds may be detected, caused by the inrush of blood into the ventricles in the mid-third of diastole and during atrial contraction, respectively. They are normally too low-pitched to be detected by auscultation.

What other ways can you investigate cardiac function?

Investigation of suspected paroxysmal arrhythmias was greatly aided by the invention in 1961 of the continuous ambulatory ECG monitor, now colloquially known after its inventor – the Holter monitor. In many patients who complain of symptoms of angina, it is very difficult to quantify just how bad their symptoms may be – one solution is exercise testing. Under medical supervision, the patient exercises to a set protocol on a treadmill whilst wired to an ECG machine. Direct correlation can then be made between myocardial ischaemia as witnessed by ST depression on the ECG trace and the patient's symptoms.

Echocardiography utilizes ultrasound to give dynamic information about ventricular wall thickness and movements, flow across valves and akinetic segments. Thallium scanning uses a radioisotope, which is taken up by myocardial muscle in proportion to its blood supply; thus well-perfused areas show up brightly on the gamma camera, whilst infarcted areas show up as holes.

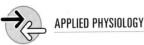
Coronary artery angiography has revolutionized pre-operative assessment of ischaemic heart disease. Access is either by placement of a transvenous catheter to give information about the right heart or arterial catheter placement, allowing angiography of the coronary arteries and exact visualization of occlusive disease, which is studied closely by the cardiac surgeon prior to coronary artery bypass grafting.

19. GASTROINTESTINAL SECRETION

How much fluid is secreted daily by the different parts of the gastrointestinal tract and how does its chemical composition vary?

The gastrointestinal tract secretes an enormous mount of fluid each day from all parts from mouth to terminal ileum, but excretes only about 150 ml per day in faeces, so whatever is secreted is almost universally resorbed.

Salivary gland secretion is between 500 and 2000 ml per day of slightly acidic (pH 6.0–7.0) saliva with a high $[K^+]$ and $[HCO_3^-]$. The concentrations of sodium and chloride are slightly lower than that of plasma. The role of saliva is to initiate starch digestion by an α amylase and also to maintain oral hygiene between meals by way of its bactericidal action. The stomach releases up to 4000 ml of highly acidic secretion daily that is usually salt-rich but obviously without bicarbonate. Gastric secretion also includes the enzyme pepsinogen, as well as small amounts of gastric lipase and amylase. Gastric cells secrete the mucus that lines and protects the stomach, and intrinsic factor necessary for vitamin B_{12} absorption.

Pancreatic secretion is alkaline with a pH of 8.0–8.5, and totals about 1000 ml per 24 hours. It is rich in sodium bicarbonate and contains enzymes for the breakdown of carbohydrates, fats and proteins. It is the acini of the gland that secrete the digestive enzymes, whilst the epithelial duct cells produce the watery bicarbonate-rich juice. They are actually under the control of separate hormone systems – the watery alkaline juice is produced in response to secretin, whilst cholecystokinin will generate the enzyme secretion from the acinar glands. Bile is released from the gallbladder, also in response to secretin, and normally totals about one litre per day rich in sodium and chloride with moderate bicarbonate content. The small bowel can secrete anything up to 10 L per day, although this is rarely actually the case; most is slightly alkaline with an isotonic composition. Virtually all is resorbed further along the small intestine, as only 1.5 L or so of liquid stool passes through the ileocaecal valve each 24 hours.

What are the biochemical abnormalities that commonly occur in a case of pyloric stenosis? Explain them

The typical biochemical upset is a hypokalaemic hypochloraemic alkalosis associated with hypovolaemia and haemoconcentration. The urine is acidic.

The gastric parietal cells generate H^+ and HCO_3^- via the carbonic anhydrase reaction; H^+ enters the gastric lumen, with chloride ions, as hydrochloric acid and the HCO_3^- enters the extracellular fluid (ECF) to be subsequently secreted into the duodenum in bicarbonate-rich biliary and pancreatic juice. Thus, when vomiting occurs with free connection between stomach and duodenum, the body loses volume, H^+Cl^-, HCO_3^-, Na^+ and K^+. The clinical problem is one of volume deficit and electrolyte disturbance rather than H^+/HCO_3^- disequilibrium. Now consider the setting of pyloric stenosis in which free connection between stomach and duodenum does not occur; vomiting will lose volume and H^+Cl^- only, causing a relative gain of HCO_3^-. The loss of H^+ drives the carbonic anhydrase reaction to produce more H^+/HCO_3^-; thus, the bicarbonate gain increases and, as renal compensation is slight, metabolic alkalosis ensues. The kidney is a sodium-preserving organ and, in the proximal tubules, as there is less chloride for sodium to be absorbed with, owing to decreased chloride from vomiting, Na^+ exchanges for H^+, giving rise to acidic urine and worsening alkalosis. As H^+ becomes scarcer, Na^+ then exchanges with K^+, giving rise to potassium-rich urine and hypokalaemia.

What is the epidemiology of this condition in the paediatric setting?

It is classically a condition affecting the male infant, usually the first-born and with an increased incidence in children of affected parents. The incidence in caucasians is about 4 per 1000. It presents at between 4 and 6 weeks with projectile vomiting, continuing hunger even after feeds, poor stools and weight loss. Dehydration and wasting is now only seen in extreme cases of delayed presentation.

Describe the diagnosis and management of a child with congenital hypertrophic pyloric stenosis

The history is usually highly suggestive of the diagnosis. Witnessing a test feed is usually enough evidence, as the baby feeds hungrily and then a wave of peristalsis can be seen to move from left to right across the epigastrium and a projectile vomit follows. The hypertrophic pylorus can often be palpated in the epigastrium as a firm olive-sized swelling. Ultrasound confirms the diagnosis. Treatment is by correction of biochemical aberrations and scheduling the child for urgent surgery in the form of Ramstedt's pyloromyotomy. Through a transverse or even periumbilical incision the pylorus is identified and the hypertrophic muscle fibres divided until the intestinal mucosa is seen to pout through the incision. The abdomen is then closed.

20. PAIN

How is pain sensed and transmitted?

Pain is sensed by free nerve endings. In the skin, they are widespread and densely packed; in most internal tissues, however, they are more widely dispersed. They react to different types of painful stimuli – thermal, mechanical or chemical – and there is often much overlap between receptors. Involved chemical mediators include bradykinin, serotonin, prostaglandins, histamine, potassium and acetylcholine. It should be noted that the body recognizes two different types of pain – acute and slow pain. Acute pain is that pain which begins within 0.1 second of the stimulus and is typified by a needle puncture of the skin. It is transmitted by Aδ pain fibres, which are small and transmit at between 6 and 30 m/s. Slow pain begins a second or so after application of the stimulus, but continues to increase over seconds and minutes. It is typified by a throbbing pain and is transmitted in large diameter C fibres at speeds of 0.5–2.0 m/s. Each type of pain fibre ends in different parts of the posterior horn grey matter before mostly crossing over and ascending in the anterolateral sensory pathway to the brainstem reticular formation before further ascending into the thalamus and higher cortical areas for processing and integration.

By what mechanisms can we modify the pain response?

Stimulation of peripheral tactile receptors, perhaps by rubbing the skin, transmits sensory input in large sensory fibres and depresses the transmission of pain signals from the locality; it is this mechanism that is invoked when footballers have linament rubbed on injuries and is probably the basis for acupuncture. In a similar fashion, TENS (transcutaneous electrical nerve stimulation) has much the same effect.

The body has an intrinsic analgesia system that allows damping down of pain signals – direct stimulation of these areas; the periaqueductal grey area of the mesencephalon, raphe nucleus magnus and part of the dorsal horn of spinal cord will block pain transmission. Implicated in this pathway are a series of opiate-like substances, which are naturally secreted, and loosely grouped as endorphins and encephalins. When these are injected experimentally into the periaqueductal grey area, they produce profound analgesia.

How do local anaesthetics work?

All local anaesthetics are esters or amides of benzoic acid and are membrane stabilizers. They plug the membrane sodium channels, prohibiting generation of an action potential and stopping transmission of sensory signals. This is reversible.

As they are non-specific membrane stabilizers, they will also stabilize other excitable tissues, such as myocardium, if inadvertently injected intravenously.

What is the safe dose of lignocaine and bupivacaine?

Maximum dosage is designed to take account of inadvertent intravascular injection; thus, in theory, a patient can have an intravenous injection of up to the maximum safe dose of local anaesthetic without side effects. As these anaesthetics diffuse into the surrounding tissue and are then gradually absorbed, and are, in general, vasodilatatory, addition of a vasoconstrictor, such as adrenaline, will slow down the rate of diffusion and consequently increase the safe maximum dose. For lignocaine, the safe dose is 3 mg/kg body weight increasing to 7 mg/kg with the addition of 1:200 000 adrenaline. 0.5 per cent lignocaine contains 5 mg/ml of lignocaine, 1 per cent contains 10 mg/ml, and 2 per cent contains 20 mg/ml. Bupivacaine has a maximum dose of 2 mg/kg or 2.5 mg/kg with adrenaline.

What happens in overdose and why is the described therapeutic range for bupivacaine much less than for lignocaine?

In systemic toxicity, all excitable tissues become membrane stabilized. The earliest features are parasthesia around the mouth and on the tongue followed by light-headedness, drowsiness and anxiety. Tinnitus is not uncommon. If untreated and serum concentrations continue to rise, loss of consciousness and convulsions supervene. Either as a consequence of this or due to a direct myocardial effect, cardiovascular collapse and cardiac arrest may follow. Bupivacaine has a tendency to be more cardiotoxic than other local anaesthetics and does not have the warning neurological signs before cardiovascular collapse occurs. Additionally, the myocardial depression tends to be more resistant to treatment compared to that initiated by lignocaine.

21. REJECTION

How do surgeons try to reduce the incidence of transplant rejection?

By choosing a donor organ that is matched for the major HLA loci, the chances of rejection are diminished and this is augmented by immunosuppressive therapy. Living related donors have a better HLA match than most cadaveric donors, with graft survival 10–15 per cent better at 1 year than cadaveric organs. Even after optimal HLA matching, outside of living twin donors, immunosuppression is needed. Originally, this consisted of steroids alone and was augmented in the early 1960s by azathioprine, which markedly increased graft survival rates. In the early 1980s, however, the introduction of cyclosporin revolutionized transplant-ation as, in combination with prednisolone or in low-dose triple therapy with both other agents, further improved graft survival has been demonstrated. Perhaps more importantly, with donor organs at a premium, cyclosporin has been able to achieve graft survival figures for poorly HLA-matched donations that approach or even equal those of highly matched organs.

What is a standard post-transplant regime?

Cyclosporin is, unfortunately in the context of renal transplantation, highly nephrotoxic and its introduction immediately after renal transplantation leads to a high incidence of primary non-function. In the immediate post-transplant period (days 0–6), the patient is immunosuppressed with anti-lymphocyte globulin (ALG) preparations, azathioprine and high-dose prednisolone. As the donor kidney recovers from the insult of cold ischaemia, cyclosporin is intro-duced at about 1 week, and the azathioprine and ALG are stopped, and the prednisolone is tailed off so that they are maintained on cyclosporin and steroids. An alternative maintenance regime is to use all three immunosuppres-sive drugs in lower doses than would be used in dual therapy and this has been shown to be equally effective.

What are the 1- and 5-year patient and graft survival figures for renal transplant?

It must be appreciated that patient and graft survival are not the same thing, bearing in mind the possibilities of renal dialysis in those for whom the graft fails. Using cadaveric grafts, the average 1-year graft survival is 85 per cent and patient survival ~90 per cent. At 5 years, these figures have fallen to 65 per cent and 80 per cent for graft and patient survival, respectively. The figures are bet-ter if living related organ donors are used, with the 1- and 5-year graft survival rates being 90 per cent and 80 per cent, respectively.

The basics of a kidney transplant procedure have remained the same since its introduction in the 1950s. Describe them

The recipient patient has an extraperitoneal approach to the iliac fossa, which is usually the opposite fossa to the side the donor organ came from. The exter-nal iliac artery and vein are isolated and controlled, and surrounding minor vessels and lymphatics dissected away. The donor organ is implanted and end-to-side anastomoses of both renal vessels to the prepared external iliac recipi-ents takes place. The artery can also be anastomosed end-to-end with the internal iliac artery. The ureter is then implanted into the bladder using a standard technique, such as the Leadbetter–Politano or extravesical antero-lateral approaches.

What are the phases of rejection and how does it present?

Three phases of rejection are described, although the distinctions are not always that clear-cut; these phases are hyperacute, acute and chronic rejection.

→ *Hyperacute rejection* begins the moment the vascular inflow is restored and is due to preformed circulating antibodies against donor-specific antigens. In the case of renal transplantation, the kidney rapidly becomes mottled and cyanotic. These antibodies fix complement, and are deposited in the small vessels of the donated organ accompanied by microthrombosis and accumulation of leucocytes in the peritubular capillaries. This should occur rarely, owing to pre-transplantation lymphocytotoxic crossmatching.

→ *Acute rejection* occurs any time from about 1 week to several months post-transplantation. Classically, it presented with a tender painful swollen graft and, in the case of renal transplantation, hypertension. However, in the cyclosporin era, this full-blown presentation is rare, and most will present at routine follow-up with graft dysfunction evidenced by deteriorating renal or liver function tests. In the setting of suspected acute rejection, biopsy of the graft organ will give definitive evidence and also some prognostic clues. Pathologically there is an interstitial infiltration of mononuclear cells, which causes tubular destruction in the kidney. There is also a vascular infiltration of mononuclear cells, which heralds a poorer chance of graft rescue. The treatment of acute rejection includes high-dose steroids and anti-lymphocyte globulin preparations.

→ *Chronic rejection* happens many months or years after transplantation, and is typified by a gradual and relentless decrease in graft function. There is collagen deposition and scarring of the interstitium and arteriolar wall thickening. Proteinuria from glomerular damage is common. It is not clearly understood why chronic rejection occurs and, as such, therapy is severely limited.

22. DIABETES

What is diabetes mellitus?

It is a condition characterized by an absolute or relative insulin deficiency. It is classified according to the need for insulin replacement therapy, and untreated gives rise to a host of complications, most of which are due to small vessel disease.

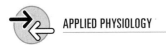

How would you diagnose and classify it?

The diagnosis may be suspected from the presentation with polyuria, polydipsia and tiredness. Alternatively, random blood or urine analysis may reveal an excess of glucose, but the definitive diagnosis is made by glucose tolerance testing.

Diabetes is defined as a fasting venous glucose >7.8 mmol/L or >11 mmol/L 2 hours after a standard glucose load. A standard glucose load is 75 g of glucose, usually represented by 353 ml of Lucozade. Impaired glucose tolerance is defined as a fasting venous glucose between 5.5 and 7.8 mmol/L or between 7.8 and 11 mmol/L 2 hours after a standard glucose load.

Type I diabetes is insulin-dependent (IDDM) and usually presents in child-hood. It may be due to a viral infection causing β-cell destruction. Type II – non-insulin-dependent diabetes mellitus (NIDDM) is usually of late onset and often familial. Treatment may vary from diet control alone, or include sulpho-nylureas or biguanides as therapy.

What special problems does the surgeon face when investigating a diabetic patient taking metformin?

Radiological investigations involving the use of contrast are contraindicated in patients on metformin because of the risk of renal impairment and precipita-tion of severe metabolic acidosis. To investigate them safely, renal function should be checked to ensure normality, and metformin withheld for 24 hours before investigation, and not recommenced until 48 hours afterwards.

How should these different types of diabetics be managed perioperatively?

Pre-operative starvation poses a problem for diabetics as their blood glucose concentrations can become seriously disordered, thus various regimes have been devised to ensure the safety of diabetic patients undergoing surgery.

NIDDM patients undergoing minor to intermediate surgery should omit their morning dose of diabetic tablets and be starved as normal. They should be operated on first on the list, if at all practicable, and then allowed to eat on return to the ward and recommence their diabetic regime as normal. NIDDM patients undergoing major surgery and IDDM patients should be started on a sliding scale. The patient is fasted but commenced on intravenous (IV) fluids and a variable IV insulin regime. Regular monitoring of blood sugar by finger-prick testing allows the rate of insulin infusion to be varied to alter the glucose concentration as appropriate. This can be continued until the patient is able to take a reasonable diet postoperatively, at which point normal diabetic therapy can be reinstituted.

A typical sliding scale – for there are many – would be as follows. The patient is infused 1 L of 5 per cent dextrose with 20 mmol/L KCl at the rate of 100 ml per hour and 50 units of human actrapid insulin are added to 50 ml of normal saline in a syringe on a syringe driver. The rate of insulin infusion is varied according to BM thus:

→ BM <4 – 0.5 ml per hour
→ BM 4–15 – 2 ml per hour
→ BM 16–20 – 4 ml per hour
→ BM >20 – review.

What perioperative complications are diabetics more prone to?

Diabetes, especially poorly controlled diabetes, predisposes to infection and wound healing can be a problem in some cases. As diabetes can cause renal damage, they are more at risk of postoperative renal failure and extreme care must be taken with fluid balance. All diabetics are at higher risk of arterial disease and, as such, complications related to this are commoner postoperatively; these include a greater risk of perioperative myocardial infarction, which may be painless due to autonomic neuropathy, risk of strokes and lower limb ischaemia. Neuropathy also leads to specific problems, such as pressure sores, especially on the heels. Obesity can be a problem, especially in non-insulin-dependent diabetics, and is associated with increased morbidity in its own right.

23. CARBON DIOXIDE

How is CO_2 transported in the blood?

It is transported in three ways. As CO_2 is 20 times more soluble in plasma than O_2, the proportion dissolved directly and carried in solution becomes significant and approaches 10 per cent, in proportion to the partial pressure. The second method of carriage is in combination with blood proteins – notably haemoglobin, as carbamino-haemoglobin – aided by the fact that deoxyhaemoglobin is a better carrier of CO_2 than oxyhaemoglobin. The majority of CO_2 is transported as bicarbonate. The reaction

$$CO_2 + H_2O \rightleftharpoons H_2CO_3 \rightleftharpoons H^+ + HCO_3^-$$

is catalysed by carbonic anhydrase in the red blood cell with the bicarbonate diffusing out of the cell. Electrochemical neutrality is maintained by an inward flux of chloride ions, known as the chloride or Hamburger shift, as hydrogen ion cannot readily diffuse out of the cell.

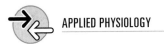
What effect does a raised CO₂ have on blood vessels?

Raised CO_2 concentrations have a moderate vasodilatory effect in most tissues, but have a marked dilatory effect on the cerebral and coronary vasculature. If CO_2 is considered as the waste product of cellular respiration, any accumulation in areas, such as ischaemic muscle, will have the effect of increasing blood flow through the area to try and reduce the tissue concentrations.

What effect does a raised metabolic PaCO₂ have on respiration?

Raised metabolic CO_2 gives rise to a metabolic acidosis because of combination with water forming carbonic acid, as detailed above. In order to attempt to correct this, the respiratory rate is increased to exhale more CO_2 and thus correct blood biochemistry. This is called respiratory compensation.

What factors control cerebral artery blood flow?

Cerebral blood flow is autoregulated. The smooth muscle of the cerebral arteries responds directly to changes in pressure gradient across the vessel wall. Thus, in most situations, the cerebral blood flow is independent of the perfusion pressure. This is true for systolic pressures of 60–160 mmHg. Autoregulation may fail, if the systemic blood pressure is outside this range, in hyperviscosity states, with raised intracranial pressure, and with changes in arterial pO_2 and pCO_2.

What factors control coronary artery blood flow?

By far the greatest proportion of coronary artery control is exerted at a local level by the heart muscle's exquisite sensitivity to local metabolite concentration. Substances implicated in the response include carbon dioxide, hydrogen ion, bradykinin and potassium. The greatest role, however, has been attributed to adenosine. When cellular oxygen levels are very low, ATP degrades to AMP and thence to adenosine, which leaches out of the cell to exert a profound vasodilatory effect. This is almost certainly not the whole story but as far as we have got so far. Neural control also plays a part; principally via sympathetic nerves as the coronary arteries have a very poor parasympathetic innervation. It should also be remembered that autonomic control of heart rate also affects coronary artery blood flow, as the duration of diastole is one determinant of flow as coronary arteries are compressed during ventricular systole prohibiting flow.

What happens to a patient with carbon monoxide inhalation?

The carbon monoxide combines with haemoglobin to form carboxyhaemoglobin, stopping normal oxygen transport. Symptoms include mental impairment, headache, nausea, vomiting and classic pink skin (usually rosy cheeked) due to the carboxyhaemoglobin. Eventually coma, respiratory distress and cardiac arrhythmias develop, leading to death if untreated. Treatment is removal from the CO source and administering high-flow oxygen; in some centres, hyperbaric oxygen therapy is also used to increase the amount of oxygen held in direct solution as a compensatory mechanism, whilst the CO is removed from the system.

24. BLOOD PRESSURE

What is blood pressure?

Blood pressure is the force exerted by the blood against any unit area of the vessel wall and is traditionally measured in millimetres of mercury. It may be expressed as a mean arterial pressure (MAP) about which there are oscillations, or more commonly as a systolic and diastolic pressure. These represent the biphasic output of the heart with high pressure on ventricular contraction and a lower pressure due to vascular recoil while the ventricles refill. As the blood pressure is closer to diastolic pressure for a greater proportion of the cardiac cycle, the mean arterial pressure is not simply an average of the diastolic and systolic pressures; it is given by the equation

$$\text{MAP} = \frac{(2 \times \text{diastolic pressure}) + \text{systolic pressure}}{3}.$$

What factors control blood pressure?

Blood pressure-controlling factors can be categorized into immediate, early and long term. Immediate factors are the central nervous system, baroreceptors and chemoreceptors. The central nervous system response occurs if blood flow to the vasomotor centre falls below 60 mmHg, at which level the centre is excited and the blood pressure is raised by sympathetic control. Baroreceptors in large arteries relay impulses to the tractus solitarius, which, as pressure increases, inhibits the vasomotor centre and excites the vagal centre, leading to the blood pressure falling. Chemoreceptors of the aortic and carotid bodies are sensitive to decreased PaO_2 and increased $PaCO_2$, which excite the vasomotor centre and raise blood pressure.

Early control mechanisms act within 30 minutes in response to changes in blood pressure. They consist of the renin–angiotensin response, stress–relaxation, capillary fluid shift, adrenaline–noradrenaline and ADH. In the renin–angiotensin system, increases in renal perfusion pressures cause less angiotensin II to be produced, causing a decrease in vascular resistance. Stress relaxation occurs as high arterial pressures cause relaxation in blood storage areas. Capillary fluid shift allows decreased capillary fluid loss with lower blood pressure allowing an increase in blood volume. Adrenaline/noradrenaline cause sympathetic vasoconstriction to raise blood pressure. ADH secretion is increased with hypotension and has a direct vasoconstricting effect, and decreases fluid loss.

Long-term control of blood pressure occurs through the renal control of body fluids. As blood pressure increases, the kidney loses more fluid and Na^+. In the long term, changes to the renal output curve develop.

Why is hypertension relevant to surgical practice?

Uncontrolled hypertension will result in cancellation of a surgical patient from theatre owing to the increased risks of cerebrovascular events and cardiac failure. Severe hypertension may rarely result in aortic dissection, particularly of the thoracic aorta, and this brings the patient to the attention of the cardiothoracic surgeons as it may need emergency surgical repair. For the majority of patients, hypertension is controlled by oral medication but the surgeon should recognize that a labile blood pressure pre-operatively may indicate widespread atherosclerosis. Diuretic treatment often gives rise to fluid and electrolyte disturbances, which should be assessed and corrected prior to embarking on surgery. Most antihypertensives are cardioprotective and should continue to be given pre-operatively with a sip of water, even when patients are 'nil by mouth'.

What causes of hypertension can be treated surgically?

Ninety per cent of people with hypertension have no obvious cause; this is idiopathic or essential hypertension. The treatment of these cases lies with the physician and his plethora of medications. Only 10 per cent of cases have a discernible cause, some of which are amenable to surgical correction and should be sought before the diagnosis of essential hypertension is accepted, particularly in young patients. Dysfunction of the adrenal gland is a potent cause of hypertension. Excess cortisol from Cushing's syndrome, driven by either a pituitary or adrenal tumour is amenable to surgical removal. Similarly, an aldosterone-secreting tumour of the adrenal gland, Conn's syndrome, may be surgically cured. Renovascular hypertension causes, by means of a reduction in juxtaglomerular perfusion, a potent stimulus to the renin–angiotensin system, causing profound hypertension. This is readily amenable to surgical treatment by excision of the stenosed segment with primary anastomosis or by radiological angioplasty techniques. Phaeochromocytoma also causes hypertension, which is usually paroxysmal, by release of huge quantities of catecholamines, causing marked vasoconstriction. Most are surgically removable.

How does the body respond to an acute fall in blood pressure due to a large gastrointestinal bleed, for example?

The body responds in such a way as to try to normalize its internal environment and maintain tissue perfusion of essential organs at a normal level, and this varies with the degree of shock. See Table 2.1.

Table 2.1 Physiological changes in response to haemorrhage

Degree of shock	Proportion of blood volume lost	Response
Class I	<15 per cent	Minimal signs and symptoms. There may be a slight tachycardia
Class II	15–30 per cent	Tachycardia increases. Tachypnoea is an early sign. Narrowing of the pulse pressure due to catecholamine-induced peripheral vasoconstriction. Anxiety may become manifest
Class III	30–40 per cent	Tachycardia, tachypnoea, a fall in systolic blood pressure and mental confusion. The skin is cool and pale as blood is diverted to essential organs
Class IV	>40 per cent	There is a marked drop in systolic pressure, diastolic pressure is often unobtainable, and urine output negligible. If >50 per cent blood volume is lost, unconsciousness ensues, and the pulse and blood pressure become unrecordable

25. PITUITARY GLAND

Describe the functional anatomy of the pituitary gland

Although named as one gland, functionally and embryologically it is two. The anterior pituitary, also known as the adenohypophysis, is derived from Rathke's pouch, an outgrowth of pharyngeal epithelium. The posterior pituitary or neuro-hypophysis is a downward projection of the hypothalamus. The adenohypophysis is connected to the hypothalamus via the pituitary portal system of blood vessels through which the hypothalamic releasing and inhibitory factors arrive at the anterior pituitary. The posterior pituitary is in direct neural connection with the hypothalamus above; indeed, the cell bodies of the neural cells of the neuro-hypophysis reside in the hypothalamus and the hormones are transported to the posterior pituitary down the axons. The anterior gland secretes six major hormones: growth hormone (GH), adrenocorticotrophic hormone, thyroid-stimulating hormone (TSH), prolactin, follicle-stimulating hormone (FSH) and luteinizing hormone (LH). The posterior pituitary secretes antidiuretic hormone and oxytocin.

What is a portal circulation?

It is a circulation that connects two capillary beds but does not receive a direct arterial supply nor drain into a venous system. The two of significance are the hypothalamic–hypophyseal and hepatic portal systems.

What is an acidophil adenoma and what are the endocrine consequences?

Cells of the anterior pituitary are often classified according to their staining characteristics, thus the cells that secret growth hormone and prolactin are known as acidophils, whilst the cells secreting TSH, FSH, LH and ACTH are classified as basophils. There are also cells with neutral staining characteristics called chromophobes. An acidophil adenoma is, therefore, a tumour of the acidophil cells. The consequences of overactivity can be viewed in two ways. Firstly, there is an excess of GH, and sometimes prolactin, which will give rise to the clinical conditions of giantism, if present before epiphyseal fusion, or acromegaly after fusion. Uncontrolled growth of an acidophil adenoma will also compress the rest of the gland and thus the patient may also suffer from hyposecretion of the basophil hormones.

What problems may result from an enlarging non-secretory pituitary tumour?

An enlarging tumour can compress normal functioning glandular tissue causing hyposecretion and a large non-secretory tumour may give rise to panhypopituitarism, with a complete absence of all anterior pituitary hormones. Owing to its anatomical location in the sella turcica, enlargement by tumour can cause pressure on the optic chiasm above leading to visual defects, such as a bitemporal hemianopia and ultimately blindness. Lateral extension can cause compression syndromes on those cranial nerves running through the cavernous sinuses. Tumours that have grown to enormous proportions may obstruct the third ventricle or protrude through the sphenoid sinuses as a pseudo-nasal polyp.

What is Sheehan's syndrome, and how does it present?

Sheehan's syndrome is pituitary infarction following a postpartum haemorrhage, symptoms are those of panhypopituitarism. Loss of libido, amenorrhoea and galactorrhoea are direct effects, secondary hypothyroidism and adrenal suppression lead to tiredness, mental slowing and mild hypotension. The classical hypopituitary patient will be pale and hairless – the 'alabaster skin' appearance.

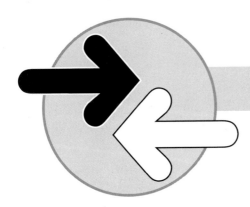

1. PANCREATITIS

What is acute pancreatitis and give a list of the common causes?

Pancreatitis is an acute inflammatory process of the pancreas with variable involvement of other regional tissues or remote organs. Acute pancreatitis is typified by severe epigastric pain radiating through to the back associated with nausea and vomiting. A raised serum amylase concentration greater than five times the normal laboratory range is the most commonly used diagnostic criterion. Elevated serum lipase is also diagnostic, and more specific, but is a rarely performed assay. In the UK, the two commonest causes of acute pancreatitis are gallstones and alcohol abuse, comprising over 80 per cent of all cases in approximately equal proportion. Other causes include:

→ anatomical abnormality – pancreas divisum, choledochal cyst
→ tumour obstructing the duct – ampullary, cholangiocarcinoma or head of pancreas carcinoma
→ drugs – oral contraceptive pill, thiazide diuretics and steroids
→ hypercalcaemia, hyperlipidaemia
→ viral infection – mumps
→ trauma – including endoscopic retrograde cholangiopancreatography (ERCP)
→ collagen vascular diseases.

How can the severity of an acute attack be assessed?

There are several validated scoring systems that can be applied to an attack of acute pancreatitis. In essence, they all attempt to identify at an early stage a severe acute attack, as studies have shown that they should be treated aggressively in a high dependency or intensive treatment unit, as the mortality is significantly higher than in mild attacks. The two commonly used systems are the Ranson criteria and the modified Glasgow criteria (Imrie).

The Glasgow criteria assesses nine variables on admission and daily throughout the first 48 hours of admission. Three positive criteria constitute severe acute pancreatitis and prognosis is related to the number of positive variables. One or two positive criteria are associated with a mortality of <1 per cent, three or four positive have a mortality of ~15 per cent, and for six or more positive criteria the mortality rate is 100 per cent. The criteria are remembered by the mnemonic 'PANCREAS' (see over).

C-reactive protein concentration will also give an accurate indication of severity; a CRP >210 in the first 96 hours of an attack also indicates severe acute pancreatitis, regardless of any other scoring.

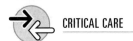
The most sensitive test for severity is an intravenous contrast-enhanced CT of the pancreas. This will delineate any areas of ischaemia and determine whether severe pancreatitis with necrosis is occurring. It is performed between days 3 and 10 of the patient's episode.

PO$_2$	<8 kPa
Age	>55
Neutrophils (WCC)	>15 × 10^9/L
Calcium	<2.0 mmol/L (corrected)
Raised urea	>16 mmol/L
Enzymes:	LDH >600 units/L, and AST >125 units/L
Albumin	<32 g/L
Sugar (glucose)	>10 mmol/L.

What are the complications of severe acute pancreatitis?

Pancreatitis has an overall mortality of 10–15 per cent, but severe acute pancreatitis has a mortality rate of around 30 per cent. In those patients who survive, there are many local complications of glandular inflammation and release of autolytic enzymes, namely, formation of phlegmons, pseudocysts or abscesses. There may be peripancreatic oedema, effusion or ascites. A phlegmon is a non-infective inflammatory mass. Pseudocyst formation is a localized encapsulated collection of enzyme-rich fluid, which is usually just necrotic sludge; it may be peripancreatic or form at some distance from the gland. Such a pseudocyst may become infected and an abscess results. Systemic complications are those organ system failures that necessitate ITU admission and can affect virtually all systems: adult respiratory distress syndrome (ARDS) and hypoxaemia are common, as is intestinal ileus and massive fluid sequestration. Metabolic derangements include hypocalcaemia, hypomagnesaemia and hypoalbuminaemia. Renal failure may ensue and cardiac arrhythmias can also occur.

After overcoming these complications, a proportion of acute pancreatitic patients will go on to develop chronicity. This is especially true where the aetiology is alcohol, mainly because many patients are unwilling, in spite of all the risks, to eschew alcohol. In those patients with gallstone aetiology, cholecystectomy is curative.

What are the current British Society of Gastroenterology (BSG) guidelines regarding pancreatitis?

The BSG has set out a series of guidelines and standards with regard to diagnosis and management that should be met in any unit treating pancreatitis in the UK. In summary they are:

→ overall mortality should be <10 per cent
→ mortality in the severe group should be <30 per cent

on laboratory references), and it becomes visible in the skin, sclera and mucous membranes at concentrations of greater than about 35–40 μmol/L.

Mechanisms of jaundice causation are as follows:

1 excessive bilirubin production from haemolytic anaemia
2 decreased hepatocyte uptake, which is rare
3 impaired conjugation, such as Gilbert or Crigler–Najjar syndromes, or severe hepatocellular disease
4 decreased hepatocyte excretion as in Dubin–Johnson syndrome or severe hepatocellular disease
5 impaired flow of bile through the biliary tree due to obstruction.

Points 1–3 cause an unconjugated hyperbilirubinaemia, 4 and 5 cause conjugated hyperbilirubinaemia, and 5 is cholestatic jaundice, often referred to as surgical jaundice.

How would you investigate a jaundiced patient?

After history taking and examination, blood should be taken for a range of laboratory tests:

→ *Haemoglobin estimation.* Anaemia may be an indicator of chronic disease or a bleeding ampullary carcinoma.
→ *White cell count.* If elevated, then cholangitis should be considered.
→ *Clotting screen.* Hepatic dysfunction disrupts clotting factor synthesis. A normal clotting screen is essential before embarking on invasive procedures.
→ *Urea and electrolytes.* Used to assess hydration and renal function as patients are at risk of hepatorenal syndrome.
→ *Liver function tests*:
  ● bilirubin – differential assays will detail conjugated and unconjugated levels
  ● alkaline phosphatase – this rises massively in obstructive jaundice
  ● ALT/AST – these tend to rise more in hepatic disease
  ● albumin – decreased in chronic disease states.
→ *Blood cultures.* Cholangitis can cause severe sepsis and cultures are essential if this diagnosis is considered.
→ *Hepatitis serology.*

How would you treat a jaundiced patient?

The initial aim of management is confirmation of diagnosis, elucidation of cause and maintenance of good hydration and urine output. The baseline imaging investigation of choice is abdominal ultrasound. This may reveal the presence of gallstones, and outline the number and position of any stones. Intrahepatic or extrahepatic duct dilatation and the level of obstruction are usually clearly seen. Ultrasound is also very good for examining the liver parenchyma for tumour, portal vein flow and porta hepatis lymphadenopathy, and may even demonstrate pancreatic masses, if overlying bowel gas permits. The septic cholangitic will need appropriate antibiotic treatment.

If it becomes clear from the ultrasound that a patient has obstructive jaundice, what is your next investigative procedure of choice?

In a case of demonstrated common bile duct obstruction, with no cause seen on the ultrasound, an urgent pancreatic CT scan is mandatory. This is to look for pancreatic lesions that would be amenable to resection. Endoscopic retrograde cholangiopancreatography should not be performed until after the pancreatic lesion is assessed. ERCP causes pancreatic inflammation, which makes subsequent imaging difficult to interpret and may occasionally make operative intervention impossible.

What are the advantages and complications of ERCP?

ERCP allows excellent demonstration of the ductal anatomy, including congenital abnormalities and the level of obstruction; it may allow brush cytology of intraluminal tumours. In addition, ERCP can be therapeutic via sphincterotomy and stone extraction, balloon dilatation or stenting. Prior to the procedure, a clotting screen should be taken and corrected, if deranged, and prophylactic antibiotics are essential.

The most important complication is ERCP-induced acute pancreatitis that occurs in up to 3 per cent of cases, although the incidence of acute, severe, life-threatening pancreatitis following the investigation is about 0.1 per cent. Despite being performed with antibiotic prophylaxis, there is an incidence of infection and septicaemia, although this risk is highest if the obstruction cannot be relieved once contrast has been injected. If therapeutic sphincterotomy is undertaken, haemorrhage may result, which can be life threatening. A small number of people may have contrast reactions. A further limitation of ERCP is the necessity of having specialist equipment and skilled endoscopists, which mean it may not be universally available.

What is this investigation, and what are the advantages and disadvantages of this test?

Figure 3.2 shows a magnetic resonance cholangiopancreatogram (MRCP). The main advantage of MRCP is that it is non-invasive. Provided the patient is not claustrophobic and can undergo MRCP, then there are no known side effects. The disadvantage of MRCP is that it is only diagnostic, and no therapeutic intervention can be performed.

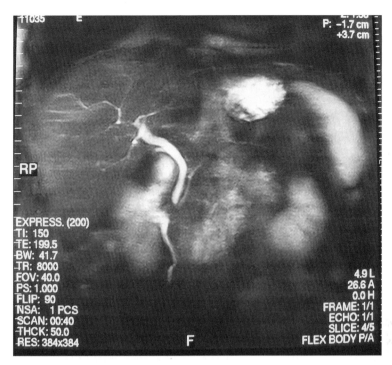

11035   E
P: -1.7 cm
+3.7 cm

RP

EXPRESS. (200)
TI: 150
TE: 199.5
BW: 41.7
TR: 8000
FOV: 40.0
PS: 1.000
FLIP: 90
NSA: 1 PCS
SCAN: 00:40
THCK: 50.0
RES: 384x384

4.9 L
26.6 A
0.0 H
FRAME: 1/1
ECHO: 1/1
SLICE: 4/5
FLEX BODY P/A

F

Figure 3.2

7. AIRWAY MANAGEMENT

What methods are there of managing a compromised airway?

A compromised airway should always be secured and the intervention needed will depend on the cause. Unconsciousness leads to airway compromise owing to loss of muscular control of the neck or tongue muscles. In these circumstances, simple emergency measures, such as jaw thrust or chin lift, will usually open the airway, and a Guedel airway or nasal airway will ensure a patent route while this is maintained.

Where definitive airway control is needed, the usual first-line treatment is by endotracheal intubation with a cuffed tube (uncuffed in children). This is usually the domain of the anaesthetist. In some cases, a laryngeal mask airway (LMA) can be used, but should be avoided in the emergency situation, since there is still a risk of aspiration with an LMA. When intubation is difficult, the anaesthetist may use a bougie to guide the tube, or even a fibreoptic laryngoscope.

In the event of an airway not being attained by these measures, then emergency surgical techniques are needed. The quickest is needle jet insufflation, using a 12- or 14-gauge cannula inserted via the cricothyroid membrane. This is connected to high-flow oxygen and a Y connector; the cycle is 4 seconds of insufflation followed by 1 second of exhalation. This technique will maintain oxygenation for around 20–40 minutes, but CO_2 levels soon rise, and this is not a definitive airway.

Definitive surgical airways are cricothyroidotomy and tracheostomy. The cricothyroidotomy can be performed as an emergency, whereas emergency tracheostomy should be avoided, if possible. Elective tracheostomy can be performed as an open technique or percutaneously using a guide wire and dilators.

A patient in A&E has a completely obstructed airway that an experienced anaesthetist cannot traverse. Describe how you would obtain an emergency airway

A cricothyroidotomy can be performed using local anaesthetic, if the patient were still conscious, or omitting it if in extremis. A fully prepared insertion tray must be ready. The patient is positioned supine with the neck extended. A 2–3 cm transverse incision is made over the cricothyroid membrane and deepened until it comes into view, the membrane is incised with a scalpel, placing the scalpel handle in the hole and turning it sideways to open the hole. A cricothyroid tube is now inserted and the patient ventilated through this, finally suturing the skin around the tube to ensure a snug fit.

In elective practice, when would you perform a tracheostomy?

The indications for elective tracheostomy are:

→ to relieve upper airway obstruction as a definitive procedure, such as in vocal cord paralysis, laryngeal tumours, chronic traumatic scarring, congenital atresias and laryngeal trauma
→ to improve respiratory function by reducing anatomical dead space and allowing regular effective aspiration of bronchial secretions
→ in respiratory paralysis, where it allows positive pressure ventilation to be used, such as elective long-term ventilation and coma
→ as a preliminary to certain head and neck surgery.

Describe the steps of an elective tracheostomy

The patient is consented and taken to the operating theatre, where, under a general anaesthetic, the patient is positioned supine with the neck extended. The neck is prepared and draped. A horizontal incision through skin and platysma is made at the level of the third tracheal ring. The strap muscles are retracted exposing the trachea and the thyroid isthmus. The isthmus is divided and oversewn for haemostasis. The tracheal rings are carefully identified and a vertical incision made through the third ring. The anaesthetist is asked to withdraw the endotracheal tube to a point above the incision. The incision is widened by removing a semicircle of cartilage on each side, and a tracheostomy tube is inserted and secured. As the tube is inserted, the anaesthetist should change the ventilator to the tracheostomy and withdraw the endotracheal tube. The wound is closed loosely around the tracheostomy.

What are the complications of tracheostomy?

Complications of tracheostomy occur at the time of creation or with tube management.

→ At the time of the procedure, bleeding from the thyroid isthmus can occur but should be controlled by oversewing.

→ Subcutaneous emphysema can occur after the tube is sited, especially if the skin is closed too tightly.

→ Blood can enter the trachea as the hole is made, leading to aspiration, and suction should be judiciously used to avoid this.

→ Infections around the tracheostomy site are not uncommon, and should be swabbed and treated as appropriate.

→ The first tube change should be performed with care, since misplacement can lead to airway compromise, but also anterior displacement can lead to erosion of the brachiocephalic vein, which is often fatal.

→ Tracheal stenosis can occur from prolonged cuff use, or with healing and scarring at a late stage.

8. RENAL FAILURE

Classify renal failure and give examples of each type

It can be easily classified into pre-renal, renal and post-renal renal failure. Post-renal failure occurs due to blockage of the passage of urine; this may be within the kidney, such as when myoglobin blocks the glomeruli or, more commonly, the blockage is extra-renal by neoplasms, calculi, prostatic enlargement, strictures or catheter occlusion. Intrinsic renal failure occurs from renal pathology, such as acute glomerulonephritis, septicaemia, nephrotoxicity or prolonged circulatory insufficiency. Pre-renal causes are the commonest type in a general surgical setting; the volume-depleted patient suffers renal circulatory insufficiency.

You are asked to see a catheterized, male, postoperative surgical patient who hasn't passed any urine for 4 hours. How are you going to assess the problem?

True anuria is generally only caused by a blocked outflow tract – commonly a blocked catheter, and so this is likely to be oliguria rather than anuria; oliguria being defined as a urine output less than 0.5 ml/kg per hour. Initially, a history is taken and the patient examined. Specific evidence of previous renal insufficiency, an enlarged bladder and the state of circulatory filling is sought. The catheter should be flushed to ensure it is not blocked. Examination of his fluid input/output charts would indicate, along with his pulse, blood pressure and pulse pressure, whether he was likely to be underfilled. All recent urea and electrolyte results should be examined and a new set requested. All information is interpreted in light of the patient's operation and operative fluid losses. In general, post-renal causes should be excluded and any evidence to suggest intrinsic renal failure is sought.

What is the management of postoperative oliguria?

In the event, the patient appeared fluid depleted increased intravenous fluids are prescribed, giving due regard to his cardiovascular status and the patient's ability to accept fluid loading. If fluid filling within the limits of clinical monitoring did not abate the oliguria, then more invasive monitoring in the form of a central venous pressure line is appropriate. With a CVP line *in situ*, a fluid challenge is given to the patient to gain an indication of the state of filling. If clinically and with CVP readings the patient is well filled but still oliguric, then the use of diuretics may be appropriate, normally in the form of intravenous frusemide. 'Low-dose renal' dopamine has not convincingly been shown to help this type of oliguric patient beyond acting as an additional diuretic. If the patient were well filled and remained oliguric after diuretics, and outflow obstruction from rare conditions, such as bilateral ureteric obstruction was excluded, then the ITU should be contacted for assistance. In the face of deteriorating renal function, as witnessed by rising urea and potassium concentrations and fluid accumulation, then renal dialysis should be considered. In patients with compromised renal function, NSAIDs should be avoided as should ACE inhibitors if possible. Gentamicin is nephrotoxic and should be changed to another antibiotic if possible.

What are the indications for renal replacement therapy?

Renal replacement therapy (RRT) is indicated in renal failure of whatever aetiology, where there is uncontrollable rising serum potassium, symptomatic uraemia or its complications, severe acidosis or pulmonary oedema from fluid overload.

How can RRT be achieved?

Available methods are haemodialysis, peritoneal dialysis and haemofiltration. In haemodialysis, the patient's blood is pumped through an artificial kidney with a dialysate to 'filter' the blood by ultrafiltration. Both hydrostatic pressure from the pump and an osmotic pressure generated from the glucose present in the dialysis fluid are used to drive the ultrafiltration process. Peritoneal dialysis allows a dialysis fluid to reside in the peritoneal cavity with exchange of metabolites by diffusion alone. In haemofiltration the patient's blood is driven through a filter by the patient's arterial pressure, and a dialysate added around the filter and diffusion of waste metabolites occurs into the dialysate – it is, in essence, a slow haemodialysis.

9. BURNS

You are called to A&E to manage a 64-year-old lady who was trapped in her room in a house fire and has suffered obvious burns including the face. Describe the first steps in your management

In a severely injured person such as this, a methodical approach is used and given the history of entrapment and facial burns the first priority is ensuring a secure airway. There should be a low threshold for intubating the patient electively as there is likely to be an inhalational component to the burn and laryngeal oedema can make emergency intubation later on very hazardous. Features that indicate likely inhalational injury are the history of fire in an enclosed space, cough, sooty sputum, facial burns, singed nasal hairs and chest signs.

Ventilation is maintained and secure intravenous access is obtained, which is needed for both fluid resuscitation and the administration of opiate analgesia. An estimate of the patient's weight is needed and an estimation of the depth and severity of burn injury.

How would you assess the extent and severity of the burns?

The depth of burn is assessed by dividing it into two categories. Partial thickness burns encompass the old descriptions of superficial and deep dermal burns. They may be blistered, red or white, but are sensate and painful. Full thickness burns are white, leathery, painless and numb. A quick approximation of burn surface area can be made using Wallace's rule of nines but, if available, the burn distribution can be plotted on a Lund and Browder chart – ensuring that the correct chart for the age of the patient is used.

The 64-year-old lady has 45 per cent full-thickness burns, including her entire anterior chest wall and encircling her right arm. She is tachycardic, tachypnoeic and hypotensive. What will you do now?

In view of the inhalational injury and the widespread burns, blood is withdrawn for FBC including PCV, urea and electrolytes, clotting, group and save, calcium, glucose and liver function tests. An arterial catheter is placed for invasive blood pressure monitoring and repeated arterial blood gas estimation. Similarly, at some stage in the initial resuscitation phase, a central venous catheter is inserted to allow monitoring of aggressive fluid resuscitation. The patient is discussed at an early stage with the regional burns unit and transfer arranged, when appropriate, which is as soon as the patient is stable enough for transport.

What resuscitation regime would you use?

Fluid resuscitation using a recognized formula is instituted. One commonly used is the Muir and Barclay formula, which gives the volume of fluid needed in addition to maintenance fluid in the first 24 hours. It is calculated as:

$$\text{Replacement fluid volume (ml)} = \text{Body weight (kg)} \times \text{burn surface area (per cent)}^2$$

and is given as Hartmann's over each of the following periods from the time of burn: 4 hours, 4 hours, 4 hours, 6 hours, 6 hours and 12 hours.

The resuscitation formula is taken to start at the time of burn; thus, by the time the patient is in A&E, they are usually well behind on fluids and this must be corrected. Other reliable formulae are Parkland or the Brooke formula. Fluid resuscitation should be initiated on any patient sustaining greater than 15 per cent body surface area burns or greater than 10 per cent in a child or the elderly.

There are no immediately available burns ITU beds in the region and your anaesthetist is becoming concerned about the increasing difficulty in ventilating her. What else would you consider?

Probable causes of the decreasing chest compliance are the effect of the inhalational injury itself causing pulmonary oedema and the constricting effect of the chest wall burns. This lady needs urgent escharotomy and, if urgent transfer to a burns unit is not feasible, then it should be performed in location – also paying attention to her arm, which will also need releasing escharotomies to prevent limb ischaemia. The plan should be discussed with the local burns centre to confirm that they agree that escharotomy should be performed rather than waiting for transfer.

What are the principles regarding urgent escharotomy of this patient's chest and arm?

If possible, escharotomies are performed in a proper operating theatre rather than in A&E. A supply of scalpel blades, a diathermy machine, a large supply of sterile swabs and crepe bandages, and a dilute solution of adrenaline are organized. Full-thickness burns requiring escharotomy are insensate and no further anaesthetic is needed. The chest wall burns are incised lateral to the nipples on both sides and transversely to release a 'breastplate' of burnt tissue to relieve the constriction. Chequerboard escharotomy gives a worse cosmetic result and is no longer in vogue. The arm is incised along the pre-axial and postaxial borders and continued on the ulnar border of the fingers, taking care to avoid the position of the digital nerves just volar to the axial plane. Liberal use of diathermy to provide haemostasis and wrapping the limbs in adrenaline-soaked swabs with firm crepe bandaging helps to decrease blood loss, which can be considerable.

What is this patient's prognosis?

Poor. A chart (Bull 1971)[1] is available relating chances of survival to age and area of burn. For this lady, there is only a 20 per cent survival chance. As a general rule, if the age and the percentage burn added together are greater than 100, then the chance of survival is poor.

10. GASTROINTESTINAL FAILURE

Define gastrointestinal failure. List the causes

Gastrointestinal failure occurs when there is insufficient nutrient absorption to maintain health and physiological function. The causes can be broadly grouped as a decrease in area, decrease in transit time, enzymatic failure, infection or one of a group of specific absorption defects.

A decrease in absorptive area may be the result of multiple surgical resections in diseases such as Crohn's disease or mesenteric thrombosis. Sometimes these patients require long-term TPN at home to survive. Resection of the terminal ileum will produce a specific defect in that vitamin B_{12} will no longer be absorbed. Coeliac disease is an autoimmune condition in which the patient is sensitive to the α-gliadin fraction of wheat gluten and villous atrophy results, which massively decreases the gut surface area. Similar histological appearances may be seen in tropical sprue, but the patient does not respond to a gluten-free diet. Inflammation of the gut wall by conditions such as Whipple's or Crohn's disease or lymphoma can also have the effect of reducing surface area.

After a gastrectomy, there may be a significant rise in transit speed that reduces enzyme mixing and decreases absorption. Similarly, in carcinoid syndrome the excess levels of 5-hydroxytryptamine and simultaneously secreted substance P cause rapid gut transit. This, however, is very rare. Chronic pancreatitis is a common cause in this country of malabsorption, as destruction of the gland decreases the amount of enzyme secretion, although steatorrhoea only occurs when >75 per cent of lipase activity is lost. Cystic fibrosis is another chronic condition that may cause pancreatic malabsorption, as the chloride

[1] Bull JP | Revised analysis of mortality due to burns. *Lancet* 1971; 7734:1133.

transport defect at the heart of the disease makes the secretions of the pancreas – and other organs – too viscid. The raised $[H^+]$ accrued in Zollinger–Ellison syndrome can, rarely, inactivate pancreatic lipase and decrease absorption.

Gut infestation with the protozoa *Giardia lamblia* may cause malabsorptive diarrhoea. Blind loop syndrome occurs with stagnation of bowel contents, which leads to an overgrowth of bacteria that has two effects: firstly, there is increased competition for vitamin B_{12} and there is a decreased absorption of this, and, secondly, there is catalysis of bile salt deconjugation impairing fat absorption. A similar effect is seen after alteration of the gut bacterial flora by broad-spectrum antibiotics. Biliary obstruction affects fat absorption by interruption of the entero-hepatic circulation of bile salts. Pernicious anaemia results in a deficiency of intrinsic factor, thus affecting vitamin B_{12} again. Disaccharidase deficiency results in an osmotic diarrhoea and electrolyte deficiency. Protein-losing enteropathy is a gut condition akin to nephrotic syndrome in which large amounts of protein are lost through an abnormally permeable intestinal wall; hypoalbuminaemia results.

What are the treatment options?

Many of these conditions have specific causes and treatment should be directed towards those, for instance, a patient diagnosed with coeliac disease should be instructed on the benefits of a gluten-free diet. Short bowel syndromes may have to be treated with permanent TPN. Insertion of an anti-peristaltic segment of gut to slow transit may be beneficial, although gambling with a length of gut in a patient with short bowel problems is a risky business and remains controversial. Sprue often responds to antibiotic therapy as will giardiasis. In cases of pancreatic enzyme deficiency of whatever cause, replacement therapy can be instituted using commercially available preparations.

If the failure is pancreatic, what may the patient describe for you?

Classically, they will describe weight loss and steatorrhoea – pale bulky offensive stools, which float and are difficult to flush away. They leave an oily sheen in the toilet pan. Steatorrhoea is defined as a daily faecal fat excretion of $>5\,g$ in a stool weight of $>60\,g$.

11. INTRAVENOUS FLUIDS

What fluid would you use to replace the loss from a nasogastric tube?

Nasogastric tube aspirate is electrolyte-rich fluid containing large amounts of potassium, sodium, chloride and bicarbonate. It should be replaced with as similar a fluid as possible, i.e. Hartmann's solution or normal saline with added potassium.

What are the constituents of 5 per cent dextrose, normal saline and Hartmann's solution?

Five per cent dextrose is a solution of 50 g of anhydrous glucose in 1 litre of water with a calorific value of 200 calories (4 cal/g). Table 3.1 shows the constituents of each (all values given as mmol/L).

Table 3.1

Osmolality	Na^+	Cl^-	K^+	HCO_3^-	Ca^{2+}	Dextrose
5% dextrose	280					5%
Normal saline	308	154	154			
Hartmann's solution	278	131	111	5	29	2

What are 'Haemaccel' and 'Gelofusin', and what are their constituents?

They are synthetic colloids that are a solution of degraded bovine gelatins, polygeline. 'Haemaccel' has the following ionic composition (all values given as mmol/L):

Na^+	Ca^{2+}	K^+	Cl^-	PO_4^- and SO_4^-
145	6.3	5.1	145	Trace

Isotonicity is maintained by the polypeptides of the gelatin. Although Gelofusin is broadly similar, it has approximately one-tenth of the concentrations of Ca^{2+} and K^+.

Explain why 'Haemaccel' stays in the circulation longer than either normal saline or dextrose

'Haemaccel' is a synthetic colloid solution that generates an oncotic pressure, whereas crystalloids, such as saline or dextrose, are salt solutions made up of small molecules that do not generate an oncotic pressure. As a result, when a crystalloid is introduced into the blood stream, it will attempt to move by osmosis to an area with a higher oncotic pressure, which is the surrounding extravascular tissues. Because colloids such as 'Haemaccel' generate their own oncotic pressure, the osmotic gradient is lower and less fluid moves out of the circulation.

What are the daily requirements of an average 70 kg man in terms of potassium, sodium, fluid volume and calories?

In general health, the average adult will ingest 50–100 mmol of both sodium and potassium, although probably slightly more sodium than potassium, and only 15 per cent or so of K^+ is retained, the rest being excreted in the urine. In the setting of intravenous fluid replacement, a daily intake of 1–2 mmol/kg body weight Na^+ and 60 mmol of K^+ will usually suffice. Assuming normovolaemia, the average daily intravenous fluid volume required for maintenance is 2500 ml. Ongoing losses from the gastrointestinal tract, pyrexia or burns must be replaced as well. Adequate nutrition in most patients can be maintained by an intake of 1800–2000 calories per day. Patients who are hypercatabolic due to disease may need more.

Describe the differences between osmolarity and osmolality. How would you make osmolar and osmolal solutions?

Osmolarity describes the concentration per litre of solvent, whereas osmolality quotes a concentration per kilogram of solution. To make an osmolar solution of a substance, dissolve the substance in 1 L of water, thus making the total volume greater than 1 L. For an osmolal solution, dissolve the substance in a small amount of solvent and then make the total volume up to 1 L – thus, the concentration in an osmolal solution is higher as the total volume is less.

12. RESPIRATORY FAILURE

What do the blood gases in Figure 3.3 show?

This is a picture of respiratory failure with a respiratory alkalosis. There is a low pO_2 and a normal pCO_2 indicating respiratory failure. Bicarbonate and base excess are normal. There is a mild alkalosis, which is due to hyperventilation in acute hypoxia.

Define and classify respiratory failure

Respiratory failure may be defined as a state where pulmonary gas exchange is impaired to give hypoxia with or without hypercapnia. Arbitrary limits for the definition of failure are $PaO_2 < 8$ kPa or $PaCO_2 > 6.7$ kPa.

Type I respiratory failure results from gas exchange problems due to lung tissue damage. Type II failure is 'pump' failure, when the system is unable to excrete the volume of CO_2 produced.

Type I failure results from increased shunt, i.e. more blood enters the left heart without being exposed to gas exchange in the pulmonary system. There is

Blood gas values		
↑ pH	7.471	(7.350–7.455)
cH_c^+	33.8 nmol/L	
pCO_2	4.55 kPa	(4.27–6.00)
↓ pO_2	6.59 kPa	(11.1–14.4)
$cHCO_3^- (P)_c$	24.6 mmol/L	
↓ sO_2	87.9 %	(95.0–99.0)
Temperature corrected values		
pH(T)	7.471	
$cH^+(T)_c$	33.8 nmol/L	
$pO_2(T)$	6.59 kPa	
$pCO_2(T)$	4.55 kPa	
Oximetry values		
ctHb	11.4 g/dl	
sO_2	87.9 %	
Hct_c	35.2 %	
Acid–base status		
$cBase(Ecf)_c$	1.2 mmol/L	
$cHCO_3^- (P,st)_c$	25.7 mmol/L	

Figure 3.3

increased respiratory rate and decreased tidal volume. Hypocarbia ensues, as the diffusion capacity of CO_2 is much greater than that of O_2. Type II failure has decreased ventilatory effort and increased dead space. There is hypercarbia and a low respiratory rate – the patient gets fatigued. Hypoxia can, in part, be attributed to carbon dioxide diluting the oxygen in the oxygen cascade. The causes of hypoventilation may be considered according to their site of action/impairment. Stroke or head injury can directly affect the higher respiratory centres, as can anaesthetic agents and opiate analgesics. Trauma, poliomyelitis, Guillain–Barré syndrome and epidural local anaesthetics all act on the spinal cord and peripheral nerves. Myasthenia gravis acts at the neuromuscular junction and can cause profound hypoventilation. Deformities or injury to the chest wall reduce the efficiency of ventilation, as do pleural effusions and pneumothoraces within the chest cavity. Constriction of the airway from tumour, asthma or chronic obstructive pulmonary disease (COPD) is the lowest site of pulmonary hypoventilation.

Explain the four types of hypoxaemia

→ *Anaemic* – hypoxaemia occurs due to inadequate amounts of haemoglobin for oxygen carriage. This may be straightforward anaemia or may also occur in situations, such as carbon monoxide poisoning, where carboxyhaemo-globin preferentially binds oxygen.

→ *Stagnant* – an effect of poor tissue perfusion either centrally from low cardiac output or peripherally from local perfusion defects.

→ *Histotoxic* – a block to the cellular utilization of oxygen is present. This is typified by the effects of cyanide inhibiting the cytochrome pathways.

→ *Hypoxic* – a broad category that includes hypoventilation, impairment of gaseous diffusion in the alveoli and V/Q mismatch.

What is adult respiratory distress syndrome?

The adult respiratory distress syndrome is pulmonary oedema with a normal central venous pressure and pulmonary artery wedge pressure, i.e. the oedema is not cardiogenic in origin. It characterizes a Type I respiratory failure and is typified by stiff lungs, diffuse bilateral pulmonary infiltrates on chest x-ray and hypoxia. There should be an identifiable cause.

What treatment strategies are available in the management of ARDS?

All types of respiratory failure are treated by increasing the concentration of inspired oxygen. Techniques such as PEEP or CPAP are utilized to recruit consolidated alveoli and hold them open, increasing the area available for gaseous diffusion.

Reversal of the inspiratory:expiratory ratio is beneficial. Prone ventilation allows alveoli previously compressed under the effect of gravity to be opened up. Nitrous oxide is a potent vasodilator and has a predilection for acting on the pulmonary circulation – its action is to dilate the pulmonary vessels near to working alveoli, thus maximizing the blood supply to ventilated lung. Newer strategies include partial liquid ventilation using perfluorocarbon compounds, which reduces the work of breathing by reducing surface tension, particularly in collapsed dependent lung areas; it also decreases lung inflammation. Some centres have used extracorporeal membrane oxygenation as a salvage method in ARDS resistant to other modalities.

13. METABOLIC RESPONSE TO TRAUMA

Describe the body's metabolic response to trauma

The metabolic response is divided into three: the ebb, catabolic or flow, and anabolic phases.

→ *The ebb phase* lasts only for a few hours from injury, and is characterized by a depression of local metabolism and reduction in energy expenditure.

→ *The catabolic 'flow' phase* soon follows, mediated by an increased catecholamine drive, which mobilizes energy reserves from adipose tissue and carbohydrate stores in liver and muscle. There is an increase in protein breakdown coupled with increasing gluconeogenesis and a parallel decrease in insulin sensitivity, thus creating hyperglycaemia. The increase in protein degradation outstrips protein synthesis, so there is marked nitrogen loss that is proportional to the pre-injury nutritional status – the largest nitrogen losses occur in previously healthy young men with major burns. In this period, no amount of exogenous protein supplementation will obviate the negative nitrogen balance and nitrogen positivity should not be attempted. This proteolysis results in muscular weakness, decreased enzymatic function, decreased immune competence and excessive hepatic gluconeogenesis. It is in this period that rapid weight loss occurs.

→ *The anabolic phase*. If recovery from the injuries occurs, an anabolic phase supervenes in which weight gain occurs, protein and fat stores are replenished and metabolic rate returns to normal. This phase may last for several months depending on the extent of the initial injuries.

Do wounds heal despite this protein breakdown?

Despite the large turnover of protein as described above, only in the worst cases of persistent malnutrition do surgical or traumatic wounds fail to heal, indicating that whatever else goes on, the wound has primacy in terms of protein manufacture.

Where does the body derive its energy from?

Hepatic stores of glycogen are readily used up and from about 24 hours after injury the energy requirements are met by triglyceride mobilization from adipose tissue. There is an increase in free fatty acid oxidation producing ketone bodies, 3-hydroxybutyrate and acetoacetate, and adaptive responses occur that allow the brain and other tissues to utilize them as energy substrates.

Describe the metabolic changes that occur in the starving patient

The changes that occur are aimed at maintaining lean muscle mass. Glycogen stores last only for about 24 hours, after which catabolic muscle breakdown begins. Metabolic rate falls, however, and protein catabolism decreases about five-fold from the 1–2 week point onwards. There is a gradual increase in fat utilization as an energy source and adaptive ketogenesis occurs; by the 3-week point, the brain can utilize ketone bodies as an energy source. Lipolysis in the early weeks is inhibited by insulin but the insulin levels fall as starvation continues. Stored triglyceride is hydrolysed for gluconeogenesis, whereas fatty acids are used as fuel or converted to ketones for fuel in the liver. There is a fall in the metabolic rate and in total body energy expenditure. The central nervous system utilizes mostly ketones and gluconeogenesis in the liver falls as protein metabolism slows. Most of the energy comes from adipose tissue, with a gradual protein loss until all available fat is used.

What kills the starving patient?

Gradual but progressive protein wasting results in muscle weakness. This weakness in respiratory muscles leads to atelectasis, pneumonia and ultimately death in the majority of people in this situation.

14. ADDISON'S DISEASE

What are the typical features of Addison's disease?

Addison's disease is adrenocortical insufficiency due to bilateral adrenal cortex destruction. The adrenal cortex secretes the mineralocorticoid aldosterone, glucocorticoids, primarily cortisol and the sex hormones.

The lack of aldosterone and cortisol results in hyponatraemia and hyperkalaemia associated with decreased mineralocorticoid activity. Stimulation of the negative feedback loop to the anterior pituitary gland results in increased serum ACTH levels.

Clinically, the patient complains of malaise, anergia and weight loss. Hypotension is marked, with 90 per cent of patients having a systolic blood pressure less than 110 mmHg and orthostatic symptoms due to hypovolaemia and sodium loss. There are usually areas of increased pigmentation, particularly the nipples, palmar creases, in the mouth opposite the molars, scars and areas of pressure, such as under bra straps, due to the increase in anterior pituitary production of pro-opiomelanocortin. This is the precursor molecule of both ACTH and melanocyte-stimulating hormone (MSH), hence the pigmentation. Plasma cortisol is low on an 8am sample and there will be elevation of plasma ACTH levels. A short synacthen test is confirmatory. The patient may complain of their symptoms for many months or even years before consideration is given to Addison's disease as a possible diagnosis – many patients are only diagnosed when they present acutely as an Addisonian crisis.

What are the common causes of Addison's disease?

→ Tuberculosis – as described in Thomas Addison's original description of the disease.

→ Autoimmune disease, which is now the commonest cause.

→ Fungal – blastomycosis.

→ Haemochromatosis.

→ Amyloidosis.

→ Sarcoidosis.

→ Metastatic carcinoma.

→ Iatrogenic – surgical removal in the treatment of Cushing's syndrome.

→ Waterhouse–Fredreichson syndrome. Meningococcal septicaemia can cause adrenocortical infarction.

Describe an Addisonian crisis and its treatment

An acute presentation may be precipitated by any intercurrent infection or situation requiring the body to mount a stress response. Acute withdrawal of the patient's normal corticoid supplements will also precipitate a crisis. The primary features are massive hypovolaemia and shock associated with headache, nausea and vomiting, weakness, abdominal pain, confusion and coma. There is usually marked hypotension. Biochemical analysis demonstrates a profound hyponatraemia, which may be as low as 115 mmol/L, hyperkalaemia and hypoglycaemia. There is often hypercalcaemia in addition. The resultant depletion of the intravascular and extravascular compartments may require enormous volumes of fluid. The major deficiencies of salt, steroid and glucose are addressed. Provided there is no cardiovascular disease, 1 L of saline is given over 30–60 minutes. If hypoglycaemic, dextrose is infused concurrently. Subsequent fluid requirements may be high and a central line should be considered for monitoring. Hydrocortisone 100 mg IV is given 6 hourly until the patient is stable. Fludrocortisone is not needed in the acute setting.

How is the diagnosis confirmed and what is the long-term treatment?

The biochemical abnormalities should strongly suggest the diagnosis and further investigation used to confirm this. A short synacthen test should prove the clinical suspicion. A standard dose of synacthen is given parenterally and plasma cortisol measured at administration and between 30 and 60 minutes later. A normal subject will demonstrate a rise in plasma cortisol, which is absent in the Addisonian patient. It is important to prohibit hydrocortisone administration for 8 hours prior to the test, as this leads to erroneous results.

The cause should be treated, if possible, such as tuberculosis or blastomycosis. Treatment is by replacement therapy, typically fludrocortisone and hydrocortisone.

The dose of glucocorticoid is judged on patient well-being and cortisol levels. Mineralocorticoid dose is assessed by blood pressure response to standing, i.e. it should not fall, and suppression of plasma renin to normal activity. Patients should be educated to increase their hydrocortisone when ill to mimic a 'stress response'.

What is secondary hypoadrenalism?

This is adrenal hypofunction due to non-adrenal causes. It occurs in hypothalamic–pituitary disease and in long-term steroid use when hypothalamic-pituitary–adrenal suppression occurs. It is tested for by the long synacthen test, with a higher dose of synacthen, and blood tests at 0, 1, 2, 3, 4, 5, 8 and 24 hours.

Thomas Addison (1793–1860) – an English physician of Guys Hospital who published his monograph on 'the constitutional and local effects of disease of the suprarenal capsule' in 1855. He committed suicide by jumping from a window shortly after retiring.

15. CARDIAC TAMPONADE

A youth is brought in to A&E having been stabbed in the 4th left intercostal space at the sternal edge. He is tachycardic and hypotensive. What is the most likely diagnosis? What is the differential diagnosis?

A pericardial tamponade is the most likely diagnosis. The other leading differential would be a tension pneumothorax. In tamponade, the pericardial blood decreases transmission of the heart sounds and they sound muffled on auscultation. There is a raised jugular venous pressure as the raised intrathoracic pressure decreases venous return, although this does not occur as dramatically as in tension pneumothorax. Hyper-resonance of the hemithorax with decreased breath sounds would point towards pneumothorax, as would tracheal deviation away from affected side. A further possibility is hypovolaemia from blood loss into a haemothorax, which would produce the same picture of shock but the breath sounds are louder due to conduction through the fluid. There tends to be an associated pneumothorax.

What is the emergency management of pericardial tamponade?

In tamponade there is a risk of an electromechanical dissociation (EMD) arrest so he needs the pericardial space decompressing. This is most easily achieved by pericardiocentesis. The skin is prepared, if time allows, and a syringe and long 12- or 14-gauge needle is inserted through the skin under the left xiphicostal angle. The needle is at 45° to the skin, aiming for the tip of the left shoulder. Suction is maintained on the syringe as the needle is advanced until the pericardium is entered. Care must be taken not to advance too far and aspirate from the ventricle. Traversing the ventricular myocardium will be signalled by ventricular ectopics and arrhythmias on the cardiac monitor. One attempt should suffice, since there is no benefit in puncturing the ventricle many times.

Describe how you would perform an anterolateral thoracotomy

The patient is anaesthetized using a double lumen endotracheal tube. The patient is in the full lateral position with the appropriate side uppermost and the body supported appropriately. The upper arm is normally supported in an arm gutter. The skin is prepared and draped and the landmarks identified. The skin incision runs from a point midway between the lateral edge of the vertebral body and the medial edge of scapula, and runs in the line of the ribs to one fingerbreadth below the tip of the scapula. The skin is incised and the underlying fat and fascia divided with diathermy. Latissimus dorsi is divided anteriorly and the anterior part of erector spinae is divided posteriorly, if more room is required. Serratus anterior should be left intact. Slide a hand up under the scapula to identify the first rib and thence count down to the sixth rib. The tissues overlying the upper portion of the sixth rib are divided using diathermy, leaving the bone intact. The periosteum is raised and a stripper used over the rib edge posteriorly and pulled anteriorly to detach the intercostals, asking your anaesthetist to deflate the lung as you go. A rib spreader is inserted and gently distracted. If more room is required, a small portion of the rib may be excised posteriorly. The thoracotomy and deflated lung now allow access to the pericardia. Care should be taken not to damage the phrenic nerve as it runs down the pericardium. Penetrating cardiac injuries from a stab wound can usually be closed directly using 'Teflon' patches to buttress the sutures. Closure after haemostasis and chest drain placement (×2) is by 0 PDS around the two previously distracted ribs, at which point the lung can be inflated. The periosteum can then be closed with the same stitch, and muscle and fascia are repaired in two layers with PDS. Subcutaneous and then subcuticular stitches are used to close the fat and skin. The chest drains are connected to an underwater seal.

16. POTASSIUM AND SODIUM

A patient of yours has a potassium of 6.9 mmol/L. In general, what are the causes of hyperkalaemia and which are commonest in surgical patients?

The commonest cause of hyperkalaemia is artefactual, caused by a haemolysed sample! Potassium is predominantly an intracellular ion and, if a sample is mishandled, cell lysis releases large amounts of potassium. Another common surgical cause is an increase of total body potassium caused by overenthusiastic potassium therapy or failure to stop potassium treatment. Severe injury, particularly crush injuries release huge amounts of potassium after reperfusion, again due to cell injury. This could be classed as a redistributive cause. A rare condition known as hyperkalaemic familial periodic paralysis is also in this category. Finally, there are renal causes of high potassium.

Potassium excretion is dependent on the amount of sodium available to exchange with; thus sodium depletion and the causes thereof will tend to cause hyperkalaemia. Any form of glomerular dysfunction can be responsible, as can any mineralocorticoid deficiency such as Addison's disease or congenital adrenal hyperplasia, where 21-hydroxylase deficiency ensures no aldosterone is synthesized. ACE inhibitor therapy has a similar effect by reduction in aldosterone secretion, owing to interference in the renin–angiotensin pathway. The classical aldosterone agonist spironalctone is, of course, used therapeutically as a potassium-sparing diuretic.

Both acidosis and hypoxia impair the Na^+/K^+ pump and cause a net gain of ECF potassium. Insulin normally enhances the passage of potassium from the ECF into the cell, but in situations of deranged glucose metabolism, such as diabetic ketoacidosis, potassium remains in the ECF space, resulting in hyperkalaemia. If glomerular function is intact, however, urinary potassium loss continues but at an insufficient rate to correct the hyperkalaemia. There is a decrease in total body potassium but a rise in serum potassium.

What are the ECG changes of hyperkalaemia?

Hyperkalaemia increases the risk of cardiac arrhythmia. Initially, there are high peaked T waves and a widened QRS complex. ST depression ensues followed by disappearance of the T waves. Cardiac arrest may supervene.

How would you treat hyperkalaemia?

Exogenous potassium therapy should be halted immediately. Calcium will temporarily antagonize the depressive effect of potassium on the myocardium, so where the potassium is grossly raised, the emergency measure of priority is the administration of 10 ml of 10 per cent calcium gluconate as a cardioprotective agent. Glucose and insulin (50 g glucose and 20 units human actrapid IV) will reduce potassium levels by driving the K^+ back into the cells. A total of 40 ml 8.4 per cent sodium bicarbonate will also reduce hyperkalaemia. The underlying cause should be sought. If it is a chronic condition, then calcium resonium orally will bind gut potassium and reduce absorption. If these measures fail and potassium continues to rise, then consideration should be given to haemodialysis.

What are the causes of hyponatraemia and hypernatraemia?

Hyponatraemia may be due to water excess or sodium deficit. Salt-deficient hyponatraemia may be caused by large sodium losses from the gut, renal salt loss in diuretic overuse, osmotic diuresis in hyperglycaemia and tubulo-interstitial renal disease. Hyponatraemia due to volume overload is uncommon in a person with normal kidneys, but postoperative overtransfusion of crystalloid is a common cause. It commonly presents in patients with heart failure, hepatic cirrhosis and nephrotic syndrome. The syndrome of inappropriate anti-diuretic hormone secretion (SIADH) occurs in conjunction with many other conditions, particularly pulmonary and central nervous system diseases. ADH secretion may also be ectopic from malignant tumours and presents with hyponatraemia with normal fluid volume.

Hypernatraemia usually occurs due to loss of water in excess of sodium. True sodium excess is very rare and is usually iatrogenic. Insufficient intake of fluids, low-sodium gastrointestinal losses, such as gastric fluid and loss from extensive burns, will all cause hypernatraemia unless adequately fluid replaced. Diabetes insipidus results in a failure to retain water and may be cranial or nephrogenic in origin.

What investigations might help you?

Investigation should include both a plasma and urinary sample for sodium analysis. This allows an assessment of whether the body is concentrating sodium or not. In volume overload, there is little sodium in the urine, whereas in sodium overload, there are usually normal to high amounts.

How would you restore a normal sodium concentration and what are the consequences if you don't?

In all cases, the underlying cause should be addressed primarily, and the sodium abnormality corrected while the primary cause is being addressed. Salt-deficient hyponatraemia should be treated by oral 'slow-sodium' or, in patients who are vomiting, by IV saline. Volume excess hyponatraemia should be treated by restriction of fluid intake and review of diuretic therapy. The clinical picture of continuing, uncorrected salt-deficient hyponatraemia is dominated by the volume depletion, whereas in volume excess hyponatraemia, symptoms are neurological as water moves into the brain cells due to falling extracellular osmolality. Symptoms are confusion and restlessness followed by drowsiness, myoclonic jerks, convulsions and coma.

Hypernatraemia should be corrected slowly using hypo-osmolar saline infusions to achieve normal sodium levels in 48 hours. Hypernatraemia is associated with volume depletion and circulatory failure. Venous thrombosis can occur, and cerebral symptoms of lethargy, drowsiness, muscle twitching and coma secondary to brain stem demyelination ensue.

17. SPLENECTOMY

What are the indications for splenectomy in the elective and emergency situations?

As an emergency procedure, splenectomy is indicated for the treatment of a ruptured spleen after trauma, which is usually a closed injury. Recently, attempts have been made at splenic conservation and repair in the trauma setting by a variety of techniques, and approximately 50 per cent of injured spleens may be saved in this manner. There is a long list of elective medical indications for splenectomy but, in essence, it should be considered as treatment for hypersplenism, splenic tumours or abscesses, for diagnosis in obscure splenomegaly, occasionally in staging or treating lymphoma or for relief of discomfort in massive splenomegaly. Hypersplenism is a combination of splenomegaly, anaemia, leukopenia or thrombocytopenia, bone marrow hyperplasia and improvement after splenectomy. This is obviously a retrospective diagnosis. Common causes of hypersplenism are haemolytic anaemia from spherocytosis or elliptocytosis, immune thrombocytopenic purpura and autoimmune thrombocytopenia. In addition, the spleen may be removed during an extended lymph node dissection during radical gastric cancer surgery (D3 gastrectomy). The spleen may have to be removed due to inadvertent iatrogenic damage during gastrectomy or left-sided colonic resection.

What are the operative risks?

Most of the risks are based on damage to neighbouring anatomical structures; thus, damage to the gastric wall, splenic flexure of colon and diaphragm are all recognized. A more serious problem is damage to the pancreatic tail. This may not be recognized at operation and can result in a subphrenic collection or high drain volumes if a subphrenic drain is left. Confirmation of a pancreatic injury can be confirmed by analysing the fluid – in such cases, the amylase concentration is grossly elevated. In cases of removal of large spleens, tears to the fragile capsule may result in significant haemorrhage and the requirement for blood transfusion is not uncommon.

What are the postoperative sequelae and risks?

In the first two days or so after splenectomy for hypersplenism, there is a rise in the blood counts of all cell lines, which in the case of leucocytes may rise to $>50 \times 10^9$/L and is often confused with the picture of sepsis by the unwary junior doctor. Propagation of clot from the ligated splenic vein in the setting of postoperative thrombocytosis may spread to include the portal vein. Underneath the diaphragm there is a raw area to which small bowel may stick and present later as small bowel obstruction; the fluid levels in such an obstruction may be misinterpreted on plain abdominal x-ray as a subphrenic abscess. If any splenic tissue is shed during splenectomy, or the trauma that precipitated it, then this tissue may hypertrophy postoperatively. In the case of the trauma splenectomy, this, or the presence of splenunculi, is beneficial but, in the elective haematological setting, this raises the possibility of recurrence of the initial problem; thus, the haematological splenectomy should prompt a thorough search of the abdomen for shed tissue and accessory spleens. There is an increased risk of certain infections postoperatively.

What prophylaxis should be considered in all splenectomy cases?

All patients, whether elective or emergency, should receive prophylactic immunization against *Haemophilus influenzae* (Hibivax), *Streptococcus pneumoniae* (Pneumovax) and *Neisseria meningitidis* strain C (Meningivax). In the elective case, this should be administered before surgery and, in the emergency setting, as soon as the patient is stable afterwards, but not while cardiovascularly unstable, as immunization can lead to further compromise. Most hospitals now also prescribe prophylactic penicillin – or a suitable alternative in allergic individuals. The duration of antibiotic use varies, from lifelong treatment to shorter periods coupled with a subsequent low threshold for antibiotic treatment, e.g. continuous antibiotics for 2 years after surgery and provision of an emergency stock to be taken thereafter when any infection supervenes.

What is overwhelmingly the greatest risk after splenectomy?

Although at greater risk of all infections, splenectomized patients are particularly at risk of overwhelming post-splenectomy infection (OPSI), with a massive pneumococcal bacteraemia and associated sepsis. The flu-like prodromal illness is followed after 2–3 days by headache, fever, malaise, coma, adrenal haemorrhage and circulatory collapse. The mortality is 50–90 per cent. Its incidence is thought to be approximately 1 per cent in trauma splenectomy patients and can be as high as 14 per cent in haematological splenectomy cases. The majority of cases occur within 2 years of operation.

Might a splenectomy affect the patient's choice of holiday destination?

After a splenectomy, patients are more susceptible to the effects of malaria as they no longer have the spleen in which to sequester infected erythrocytes; thus, they have a much greater parasitaemia. Splenectomized patients may well be advised to avoid malaria endemic areas.

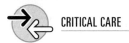

18. DRUG TOXICITY

Gentamicin is a commonly used drug in the septic surgical patient. How does it work and what are its common side effects?

Gentamicin is an aminoglycoside antibiotic. It inhibits protein synthesis in bacterial ribosomes and RNA to DNA translation. This is bacteriostatic, yet the aminoglycosides are also bactericidal, although the mechanism is obscure. Important adverse effects include hypersensitivity reactions with 5 per cent of patients developing a skin rash, auditory and vestibular dysfunction leading to dizziness and acute renal impairment due to tubular damage, especially in patients with pre-existing renal disease.

Poor renal function is common in the elderly surgical patient as is the use of non-steroidal anti-inflammatory drugs and ACE inhibitors. Why is it wise to avoid NSAIDs in renal impairment?

Non-steroidal anti-inflammatory drugs should be avoided because of their effect on prostacyclin synthesis. By inhibiting the cyclo-oxygenase pathways, prostacyclin production is decreased and prostacyclin-dependent renin release is inhibited. The resultant hyporeninaemic hypoaldosteronism, coupled with decreased glomerular perfusion pressure will worsen renal impairment. There is also a risk of acute tubulo-interstitial nephritis, which occurs as a cell-mediated hypersensitivity to some NSAIDs and results in interstitial oedema, inflammatory cell infiltrates and a further worsening of renal function.

Why is it wise to avoid ACE inhibitors in renal impairment?

ACE inhibitors have a significant risk of first-dose hypotension. Serious hypotension can result in acute renal failure, especially if there is already a degree of renal impairment. Angiotensin II is a potent vasoconstrictor, which tends to act to a greater degree on the efferent than the afferent glomerular arterioles; this serves to increase glomerular perfusion pressure and maintain renal function. Inhibition of angiotensin II production, therefore, has obvious consequences.

What is the difference between cyclo-oxygenase inhibitors and NSAIDs?

The recent discovery of two isoenzyme forms of cyclo-oxygenase (COX), and the differentiation of the function and disposition of each led to the synthesis of specific COX-2 inhibitors. COX-1 alone is found in the gastric mucosal cells and its prostaglandin products are protective for the mucosa. NSAIDs inhibit both COX-1 and 2, reducing inflammatory products but also reducing gastroprotective prostaglandin synthesis and predisposing to gastric ulceration. Specific COX-2 inhibitors maintain the anti-inflammatory and analgesic effects of NSAIDs, but also retain a gastric protective action. The incidence of major gastrointestinal bleeding, which is estimated at between 2 and 4 per cent per year, has limited the use of NSAIDs. The new COX-2-specific drugs have enabled analgesia and an anti-inflammatory effect with decreased gastrointestinal risk.

How does warfarin work as an anticoagulant and how is it monitored?

The synthesis of clotting factors II, VII, IX and X, as well as the anticoagulant factors Protein C and S, occurs within the liver and is vitamin K dependent. Warfarin acts by preventing the γ-carboxylation of the glutamic acid residues necessary for calcium binding. Without these residues, they cannot bind to anionic phospholipid surfaces and the coagulation complexes cannot be assembled. It is monitored by using the international normalized ratio (INR), which compares the patient's prothrombin time with a control sample, e.g. if the patient sample has a prothrombin time twice that of the control, the INR is 2.

How does heparin work as an anticoagulant and how is it monitored?

Heparin is a mucopolysaccharide that works by enhancing the activity of antithrombin on both thrombin and other coagulant proteins of the intrinsic pathway, particularly Factor Xa. The newer low molecular weight heparins have an increased anti-Xa to antithrombin activity ratio and give rise to more predictable anticoagulation. It can be monitored by measuring the activated partial thromboplastin time (APTT).

Draw the clotting cascade

See Figure 3.4 on page 96.

19. PULMONARY ARTERY FLOTATION CATHETERS

What information does a CVP line give and what is it extrapolated to mean?

A CVP line is situated in the lower end of the superior vena cava or the right atrium and records right atrial pressure. This is extrapolated to equal left atrial pressure, and further interpreted to represent left ventricular pressure and filling.

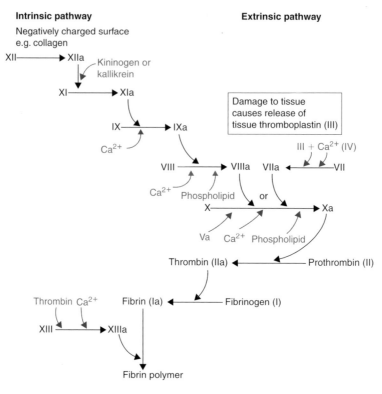

Intrinsic pathway

Negatively charged surface
e.g. collagen

XII ——————→ XIIa
Kininogen or
kallikrein

XI ——————→ XIa

IX ——————→ IXa
Ca^{2+}

Extrinsic pathway

Damage to tissue
causes release of
tissue thromboplastin (III)

$III + Ca^{2+}$ (IV)

VIII ——————→ VIIIa   VIIa ◄——————VII
Ca^{2+}
Phospholipid   or
X ——————————————————→ Xa
Va Ca^{2+} Phospholipid

Thrombin (IIa) ◄—————— Prothrombin (II)

Thrombin Ca^{2+} Fibrin (Ia) ◄—————— Fibrinogen (I)

XIII ——————→ XIIIa

Fibrin polymer

Figure 3.4 The clotting cascade. Cofactor requirements are shown in grey.

In what circumstances is this extrapolation invalid?

If the right and left heart are not functioning synchronously, then this will be invalid and some other method of assessing left heart function is needed. This is often the case, since the function of right and left hearts is marked differently.

What other invasive monitoring technique might you consider using?

In such an instance, a pulmonary artery flotation catheter (PAFC) or, in common parlance, a Swan–Ganz catheter could be used.

How is a PAFC passed?

An internal jugular route is most commonly used to gain central access and a standard Seldinger technique is used to pass the PAFC cannula, which is larger than a normal central venous line. The PAFC is connected to the transducer and the balloon at the tip of the catheter inflated with air; this allows it to be floated through the heart and into position in the small pulmonary vessels beyond the right ventricle. The transducer trace allows a continuous assessment of the location of the catheter as it progresses through the right heart and into the pulmonary vasculature.

Draw the pressure waves as a PAFC is passed

See Figure 3.5.

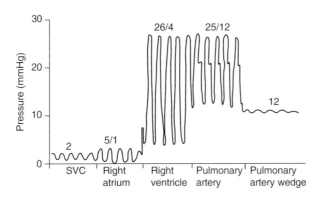

Figure 3.5 Pressure waves seen on passing a pulmonary artery flotation catheter. Approximate normal values are given above each waveform.

What conditions must prevail for the PAFC readings to be valid?

A PAFC, as its name suggests, measures the pressure in the small vessels of the pulmonary artery system. As there are no valves between it and the left atrium, its pressure recording is deemed to represent left atrial pressure, and thus is extrapolated to left ventricular pressure and filling. For these assumptions to be valid, there must be no obstructions between the catheter and the left atrium, so that it is truly a continuous column of blood; there must be no flow, as that would indicate a pressure gradient and invalidate the readings.

What variables does a PAFC actually measure and which are derived?

The PAFC can also measure the temperature of the blood and is used to measure changes in temperature in order to calculate cardiac output. Injection of a known volume of cold water through the catheter will cool the blood and the degree of temperature change is proportional to the rate of flow of blood past the thermistor, which allows calculation of cardiac output. It also allows true mixed venous blood sampling, which in turn allows calculation of oxygen delivery and uptake; other derived variables include the systemic vascular resistance.

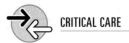

20. OXYGEN DELIVERY

In what ways can oxygen be delivered to the patient?

The patient can breathe room air as normal with an inspired oxygen concentration of 21 per cent. Increased concentrations can be inspired using a mask system attached to an oxygen supply, but this gives a very variable concentration of inspired oxygen (FiO_2) owing to a dilutional effect of the oxygen escaping around the mask. High air flow oxygen entrainment (HAFOE) uses the Venturi principle with a high-flow low-pressure system to suck in oxygen to give a known FiO_2. A reservoir bag uses the oxygen in the bag effectively to 'dilute' the inhaled mixture, increasing FiO_2. To deliver FiO_2 greater than 40 per cent reliably, endotracheal intubation and ventilation is required. It should be noted that prolonged exposure to FiO_2 greater than 80 per cent is injurious to the lung. Hyperbaric oxygen therapy also occasionally impinges on surgical practice in cases such as necrotizing fasciitis. It delivers 100 per cent oxygen at greater than 1 atmosphere of pressure in specially constructed tanks.

What is CPAP and what are its indications?

It stands for continuous positive airway pressure. Patients with impending respiratory failure may be helped by this technique, which uses a one-way valve in a very closely applied facemask. As the patient expires, gas is expelled through the valve until a certain pressure is reached, after which no further gas is allowed to escape. This has the effect of always maintaining a positive pressure in the airways – as the name suggests – preventing collapse of alveoli, and even recruiting previously collapsed ones. It is the stage of respiratory management before intubation and ventilation, but many patients find it very uncomfortable and are unable to tolerate the mask. There are also problems with the mask causing pressure necrosis of the face particularly over the nasal bridge.

If the patient requires ventilation, what modes of ventilation are you familiar with? Describe what parameters the ventilator can be set to

The patient can, of course, be allowed to ventilate spontaneously, but this is not common in the ITU setting. The commonest mode is intermittent positive pressure ventilation (IPPV), also known as continuous mandatory ventilation (CMV). In this mode, there is no patient interaction and the gas mixture is forced into the lungs at regular intervals, which has important physiological consequences. In normal breathing, there is a negative intrathoracic pressure in inspiration, whereas in IPPV the reverse is true, as there is a positive pressure in both inspiration and expiration. This has the effect of compressing the great vessels and impeding venous return, in turn reducing cardiac output. In this setting, a patient with borderline right heart function may well be tipped into right ventricular failure; conversely, it may help left ventricular failure by assisting the squeeze of blood into the aorta. The machine can be set to give a set number of breaths per minute and to deliver either a set volume of gas or to provide gas at a given pressure or a given flow rate. One can also set the ratio of duration of inspiration to expiration and this can be varied according to the clinical need in ARDS or asthma, for example. Synchronized intermittent mandatory ventilation (SIMV) allows the patient to do some of the work. The ventilator is set to the lowest acceptable parameters and, if the patient does not breathe, the machine will cut in and perform that breath instead; it is used as a weaning tool. Pressure support ventilation (PSV) allows the patient to breathe on their own, without a set respiratory rate but, if the patient's breath does not reach a pressure trigger point, then the ventilator will aid the breath – another weaning tool.

What is PEEP and autoPEEP?

PEEP stands for positive end expiratory pressure. As air leaves the lungs in expiration, the alveoli will tend to collapse. In normal lungs, surface tension keeps the alveoli open and allows inflow of gas with the next breath. In the situation of poor respiratory function, alveoli will tend to collapse at the end of a breath. By setting the ventilator to a certain PEEP level, as the airway pressure falls, the closure of a valve in the circuit will not allow the pressure to fall back below that level – or to a negative pressure as happens in physiological ventilation – thus splinting the alveoli open. The stiffer the lungs, the higher the level of PEEP needed to achieve this aim. In acutely ill asthmatics, the pressures in the airway are so high that they are still exhaling when the next breath starts, thus splinting the airway open – so called autoPEEP.

21. LARGE BOWEL OBSTRUCTION

How does the presentation of mechanical large bowel obstruction differ from that of small bowel obstruction?

Large bowel obstruction tends to present with a longer history than small bowel obstruction, since there is more capacity for expansion. Indeed, the patient may not initially realize they are unwell. Vomiting is a late feature, whereas absolute constipation may have been present for several days. The abdominal distension is rarely painful and there is an absence of colic. Pain may become a feature as perforation becomes imminent. The abdomen is often dramatically distended, more so than with small bowel obstruction. Because of the different aetiologies, symptoms may have been present for much longer periods of time.

What are the commonest causes of large bowel obstruction in the UK?

By far the most common cause in the UK is colorectal cancer. Other causes include diverticular disease with stricture or inflammatory mass, intussusception, band adhesions, postoperative adhesions, hernias, inflammatory strictures, such as in colonic Crohn's disease, bolus obstruction, such as in faecal impaction, atonic colonic segments, which may be either congenital or acquired, and extracolonic malignancies.

On the AXR, if you see gas in a distended large and small bowel, what are the implications?

It is a sign that the ileocaecal valve is incompetent, allowing backflow of gas into the small bowel; it functions as a 'safety valve' and stops the formation of a closed loop obstruction, but only occurs in 10 per cent of cases.

What does the AXR in Figure 3.6 show and what is your worry?

This film shows a closed-loop large bowel obstruction. The loop is closed between the obstructing tumour and a competent ileocaecal valve. Because of the larger diameter of the caecum, the gas in the colon will preferentially cause distension here first. With increased distension, the caecum can reach bursting point. Perforation of an obstructed colon should not be allowed to occur, if at all

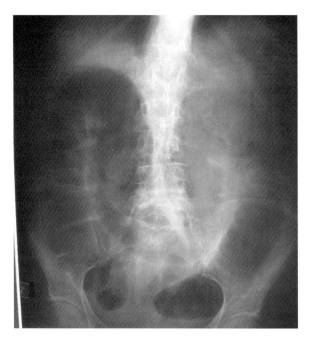

Figure 3.6

possible, owing to the high mortality associated with faecal peritonitis. This gives rise to the surgical saying 'Never let the sun go down on a closed loop obstruction'.

How would you manage the patient with the above condition and what does increasing right iliac fossa tenderness imply?

Patients with large bowel obstruction are almost inevitably dehydrated and require resuscitation in the form of intravenous fluids, initially normal saline or Hartmann's, at a rate dependent on the degree of volume depletion and oxygen via a facemask. Decompression of the upper gastrointestinal tract by passage of a nasogastric tube is often helpful and a urinary catheter is essential for monitoring of fluid balance and as a guide to the adequacy of tissue perfusion. Blood is withdrawn for crossmatch, U&E, FBC, LFT and clotting. An emergency contrast enema is arranged to confirm obstruction and identify the level. If a contrast enema were not available, an abdominal CT scan is the next investigation of choice.

Increasing right iliac fossa tenderness suggests an increasing likelihood of caecal perforation, which should serve to expedite any remaining investigations. At this stage, a low threshold for taking the patient to theatre for laparotomy is appropriate.

How would you treat an obstructed sigmoid cancer?

The interventions to choose from would be:

→ stenting as a bridge to surgery or as palliation
→ Hartmann's procedure
→ resection and primary anastomosis
→ resection and primary anastomosis and defunctioning stoma.

Currently, most colorectal surgeons would perform a resection where possible with a primary anastomosis. The procedure can be performed with or without on-table colonic lavage. This may be facilitated by primary stenting to decompress the distended bowel and allow formal pre-operative staging and bowel preparation prior to definitive resection. Proximal defunctioning is dictated by both personal preference and the appearances at surgery.

22. ANAESTHESIA

What constitutes general anaesthesia?

General anaesthesia is the triad of muscle relaxation, reversible loss of consciousness and blockade of painful stimuli.

What alternatives are there to a general anaesthetic when performing surgery?

Alternatives to general anaesthesia depend on the site and duration of surgery. The options are as follows.

→ *Spinal anaesthesia*. Local anaesthetic and analgesic agents are injected directly into the spinal canal, creating a level of anaesthesia below (see Figure 3.7).

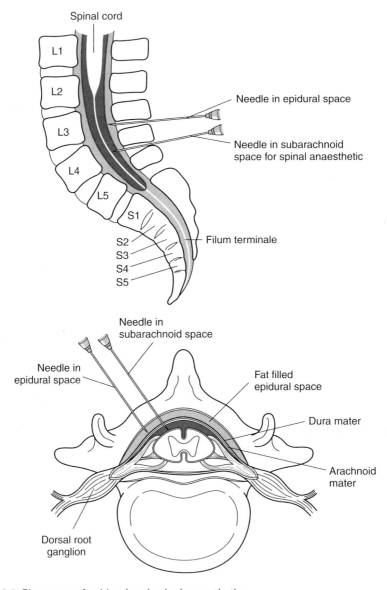

Figure 3.7 Placement of epidural and spinal anaesthetics.

→ *Epidural anaesthesia*. A catheter is inserted into the epidural space and local anaesthetic mixtures infused to give anaesthesia and later postoperative pain relief (see Figure 3.7).

→ *Epispinal*. A combination of both spinal and epidural techniques.

→ *Regional nerve blocks*. These can be used to operate on specified territories, such as a brachial nerve block for the upper limb, an ankle block for the foot, or perhaps most commonly a digital nerve block for operating on fingers and toes.

→ *A Bier's block*. A regional technique using intravenous prilocaine to anaesthetize a limb that is under tourniquet to prevent systemic spread of local anaesthetic agent.

→ *A field block*. Injection of local anaesthetic around the required area in a ring creates a central area of anaesthesia, and is often used for 'lumps and bumps' surgery.

→ *Topical*. Local anaesthetic agents will act topically. Cocaine paste in nasal surgery, amethocaine drops for corneal anaesthesia, and EMLA (eutectic mixture of local anaesthetics) for skin anaesthesia are examples.

How is anaesthesia induced?

Anaesthesia is induced after pre-oxygenation by the use of an induction agent. In adults, an intravenous induction agent, such as sodium thiopentone or propofol is usually used, whereas in children, gas inhalation is often used, typically with isoflurane or the newer, less pungent sevoflurane. The induction agent, when given intravenously, is short acting, but a sufficient dose is given to induce anaesthesia within 30 seconds and allow an airway to be secured, after which inhalational agents may be used to maintain anaesthesia.

What types of muscle relaxants are there?

They are either depolarizing or non-depolarizing. The only depolarizing blocker in clinical use is suxamethonium, which is two acetylcholine molecules stuck together; this acts at the motor end plate and spontaneously reverses under the action of pseudocholinesterase after about 5 minutes. The non-depolarizing relaxants are based on the original properties of curare, a neuromuscular poison popular in the Amazonian jungle; its latter-day derivatives include atracurium, vecuronium and pancuronium, although there are others. These do not reverse spontaneously, except atracurium, which undergoes Hoffman degradation, and need to be reversed by neostigmine, which is administered with glycopyrolate or atropine to prevent accumulation of acetylcholine elsewhere causing problems.

How does lignocaine work?

Lignocaine works as a local anaesthetic by decreasing the transient increase in sodium permeability of excitable membranes, which increases the threshold for electrical excitability. It also works as a class I anti-arrhythmic by slowing the rate of depolarization of the cardiac action potential, thus suppressing cardiac automaticity. Depolarization is slowed and action potential duration is shortened with minimal shortening of the refractory period. Thus, the proportion of time for which fibres are refractory is increased.

What is an LMA?

It stands for laryngeal mask airway, which is a relatively new device. It is placed without the use of a laryngoscope and lies across the larynx to provide a relatively secure airway; however, it does not protect completely against aspiration problems.

23. OPTIMIZATION

How would you try to optimize the following patients?

A 78-year-old man with longstanding COPD and a BMI of 31 who has smoked 25 cigarettes/day for half a century who needs a right hemicolectomy for cancer?
The main worries are his weight and his poor respiratory function. He should be encouraged in the strongest possible terms to stop smoking. Pre-operative physiotherapy and bronchodilators may help. Pre-operative spirometry, including flow-loop analysis, and reversibility studies are arranged. A pre-operative blood gas would be useful to act as a baseline for postoperative samples, when respiratory assessment may be required. Attending to his weight is trickier, as a reduced calorie intake before a cancer resection is not optimal, nor is significant weight loss possible before urgent surgery, thus his weight is not addressed in this instance; if he were undergoing surgery for a non-malignant condition, dietetic advice should be arranged to try and reduce his BMI.

A 62-year-old man, who had his second myocardial infarction 6 weeks ago, who requires a partial gastrectomy for carcinoma?
This patient is at huge risk of cardiovascular morbidity and he should be warned of the substantial mortality risk of undergoing what is essential surgery so soon after a myocardial infarction. The mortality risk of undergoing general anaesthesia for major surgery within 3 months of a myocardial infarct is around 50 per cent. Discussion with the patient and anaesthetist is arranged, and the surgical risks explained, and also the risks of waiting a further 6 weeks to reduce the anaesthetic

risks. When surgery is an acceptable risk to all concerned, he should be admitted pre-operatively to HDU or ITU, and a pulmonary artery flotation catheter considered so that cardiac output and oxygen delivery can be optimized. Pre-operative echocardiography should be performed to assess ventricular function and advice obtained from a cardiologist regarding the need to arrange a cardiac thallium scan to further assess function.

A cachectic 56-year-old with dysphagia about to undergo an oesophagogastrectomy for a lower third tumour?

Dietician review is arranged, and his oral intake maximized prior to surgery. This may be possible using nutritionally balanced high-protein drinks, but may not be possible because of his dysphagia. This is one of the occasions where pre-operative parenteral nutrition may be appropriate. He is in a poor nutritional state already and, during surgery and for several days thereafter, he is going to be hugely catabolic. At surgery, a feeding jejunostomy can be placed but, prior to surgery, TPN may help steady the decline in his nutritional status. Surgery should not be delayed because, although TPN can help prevent further decline, there is no evidence that it is beneficial in restoring nutritional parameters to normality when given pre-operatively.

A 45-year-old smoker of 20 cigarettes/day about to have a small bowel resection for Crohn's disease?

His nutritional status is assessed, since a poor nutritional state is not uncommon in Crohn's disease, and this may affect the surgical options. If nutrition is poor, oral supplements or TPN feeding pre-operatively and postoperatively may be required. The patient must be advised to stop smoking, since not only are general complications higher in smokers, but Crohn's disease-specific complications, including recurrence, are higher. He should, of course, have an ECG and chest x-ray. He should also be counselled, consented and marked for a stoma in preparation for this possibility.

24. CLOSED HEAD INJURY

In a closed head injury, what are primary and secondary brain injuries?

A primary brain injury is one that is caused at the time of injury. A number of mechanisms may be involved. The cortex may be injured directly as it impacts against the skull vault or projecting areas of the skull base, such as the wing of the sphenoid, shearing forces during acceleration/deceleration may sever axonal connections causing diffuse axonal injury or laceration of subdural veins giving rise to haematoma; if smaller vessels are injured, cerebral petechial haemorrhages result.

A secondary brain injury results from subsequent hypoxia or infection after the initial injury. This may be due to:

→ pressure from haematoma or brain herniation
→ regional ischaemia from major vessel compression
→ global ischaemia as a result of reduction in cerebral perfusion owing to the rise in intracranial pressure
→ hypoxic hypoxia due to associated airway or chest problems
→ anaemic hypoxia owing to blood loss from associated injuries.

How may conscious level be graded?

The Glasgow Coma Scale (GCS) allows a rapid and objective assessment of conscious level that is universally accepted. It assesses three parameters: verbal response, eye opening and motor response. It gives a score out of 15 and is broken down as follows.

→ *Eye opening*:
- 4 – spontaneously
- 3 – to speech
- 2 – to pain
- 1 – not at all

→ *Motor response*:
- 6 – obeys commands
- 5 – localizes pain
- 4 – withdraws from pain
- 3 – abnormal flexion to pain
- 2 – extension to pain
- 1 – no response

→ *Verbal response*:
- 5 – orientated
- 4 – confused conversation
- 3 – inapproriate words
- 2 – incomprehensible sounds
- 1 – no verbalization.

A GCS of 8 or below is an indication for intubation for airway protection. Coma is defined as not obeying commands, not uttering intelligible words and not opening the eyes.

What factors influence intracranial pressure?

The skull is a fixed volume box and the pressure within, the intracranial pressure, is due to the relative volumes of its contents – brain (85 per cent), cerebrospinal fluid (CSF; 10 per cent) and blood (5 per cent). Increases in the volume of one component without corresponding decrease in another will raise the ICP.

Why is limiting the ICP so important?

$$\text{Cerebral perfusion pressure (CPP)}$$
$$= \text{Mean arterial pressure} - (\text{ICP} + \text{CVP})$$

Cerebral perfusion pressure is the driving pressure that pushes blood around the cerebral circulation. The intracranial compliance curve shows that, up to a given point, a rise in intracranial volume is compensated for and a constant ICP and, therefore, perfusion pressure is maintained. This is cerebral autoregulation. After the compensatory mechanisms are saturated, a small increase in volume results in large rises in pressure. Thus, a rise in ICP will, in general, mean a fall in CPP, which will cause global hypoxia to an already injured brain. One of the basic tenets of managing a closed head injury is to control ICP, so that CPP is maintained at adequate levels to prevent secondary brain injury.

What measures may be instituted to control ICP?

There are only three variables, brain, CSF and blood, that can be manipulated. The volume of the brain itself is difficult to alter, although some of the cerebral oedema can be minimized by the use of osmotic diuretics, such as mannitol in a dose of 1 g/kg as an intravenous infusion over 30 minutes. Carbon dioxide is a potent vasodilator and will increase the volume of the vascular compartment; superficially it may appear to be beneficial to increase cerebral blood flow, but the increased blood volume actually raises ICP and, therefore, lowers CPP. Whilst studies have not shown any benefit from hyperventilating head injured patients to subnormal $PaCO_2$ levels, possibly due to altered vascular reactivity in injured brain tissue, hypercapnia should definitely be avoided; aiming for $PaCO_2$ levels of low normal is appropriate. Increased cerebral metabolic activity demands increased oxygen delivery and will, therefore, raise ICP; thus, sedation, avoidance of fitting by prophylactic anticonvulsants, avoidance of hyperthermia, or even mild surface cooling and avoidance of hyperglycaemia with its concomitant accumulation of lactic acid in this anaerobic environment, are all beneficial in controlling ICP and maintaining cerebral perfusion.

ICP may be measured directly by placement of an intraventricular catheter, which has the added advantage that CSF can be withdrawn therapeutically.

25. HYPOVOLAEMIA

A patient with small bowel obstruction is oliguric, tachycardic and hypotensive. Outline your initial thoughts as you approach the bedside

Patients with small bowel obstruction can sequester many litres of electrolyte-rich fluid in their distended bowel causing hypovolaemia; there is a resultant oliguria owing to decreased renal perfusion pressure and a tachycardia in an attempt to maintain cardiac output. Volumes of sequestered fluid are often underestimated, and fluid replacement may be insufficient and occasionally of the wrong type. After assessing the patient to ensure no other cause of circulatory collapse has been missed, and the sufficiency of fluid therapy assessed, fluid resuscitation of the patient with crystalloid containing potassium is initiated. A recent set of electrolyte results should available.

How will you monitor the adequacy of your fluid resuscitation?

In the first instance, monitoring is clinical and is by repeated observation of vital signs for evidence of improvement. If the patient is not catheterized, then they should now be catheterized. If fluid resuscitation within the limits of clinical monitoring were insufficient, then central venous pressure monitoring should be initiated to assist fluid management.

How do you place a CVP line – and what is a normal CVP?

The two common routes for placement of central venous lines are via the right subclavian vein or the right internal jugular vein. The right subclavian route will be described.

The procedure is explained to the patient and consent obtained, if practicable. The patient is attached to a cardiac monitor. The central line is flushed down each port with saline and three-way taps attached to each lateral lumen. The patient is positioned supine with the head turned fully to the left. The bed is tilted head down. The area of the right neck and anterior chest is widely prepared with skin antiseptic and draped to reveal the area beneath the mid-clavicle. After infiltration with local anaesthetic, a large-gauge needle with attached syringe is advanced through the skin immediately beneath the clavicle at its junction of middle and lateral thirds. The needle is advanced with suction on the syringe, aiming for the suprasternal notch at about 30° to the skin. As the needle advances, it will enter the subclavian vein and venous blood can easily be withdrawn into the syringe. Many sets now have hollow-barrelled syringes so that a guide wire can be passed directly down through the syringe and needle to enter the vein. The guide wire is passed to a sufficient length to enter the lower superior vena cava. The needle is withdrawn. The skin at the point of entry is nicked with a blade and a dilator is passed over the wire to enlarge the track through the soft tissues. The central line is then passed over the wire into the subclavian vein. When sufficient length has been passed, the guide wire is withdrawn. The channels – usually three – are aspirated, flushed and heparin/saline locked. The catheter is then securely sutured in place and covered with a transparent occlusive dressing. A chest x-ray is organized to check catheter placement and to check for complications, after which the line may be used. If advanced too far, it is a simple job to withdraw it by the appropriate amount and resecure it. A normal CVP reading is between 8 and 10 cm water, although an absolute value is not as important as trends in the readings.

What are the complications of central line placement?

They are either acute or delayed. Acute complications include misplacement, pneumothorax, haemothorax, cardiac arrhythmias and bleeding into the mediastinum or neck. The primary delayed complication is that of infection, as these lines provide an easy portal for ingress of bacteria; patients should be nursed with meticulous care.

How can you tell if your patient is adequately resuscitated now you have a central line?

See Figure 3.8. The patient should be fluid challenged. After reading the CVP, a bolus of 200 ml of crystalloid is infused and the CVP rerecorded. Three patterns occur as shown in the figure. In A, the CVP rises a little and then goes back to its previously low value, denoting continued hypovolaemia. In C, the CVP rises and stays high – this indicates overfilling. A CVP that rises and then after 15 minutes or so settles down to a normal value is indicative of normovolaemia (B).

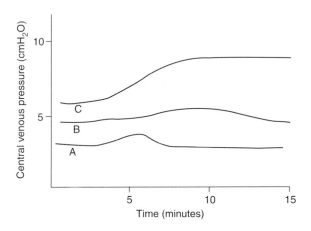

Figure 3.8 Central venous pressure response to a fluid challenge.

If venous access was very difficult, you might be called upon to perform a 'cut down'. Which are the two commonest sites used and describe the procedure?

The two commonest sites are the long saphenous vein at the ankle and the brachial vein in the antecubital fossa. The long saphenous is used most commonly. The vein is constant at the ankle, being located 2 cm above and anterior to the tip of the medial malleolus. After skin preparation and local anaesthetic, if time permits and the conscious state of the patient dictates, a small transverse incision is made in the skin directly over the vein. The vein itself is freed from surrounding tissue by gentle dissection with a haemostat and the vein lifted free. Two ties of 0 silk are passed beneath the vein. The proximal one is looped and left free, whilst the distal one is used to ligate the vein. Using the proximal one to elevate the vein, a nick is made in the anterior surface and the catheter is threaded into the vein and securely tied in place by the second thread.

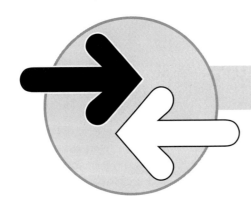

1. CARPAL TUNNEL RELEASE

What is the carpal tunnel and to what is the flexor retinaculum attached?

The carpal tunnel is a space on the ventral surface of the wrist between the bony gutter of the concave carpus and the overlying flexor retinaculum. The retinaculum is a strong fibrous band attached proximally to the tubercle of the scaphoid and the pisiform bone and distally to the hook of hamate and tubercle of the trapezium.

What are the contents of the carpal tunnel?

Figure 4.1 The contents of the carpal tunnel.

See Figure 4.1. The four tendons of flexor digitorum profundus tendons are seen lying one beside the other posteriorly, with those of the flexor digitorum superficialis arranged as two pairs anteriorly. The tendons of flexor pollicis longus and flexor carpi radialis lie lateral to the long finger flexors and the median nerve is the most superficial content of the tunnel.

What are the causes of carpal tunnel syndrome?

The causes of carpal tunnel syndrome are those conditions that increase the pressure within the tunnel and compress the median nerve. They include:

→ rheumatoid arthritis
→ myxoedema

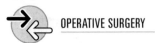

→ pregnancy
→ tumour
→ acromegaly
→ hypothyroidism
→ amyloid – due to infiltration of the flexor retinaculum
→ trauma – an acute carpal tunnel syndrome can occur and is a recognized complication of Colles fracture.

Is the ulnar nerve ever involved in a carpal tunnel syndrome?

Never. The ulnar nerve does not lie within the carpal tunnel and cannot be affected by a carpal tunnel syndrome *per se*. It can, however, suffer similar compression syndromes within the ulnar nerve canal (of Guyon) associated with an injury to the wrist or be coexistent with a carpal tunnel syndrome.

How would you perform a carpal tunnel release?

The arm is laid out, fully supinated on an arm board, and prepared and draped to expose the whole hand, which is held flat by a 'lead hand' retractor. A skin incision is made beginning 3 cm distal to the distal wrist crease to just proximal to the level of the first web space. The incision lies just lateral to the palmaris longus tendon and aims for the ulnar border of the ring finger. A West's self-retaining retractor holds the skin apart and reveals the retinaculum beneath. A Macdonald's elevator is slid immediately beneath the retinaculum, allowing it to be safely divided – the band is cut until the palmar arch becomes visible beneath and the palmar fat pad is seen. Haemostasis is achieved and the skin closed with interrupted nylon sutures and completed with a firm dressing.

What structures must the surgeon constantly be aware of?

The two structures that a surgeon must always bear in mind and avoid are the palmar cutaneous branch of the median nerve and the recurrent motor branch of the median nerve. The former passes superficial to the retinaculum, on the radial side of palmaris longus, and supplies sensation to the skin of the thenar eminence. The recurrent motor branch leaves the median nerve on its lateral side as it emerges from the carpal tunnel to turn back on itself to give motor supply to the thenar muscles.

Are there any other techniques in use for carpal tunnel release?

Recently, an endoscopic method of flexor retinaculum division has been devised. Although this initially utilized a two portal technique, some surgeons are now performing a single portal procedure. It remains a tool of the experienced hand surgeon and is not in routine use.

2. APPENDICECTOMY

Describe how you would perform an appendicectomy in a 24-year-old woman

Informed consent should be obtained before the procedure, warning her specifically that she will end up with a scar, of the risks of infection and of the possibility that the appendix might be normal. The patient is positioned supine under general anaesthetic with an endotracheal tube. The abdomen is prepared with povodone-iodine from umbilicus to pubis, and draped to expose the right lower quadrant including the right anterior superior iliac spine (ASIS) and the umbilicus and midline.

The skin is incised using a Lanz incision centred on a point two-thirds of the way from the umbilicus to the right ASIS, remaining in the line of the skin creases. Using cutting diathermy, the subcutaneous fat and Scarpa's fascia is divided down to the external oblique aponeurosis aided by the insertion of a self-retaining retractor. Having incised the aponeurosis in the line of its fibres, the underlying internal oblique and transversus abdominis muscles are split in the line of their fibres using clips to reveal peritoneum beneath. Picking up peritoneum between two clips and ensuring there is nothing stuck to it, the peritoneum is opened with a knife and the opening extended in the line of the skin incision with scissors. Note is made of any free fluid or pus that was evident and a swab taken for culture. An attempt is made to identify the appendix by sweeping inside the peritoneal cavity with a finger and, if able, the appendix is delivered into the wound; otherwise the taenia are followed on to the caecum and downwards to the area of the ileocaecal valve where the appendix should lie, enabling delivery of the whole appendix into the wound.

The appendix is held between Babcock's forceps and the mesoappendix divided between clips to free the appendix to its base, then a straight crushing clamp is applied across the base and replaced slightly more distally. After ligation of the appendix base, it is removed flush to the clamp. The pouting mucosa of the appendix base is diathermized and the abdomen washed out with saline. The peritoneum is closed with continuous vicryl, the muscular layers with vicryl and subcuticular monocryl to skin.

At operation you remove a 'lilywhite' appendix. What do you do now?

If the appendix appears unlikely to be responsible for the patient's pain, then a search for other possible causes is made. In a young girl, palpation of the right ovary and tube would be essential and withdrawal of the terminal ileum to palpate for thickening, which might indicate Crohn's ileitis or a tuberculous ileitis, depending on the patient's background. The last metre of the small bowel is examined, taking note of any mesenteric lymph nodes. If all were negative, cholecystitis is excluded by direct examination of the gallbladder. If no cause for the pain is identified, the abdomen is closed.

On further examination, you discover an inflamed mass on the antimesenteric border of the ileum about 60 cm from the ileocaecal valve. What is it likely to be? Describe its embryological origin

It is likely to be a Meckel's diverticulum. This is a true diverticulum that is an embryological remnant of the vitellointestinal duct. It is said to be present in 2 per cent of the population, 2 inches long and sited 2 feet from the ileocaecal valve on the antimesenteric border of the ileum.

How may Meckel's diverticulum present?

It may be found incidentally at laparotomy or it may present clinically with the following.

→ *Diverticulitis* – obstruction of a narrow neck may result in an acute inflammation, which may be clinically indistinguishable from acute appendicitis.
→ *Intussusception* – the diverticulum may invert and become the focal point of an intussusception, presenting as intestinal obstruction.
→ *Obstruction* – a remnant band joining the tip of the diverticulum to the umbilicus may be the band around which the small bowel twists and obstructs.
→ *Haemorrhage* – one in six Meckel's contain ectopic gastric mucosa capable of acid secretion and this may cause peptic ulceration, which can bleed.
→ *Perforation* – ectopic gastric acid secretion can lead to ulceration and perforation downstream from the Meckel's.
→ *Littre's hernia* – a very rare presentation, with the Meckel's present in an inguinal or femoral hernia.

If an inflamed Meckel's diverticulum were found during appendicectomy, how should it be dealt with?

As it is inflamed, the Meckel's diverticulum is resected with a short segment of adjacent normal bowel and a primary single layer extramucosal anastomosis is performed.

Would your treatment be different if the lesion were not inflamed?

If the Meckel's diverticulum was not inflamed and looked blameless, it should be left alone. Some surgeons would resect a normal Meckel's, if it had a particularly narrow neck that might later obstruct.

Johann Friedrich Meckel The Younger (1781–1833). Third in a family line of Pro-
fessors of Anatomy and Surgery in Halle, Germany. He described this diverticulum
in 1809, although Lavater had previously done so in 1699. He also described the
first branchial cartilage.

Alexis Littre (1658–1726). Surgeon and anatomist of Paris who described this hernia
in 1700, 81 years before Meckel (who named its content) was born.

3. FEMORAL HERNIA

Define a 'hernia'

A hernia is the abnormal protrusion of a viscus or part of a viscus through an
opening in the walls of its containing cavity.

Describe three different approaches to the surgical repair of a femoral hernia

The three general approaches to femoral hernia repair are the high approach, typified by the McEvedy approach, the inguinal approach, such as the Lotheissen
technique, and the low/crural approach of Lockwood (see Figure 4.2). The
McEvedy operation utilizes a vertical skin incision over the lateral aspect of the
lower rectus sheath, the rectus muscle is retracted medially revealing the peritoneum. From this extraperitoneal position, the sac can be withdrawn and the
peritoneum opened, if necessary, for resection of bowel. The Lotheissen operation
begins as one would for an inguinal hernia repair and divides the posterior wall of
the inguinal canal to reveal peritoneum, which is then opened. The contents of
the femoral sac can now be reduced and inspected directly. Great care must be
taken to perform an immaculate repair of the inguinal canal, otherwise you will
have exchanged the patient's femoral hernia for an inguinal one! The low
approach uses an incision over the bulge in the groin itself and the layers over the
hernia are divided until the sac is encountered. The sac is opened, and, if necessary, the femoral ring dilated to facilitate access to the bowel and to return it to
the abdominal cavity. If further access is required, the inguinal ligament can be
divided, but must be meticulously repaired.

After any of these approaches, steps should be taken to narrow the femoral
ring to prevent recurrence. Three non-absorbable sutures placed between the
pectineal line and the underside of the inguinal ligament are usually adequate to
narrow the ring without risking compression of the femoral vein. Alternatively
a plug of prolene mesh can be used to seal the femoral ring.

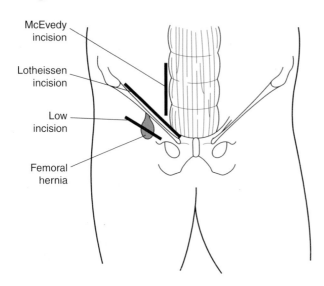

McEvedy
incision

Lotheissen
incision

Low
incision

Femoral
hernia

Figure 4.2 Surgical approaches to a femoral hernia.

Which approach would you use for an elective femoral hernia repair?

In an elective femoral hernia repair or one in which I felt that the chances of strangulation were low, I would use the low approach and place my skin incision over the bulge of the hernia in the line of the inguinal ligament.

What would you do if clinically there were dead bowel in the hernia?

The disadvantage of the low approach is that devitalized bowel can rarely be delivered through the low approach to allow resection. In this instance, a laparotomy through a lower midline incision can be performed, reducing the hernia from within the abdomen. This would then allow a full assessment of bowel viability. If necessary, the dead bowel is resected and a primary anastomosis of the two healthy bowel ends is performed. After a thorough peritoneal washout, the abdomen is closed as a mass closure and then the groin wound repaired. Postoperative management is as for any other small bowel resection.

What important but inconsistent structure may be at risk in a femoral hernia repair?

An accessory obturator artery is present in about 50 per cent of patients and has an aberrant medial course in about half of those, where it runs along the posterior part of the lacunar ligament, medial to the hernial sac. Division of the lacunar ligament (Hay–Groves manoeuvre) to dilate the femoral canal potentially to perform a bowel resection through a single incision is fraught with danger.

Georg Lotheissen (1868–1941). Austrian surgeon of the Kaiser Franz Joseph Hospital in Vienna who described his approach to the femoral hernia in 1898, 22 years after Thomas Annandale.

4. NEPHRECTOMY

Outline the various operative approaches to the kidney for nephrectomy

There are several different approaches to the kidney and, whilst it can be a matter of personal choice for the surgeon, the choice of approach is in some cases influenced by the indication for nephrectomy. In cases of renal trauma or for large renal cell carcinomas, an anterior abdominal approach is probably best as it allows early control of the vascular pedicle. Alternatively, a posterior approach through the bed of the 12th rib can be used with the patient positioned laterally and the table 'broken', i.e. with the centre of the table higher than both feet and head ends. A laparoscopic approach, usually by the retroperitoneal route, for both benign and malignant disease is being increasingly used with good results.

Describe the operative steps in performing a radical nephroureterectomy

The patient is positioned supine with the legs in Lloyd Davis supports and, before the abdominal procedure is begun, a cystoscopy is undertaken. At cystoscopy, the involved ureter is circumscribed with point diathermy and the cystoscope replaced by a urinary catheter. The ureteric defect does not need formal closure. The abdomen is prepared and draped for a laparotomy. The abdomen is opened via a midline, paramedian or transverse incision placed on the appropriate side and a full laparotomy undertaken. The peritoneal reflection lateral to the colon on the given side is divided and the colon retracted medially revealing the perinephric fat beneath. The renal artery is clamped followed by ligation and division of the renal vein, taking care to identify the accessory renal veins that are often present. Similarly, if the kidney does not 'deflate' after renal artery clamping, then the surgeon must search for and clamp the secondary arterial inflow. After division of the renal veins, the arterial supply is transfixed and divided. At this stage, the kidney is held only by the ureter and the tissues behind the kidney. In a simple nephrectomy, for chronic infection or renal cell carcinoma, the ureter can simply be divided at a convenient point and the kidney gradually dissected off the posterior tissues by gradual medial mobilization. If the procedure is for transitional cell carcinoma, then the entire ureter must be removed. The ureter is now freed along its course by blunt dissection to the previously isolated distal end, and the specimen removed and sent for histology.

Does tumour invasion from the kidney into the inferior vena cava render it inoperable?

Not necessarily. Renal cell carcinoma may often extend along the renal vein, into the IVC and even into the right atrium, but this does not necessarily make it inoperable. The extent of tumour migration should be determined by CT scanning and angiography pre-operatively, and surgery planned appropriately. If there is spread close to or into the IVC, then it can be excised by excluding the tumour using a vascular clamp and resecting it with direct closure or vein patching. If the segment involved is long, then resection and interposition grafting may be feasible. Extensive tumour migration such as this should be discussed prior to surgery with a vascular surgeon, who should be available to assist in the procedure.

You are called to perform an emergency nephrectomy on a man who has suffered blunt abdominal trauma. What investigation will you request to see before removing the kidney?

Before removing a kidney for blunt trauma, the films of an IVP or contrast CT scan should be seen before proceeding. This is to ensure that the patient has a functioning contralateral kidney as shown by contrast excretion on the films. Congenital single kidneys occur in 1 per cent of people and many other people lose a kidney to pyelonephritis or for living donor transplant. If no such films are available, an on-table IVP can be performed. Although they are very easy to perform in the trauma situation after the trauma series x-rays, they are often forgotten. Injection of 50 ml of intravenous contrast and a single abdominal radiograph is sufficient to demonstrate function.

What is the grading system for blunt renal trauma?

→ Type I – minor contusion only
→ Type II – minor parenchymal laceration without collecting system involvement
→ Type III – major laceration with collecting system involvement
→ Type IV – renal pedicle injuries.

Type I and II injuries should be managed conservatively by bed rest until macroscopic haematuria settles. In Type II injuries with an associated capsular tear, prophylactic antibiotics should be given, as there will inevitably be extravasation of urine. Type III injuries do equally as well by either conservative or operative management, and the conservative approach is to be preferred, although drainage of an urinoma is occasionally required. Type IV injuries almost always require surgical management.

5. VASECTOMY

How would you counsel a man before obtaining consent for vasectomy?

The four main specific points to raise with regard to vasectomy are as follows.

→ The operation should be considered irreversible. Reversal of vasectomy is a procedure not widely available on the NHS and has mediocre results, which get worse as the time since the original vasectomy lengthens.
→ Conversely, there is a risk of spontaneous failure. For reasons unknown, a small number of men – of the order of 1 in 2000 – spontaneously rejoin and recanalize the divided vas deferens. In a few cases, this is enough to restore fertility.
→ The incidence of postoperative pain. This varies from study to study but was up to 22 per cent in one series. In many men this will be mild, self-limiting discomfort but the spectrum does include patients whose chronic, severe, unremitting pain is only abolished by vasectomy reversal.
→ The need for continued contraceptive precautions until two clear sperm samples have been analysed at 8 and 12 weeks post-procedure. If these samples are not clear, then continued precautions must be maintained until clearance is achieved.

Aside from these specific points, the procedure should be explained to him, and the pros and cons of general versus local anaesthesia and general points discussed, such as bruising and wound infection that are relevant to any surgical procedure.

Describe how you would carry out the procedure

With the patient supine, the external genitalia are prepared with an aqueous antiseptic solution and draped. Palpation of the cord through the scrotal skin allows identification of the vas deferens. Local anaesthetic, such as 1 per cent plain lignocaine, is infiltrated over the vas. The vas is manoeuvred to lie just below the skin and is held there by securing it and the overlying skin in a Babcock's forceps. The skin is incised and the vas freed from the surrounding cord by incision of the investing layers until the glistening white surface of the vas is clearly seen. The Babcock's forceps are now transferred to encircle the vas alone, which is cleared of its coverings for 3 cm or so. It is then clipped and at least 2 cm of vas excised and sent for histology. The two ends are turned over upon themselves and tied. The ends of vas are returned to the scrotum and the small skin incision closed with a single haemostatic stitch of vicryl. The procedure is repeated on the other side.

What are the common postoperative complications?

The commonest complication is a scrotal haematoma, which usually settles with conservative management and a firm groin support. Other than pain, the less common but more important complication is failure. If a patient persistently fails to provide clear samples, then the histology of the removed tissue should be sought. Occasionally, junior surgeons excise tissue other than vas, which is the justification of histological examination of the specimens. If the procedure has failed for whatever reason, then the scrotum should be re-explored by an experienced surgeon under general anaesthesia and the procedure performed again.

How successful is vasectomy reversal?

The short answer is not very. It is more successful when performed soon after the original vasectomy. At 5 years post-vasectomy, the success rate of reversal is so low as to negate attempting it. Whilst about 35 per cent achieve patency and sperm flow after a reversal at 3 years post-vasectomy, only a much smaller percentage achieve fertility.

6. BURR HOLES

A patient with a closed head injury has a CT-proven right temporal extradural haematoma. He is *in extremis* and will not survive transfer to a neurosurgeon. Describe what you would do

After discussion with the regional neurosurgical unit, an emergency right temporal burr hole to relieve the rising intracranial pressure is performed. Assuming the patient is already intubated and ventilated, the patient is positioned supine with the neck extended and the head supported on a head ring. If time allows, the head is shaved completely, otherwise a 10 cm square area is shaved over the site of the planned burr hole. Head shaving can be omitted if time is particularly pressing. The burr hole should be sited two fingerbreadths in front of the tragus of the ear and three fingerbreadths above, which should correspond to a point above the mid-point of the zygomatic arch. A vertical incision in the skin is made and continued through temporalis fascia and muscle, a self-retaining retractor is then inserted which aids haemostasis from the skin edges. The periosteum of the skull is incised and elevated. A Hudson brace is used to drill through the skull and when the drill starts rocking erratically it indicates that the inner table has been breached. At this point change the drill to a burr and continue to enlarge the hole in the skull. The extradural clot will now begin to extrude itself through the hole and regular irrigation with saline will ease its passage. Any bleeding points are coagulated using the bipolar diathermy machine, and this may include the middle meningeal artery itself. With the immediate pressure removed and haemostasis achieved, the burr hole is covered with a dry dressing and urgent transfer arranged to the neurosurgical unit for definitive management.

Where would you site frontal and occipital burr holes?

See Figure 4.3. A frontal burr hole is situated in the mid-pupillary line, level with a point 13 cm back from the nasion, which should coincide with the coronal suture line. Emergency occipital burr holes are rarely needed, as posterior fossa haematomas tend to accumulate more slowly. The occipital burr hole should be sited over the posterior fossa two fingerbreadths from the midline.

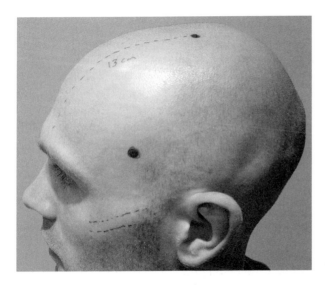

Figure 4.3 Siting of frontal and temporal burr holes.

How could you enlarge these holes?

An initial burr hole may be enlarged by using a larger sized burr, but this is rarely adequate and craniectomy by nibbling the edges of the hole with bone nibblers is the usual practice. An experienced operator may choose to convert the burr hole into the starting point for raising a bone flap and convert it to a formal craniotomy – but this should not be encouraged outside of a neurosurgical centre.

What are the usual causes of temporal extradural and subdural haematomas?

Classically, extradural haematomas are caused by disruption of the middle meningeal artery, a branch of the maxillary artery, as it runs beneath the pterion – the weakest part of the skull. Subdural haematomata arise from rupture of the veins traversing the subdural space and, as such, are often harder to find and control.

7. HEMIARTHROPLASTY

What are the commonly used approaches to the hip joint?

The hip joint can be reached by a variety of approaches depending upon the specific operation contemplated. The two commonest, however, are the anterolateral (Hardinge) and anterior (Smith-Petersen) approaches. In the Hardinge approach, the patient is placed lateral, or supine with a sandbag under the buttock. The skin incision curves down and backwards to the greater trochanter, and then down the axis of the thigh. Tensor fascia lata is divided and held apart with a self-retaining retractor over the greater trochanter and gluteus medius is divided off the front to expose the joint capsule beneath. The Smith-Petersen approach disconnects the tensor fascia lata and gluteal muscles from the iliac crest to gain access to the joint capsule. The posterior approach is quick and easy, and provides excellent access, but has an increased risk of dislocation after surgery, hence it is unpopular with many surgeons. In the lateral position, skin and tensor fascia lata are incised, the hip is internally rotated and the presented short external rotators divided and folded back to protect the sciatic nerve, which is close by. The capsule is now presented.

A 76-year-old lady has fallen and sustained the injury shown in this x-ray (Figure 4.4). Describe and justify your management plan and describe the procedure you would perform

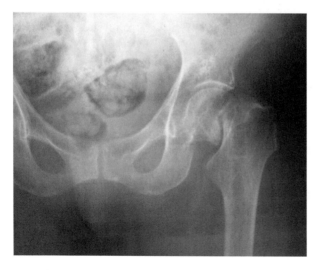

Figure 4.4

This is an intracapsular fracture of the femoral neck. An intracapsular fracture in a lady of this age is liable to compromise the blood supply severely to the femoral head with a significant risk of avascular necrosis if the head is left *in situ*. A procedure to replace the femoral head is indicated. This may be hemiarthroplasty (cemented or uncemented), insertion of a bipolar prosthesis or a total hip replacement. The decision as to which procedure to undertake largely depends upon the wear that the prosthesis is likely to undergo. This takes into account many factors, such as the pre-fall performance status of the patient, coexisting morbidities and estimated longevity of the patient. In a lady of this age, an uncemented hemiarthroplasty would be a suitable prosthesis.

The operation is conducted under general anaesthetic. The patient is positioned according to the surgeon's preferred approach to the hip joint. If a modified Hardinge approach is to be used, the patient should be in the lateral position with the injured leg uppermost. The skin and tensor fascia lata are incised, and the gluteus medius tendon divided, leaving the posterior half attached to the greater trochanter. This now gives access to the femoral neck and capsule, which is divided. The neck is then cut with a power saw and the leg externally rotated to allow the femoral head to be removed from the acetabulum. The head is then sized and the acetabulum washed out. The femoral shaft is prepared by reaming and a trial reduction attempted. If all is well, the Austin Moore prosthesis is hammered home so that it rests on the calcar femorale. The hip is reduced, stability checked and the muscles then reattached sequentially before closing skin. An x-ray is required the following morning to check the position.

Would you consider any other procedure if the injury were more distal?

If the fracture were extracapsular, i.e. the blood supply to the femoral head is liable to be intact, then the fracture would be suitable for an open reduction and internal fixation with a dynamic hip screw or cannulated AO screws.

What are the complications of hip hemiarthroplasty?

The age and associated morbidities of the patients undergoing hip hemiarthroplasty mean that there are often significant problems. Operation-specific ones include peri-prosthetic fracture, infection, and loosening and migration of the prosthesis. Any hip replacement has a risk of dislocation. Non-specific problems arise because these, often elderly, patients lie immobile in bed for long periods of time and may succumb to orthostatic pneumonias, deep venous thrombosis and pressure sores. All these can be ameliorated or prevented by good nursing care and early mobilization with aggressive physiotherapy, which is the norm in most orthopaedic units now. In spite of this, a fractured neck of femur is a pre-terminal event in many elderly patients and only 50 per cent will be alive 6 months after their fall.

Marius Smith-Petersen (1886–1953). Orthopaedic surgeon from Boston, USA, who in addition to describing his approach to the hip joint devised a flanged nail for open fixation of femoral neck fracture – the first to do so.

8. CATHETERIZATION

How would you insert a urinary catheter into a male patient?

The procedure is explained to the patient, who should be supine on a bed or trolley at a comfortable height, with the bedclothes folded down and his legs parted. The equipment is laid out on a sterile field and the catheter balloon checked. The procedure is an aseptic technique and begins with cleaning of the glans penis with aqueous antiseptic. Whilst holding the penis with the foreskin retracted with a swab in the left hand, sterile lignocaine gel is instilled into the penile urethra and it passes the prostate by gentle massage. The end of the sterile bag in which the catheter is covered is removed and the catheter is passed into the penile urethra with the penis held straight up and the catheter advanced. At the level of the prostate gland, the penis is lowered into a 'straight line' as this often aids passage through the prostatic urethra. The catheter is inserted fully and the balloon inflated with 10 ml of sterile water. The catheter is then connected to a collection bag and reassurance gained from the appearance of urine into the system. When placed for relief of urinary retention, the residual volume drained is noted. The foreskin is replaced over the glans penis to prevent paraphimosis formation.

If the urethral catheter does not pass easily, what options are open to you?

The common causes of failure to pass a urethral catheter are meatal or urethral stricture or, more commonly, inability to negotiate the curves of the prostatic urethra in the elderly patient with prostatic hyperplasia. In that instance, an experienced hand may be able to pass the catheter using a sterile introducer, which, passed down into the catheter, provides more rigidity to aid negotiation of the prostate. It runs the risk in inexperienced hands of creating holes and false passages into the prostate gland. The easier option in most cases of failure of the urethral route is to insert a suprapubic catheter (see Figure 4.5).

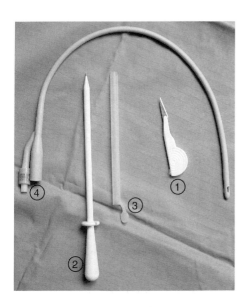

Figure 4.5 A suprapubic catheterization kit.
1, blade; 2, trochar; 3, sheath; 4, catheter.

How would you pass a catheter by the suprapubic route?

After explanation and with the patient in the same position as described above, the lower abdomen is palpated and percussed to confirm a full bladder. The lower abdomen is prepared with aqueous antiseptic solution. Using a syringe of plain lignocaine, the skin and then the tissues below are anaesthetized in the midline, three fingerbreadths above the pubic symphysis in an area of dullness to percussion previously identified. If the patient is slim, the anaesthetic needle may actually enter the bladder, which can be confirmed by aspiration of urine. After making a small nick in the skin with a scalpel blade, push the trocar and sheath from the suprapubic set through the skin hole and into the bladder, which is greeted by a rush of urine. Remove the trocar, pass the catheter through the sheath and inflate the balloon. The sheath can now be removed and a dressing applied around the entry point of the catheter, which is connected to a collection system in the usual way.

9. INGUINAL HERNIA REPAIR

Omitting details of preoperative preparation, describe in detail the repair of an indirect inguinal hernia

A skin incision parallel to and 2 cm above the medial half of the inguinal ligament, or in a suitable skin crease, is made and extended slightly beyond the pubic tubercle. Subcutaneous tissue and Scarpa's fascia are divided until the aponeurosis of external oblique is identified and opened in the line of its fibres, revealing the spermatic cord beneath. Care is taken to protect the ilioinguinal nerve, whilst the cord is mobilized by blunt dissection at the level of the superficial ring and then encircled by a hernia ring. The sac of an indirect hernia will lie anterosuperiorly on the cord and it should be carefully dissected free after division of the overlying cremaster muscle. With the sac isolated down to the neck at the deep ring, where the limit of dissection is marked by the pre-peritoneal fat, it is opened between clips and the contents inspected. If a simple hernia, the redundant sac is twisted, ligated at the deep ring and excised, after which the stump is returned to the peritoneal cavity.

A polypropylene mesh is now cut to shape and anchored to the pubic tubercle with a synthetic non-absorbable suture. The mesh should be cut so that it protrudes medially from the tubercle for 2 cm to prevent medial recurrence. The lower edge is then sutured to the edge of the inguinal ligament, taking care not to include the external oblique fibres. At the deep ring, the mesh is split longitudinally to 'fish-tail' around the cord as it passes through the ring and is secured to reduce the size of the ring to obviate recurrence. A few tacking sutures then secure the upper border of the mesh on to the muscle of internal oblique under cover of the elevated external oblique fibres. External oblique is then closed over the mesh using vicryl and the skin closed with an absorbable subcuticular stitch. The wound may be infiltrated with local anaesthetic, if performed under general anaesthetic.

What is the underlying defect that is addressed in an inguinal hernia repair?

The described methods of open inguinal hernia repair are legion and all the successful ones address the common basic problem, which is a weakness/failure of the transversalis fascia to maintain the integrity of the posterior wall of the inguinal canal.

What other methods do you know for hernia repair?

The most commonly employed method other than the mesh repair described above is the Shouldice repair. This method divides and then double breasts the transversalis fascia using a non-absorbable suture – originally stainless steel wire – to reinforce the posterior wall of the inguinal canal. The Bassini repair is currently out of favour, but is one of the oldest methods and involves approximating the arching fibres of the conjoint tendon to the inguinal ligament. The Stoppa method involves using a plug of mesh to fill the excess space of the deep inguinal ring via an extraperitoneal approach. Before mesh was readily available, many surgeons performed a darn repair, placing a darn of non-absorbable suture between the inguinal ligament and the conjoint tendon, which is where the mesh now rests.

What route might be preferable when dealing with a recurrent hernia?

Recurrent and bilateral hernias are ideal cases to be repaired laparoscopically. By avoiding the scarred and distorted anatomy of an anterior approach in a redo procedure, many complications can be avoided. The laparoscopic method can be performed either transperitoneally or pre-peritoneally.

When obtaining consent for open repair of a recurrent hernia in a man, what will you specifically mention?

Reoperating through the scarred tissue and distorted anatomy following surgery, particularly if a mesh has been used, leaves many structures prone to inadvertent damage. In some cases, the only way to achieve a sound repair is to sacrifice the cord and testicle, so informed consent includes consent for orchidectomy. In addition, the patient must be warned about persistent groin pain, which has an incidence of 2–3 per cent, damage to the ilioinguinal nerve, which is common, and the possibility of testicular atrophy following damage to the testicular blood supply. Informed consent should also include a discussion of the alternative treatments, which in this case should specifically detail the laparoscopic approach.

10. MALE GENITALIA

What are the medical indications for circumcision?

The medical, as opposed to religious, indications are few in number and undoubtedly large numbers of unnecessary circumcisions take place. The main indications are true phimosis, balanitis xerotica obliterans and carcinoma of the prepuce. Occasionally, an emergency circumcision or dorsal slit is required for a paraphimosis that will not reduce by any other method.

Describe your method of performing the operation

The patient is laid supine under general anaesthesia. The external genitalia are prepared with aqueous antiseptic and draped. The prepuce must be retracted and the glans beneath cleaned also. Two straight artery forceps are applied side by side on the dorsum of the foreskin and scissors used to divide the foreskin between the two clips to a level just below the corona. The incision is then continued circumferentially in either direction around the penis keeping 0.5 cm or so below the corona until the incisions meet at the frenulum. The frenulum is picked up in a clip and the redundant foreskin excised. The frenulum and its artery are transfixed. Bleeding vessels can either be clipped and tied, or coagulated with bipolar diathermy. After obtaining haemostasis, the ridge of skin below the corona and the free edge of foreskin remaining down the shaft are opposed with interrupted absorbable sutures. The penis is loosely dressed in paraffin gauze and then dry gauze.

Is there an alternative method in children?

No. Commercial devices such as the 'Plastibell' have proved to be unsuccessful. Amputation of the stretched foreskin, as performed previously, is negligent.

What methods of postoperative pain relief can be useful after circumcision?

All circumcisions should be performed with either a caudal or penile block *in situ*, which makes the early postoperative period more comfortable. Insertion of a non-steroidal anti-inflammatory suppository just before the end of the anaesthesia will also give good analgesia for the first 12 hours or so; thereafter oral analgesia can be taken. Other methods of analgesia, such as PCA and epidurals should not be necessary after this procedure.

What types of hydroceles are recognized? What are the clinical findings of a hydrocele?

A hydrocele is a collection of fluid in some part of the processus vaginalis. Hydroceles can be divided into primary, i.e. idiopathic, or secondary, i.e. those that occur secondary to testicular pathology.

The different types are dependent on which parts of the processus remain patent:

→ *congenital* – the processus remains patent into the peritoneal cavity
→ *infantile* – the processus obliterates only at the level of the deep ring
→ *vaginal* – the fluid collects only around the testis; this is the commonest type
→ *hydrocele of the cord* – the fluid is in an isolated collection around the cord; this is the rarest type.

On examination of the scrotum, a soft swelling is felt which is separate from the testis. It brilliantly transilluminates.

When is it worth organizing an ultrasound in the routine assessment of a hydrocele? Would you aspirate the hydrocele in clinic?

The diagnosis of hydrocele is usually straightforward and rarely requires an ultrasound for diagnostic purposes. One cause for a hydrocele, however, is a testicular tumour and, if there is a suspicion of a tumour-associated hydrocele, or the testis cannot be adequately assessed clinically because of the hydrocele, then ultrasound examination is warranted. Provided there is no suspicion of malignancy, aspiration of the hydrocele will allow examination of the testicle without hindrance. Aspiration of a tumour-related hydroceles risks seeding of malignant cells to scrotal skin and thus involves a different lymphatic field. Aspiration as a treatment option is limited, as the fluid will inevitably re-accumulate.

Describe the operative treatment of a hydrocele

A Jaboulay procedure would be appropriate. The scrotum is opened and the hydrocele sac incised longitudinally and then everted. Any redundant sac is excised and the remnants of tunica are sutured together behind the cord. The scrotum is closed using haemostatic absorbable sutures. A firm athletic support is worn. The patient is warned that the scrotum may feel boggy, as the hydrocele fluid is now being drained via the scrotal lymphatics, although this tends to settle down over time.

Lord described an equally simple procedure for hydroceles, whereby the tunica is plicated into a ruff and sutured to the epididymo-testicular junction. Lord's procedure works well for small to medium-sized hydroceles.

Matthieu Jaboulay (1860–1913). French surgeon in the city of Lyons who also made early but unsuccessful attempts at renal transplantation using animal organs.

11. RIGHT HEMICOLECTOMY

What operation would you perform for a cancer of the caecal pole?

A caecal tumour should be treated by a right hemicolectomy with an ileocolic anastomosis.

What is a laparotomy and how would you perform one?

Laparotomy is the systematic examination of the abdominal cavity and its organs. It is technically an investigation. There are many ways to perform a thorough laparotomy, and it matters little in which order the abdominal organs are examined as long as all organs are inspected every time. One scheme is as follows.

The peritoneum is opened and any escaping gas, foul odour or fluid is noted. The solid viscera and associated organs are then palpated, that is, the liver and gallbladder, spleen and pancreas, which is palpated through the back wall of the stomach. The gastrointestinal tract is then examined – oesophagus, stomach, duodenum, duodenojejunal flexure, the entire small bowel, the appendix, colon, rectum and omentum. The retroperitoneum, including the kidneys, can be seen and the aorta palpated. In a woman, the cervix, uterus, tubes and ovaries are felt and, in a man, the base of the prostate is felt through the bladder. The bladder itself is palpated in either sex to complete the examination.

Describe the steps of a right hemicolectomy

The abdomen is entered by a midline, right paramedian or right transverse incision. A thorough laparotomy is performed, paying particular attention to any evidence of hepatic, peritoneal or mesenteric deposits. The tumour is assessed for mobility and resectability before examining the rest of the colon, bearing in mind that synchronous tumours occur in 3 per cent of cases. Assuming the tumour is resectable, the lateral peritoneal reflection is incised using scissors or point diathermy. The right colon is gradually dissected free and turned medially, taking care not to pull up on the right ureter. The plane of dissection should aim to leave the gonadal vessels behind lying on Gerota's fascia. Care must be taken at the hepatic flexure, not only because of the liver but because of the duodenum that lies directly beneath the colon at this point. The greater omentum is freed from the right half of the transverse colon. The line of division of the transverse colon depends in each case on the exact disposition of the vessels. The aim is to remove the territory of the right colic artery and the right branch of the middle colic artery, leaving the left branch of the middle colic artery intact. The ileocolic artery should be taken close to its origin as a high tie. The peritoneum over the mesentery is incised to a suitable point of division of the ileum approximately 15–20 cm from the ileocaecal junction. The mesentery and transverse mesocolon are then divided between clips and ligated until the resection specimen is tethered only at either end. Soft and crushing clamps are applied and the bowel transected between them. The colon is cleaned out with betadine-soaked swabs and the blood supply to the bowel ends is inspected and, if adequate, a sutured anastomosis is performed in an end-to-end manner. A stapled 'functional end-to-end' anastomosis may also be fashioned. The non-crushing clamps are removed and thorough haemostasis achieved. The defect in the mesentery is closed with an absorbable suture such as vicryl. The abdomen is closed using 1 PDS or similar in a mass closure technique with subcuticular vicryl to skin. The patient should have one dose of prophylactic antibiotics and should receive a low-molecular-weight heparin as DVT prophylaxis, unless specifically contraindicated.

What structures are specifically in danger during this procedure?

During mobilization of the right colon the right ureter, gonadal vessels and kidney and the duodenum are all in particular danger and specific care should be taken to avoid injury to them.

Describe in detail how you would construct your anastomosis

By choice, a hand-sewn, interrupted, single-layer, extramucosal end-to-end anastomosis is performed. The anastomosis is made using 3/0 PDS sutures. With the two pieces of bowel laid end to end without undue tension, the first stitch is at the mesenteric border passing extramucosally on both segments. This suture is clipped. A similar stitch is now placed at the antimesenteric borders and clipped. A third suture is placed half way between the two and clipped. This method takes advantage of the fact that both ends of bowel are usually highly mobile and will be able to be turned over to complete the back wall in a similar fashion. Extramucosal sutures are then placed, tying them along the length of the bowel 5 mm apart and bearing in mind that there may be a need to adjust the stitch placement to accommodate any size discrepancy. Once the anterior layer has been completed and checked to ensure that there are no large gaps, the bowel is flipped over and the procedure repeated for the remaining free bowel. The two corner sutures are tied finally, and the anastomosis checked for lumen size by squeezing between finger and thumb, and for leaks by squeezing small bowel content through the anastomosis.

What would your postoperative instructions be?

Instructions would be to allow the patient to drink 30 ml of water an hour as soon as he wants after he comes round from his operation. He should continue DVT prophylaxis whilst in hospital, but should not need any further antibiotics unless there was enteric soiling during the procedure. On the first postoperative day, he can drink free fluids as tolerated and start a light diet when he feels able. If he becomes nauseated, then he should reduce his oral intake. Most patients are ready for discharge home between 5 and 8 days after surgery.

12. DISLOCATED SHOULDERS

What abnormality is seen in the x-ray shown in Figure 4.6 on page 134?

This is an anterior dislocation of the shoulder.

What might you see on assessing the patient clinically?

The patient will complain of pain and loss of movement in that shoulder. They may sit holding their dislocated arm with the other, lest it move. The elbow is unusually prominent as the normal alignment of the arm is lost. When viewed

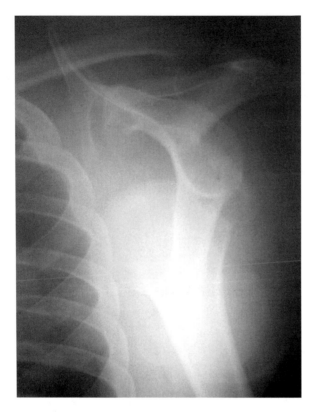

Figure 4.6

from the front, an anterior swelling and lateral flattening of the shoulder – sometimes best seen from above – are usually obvious.

Name two other types of shoulder dislocation. How common are they?

The other two sorts are posterior and vertical dislocations. The first is rare and the latter extremely rare. In the posterior dislocation, said to be commoner after electric shocks or epileptic fits, a posterior bulge may be noticeable and external rotation severely limited. The anteroposterior x-ray may appear normal and the diagnosis usually requires an axillary view x-ray, which shows the head of the humerus resting on the posterior glenoid lip. A vertical dislocation, known as luxatio erecta, is noticeable by the fact that the patient's arm is held vertically above the head; the humeral head is below the glenoid.

How would you reduce an anterior dislocation? List the options and describe your tried and trusted method

The options include postural reduction – best in those patients under the influence of drink or analgesics, Kocher's method or the Hippocratic method, which involves leverage with the stockinged foot in the axilla to manipulate the head of the humerus. It is rarely performed nowadays because of risk of axillary nerve damage. The preferred method is that of Kocher. With the patient supine and under either general anaesthesia or analgesia with sedation, the flexed elbow is abducted and rotated externally, to relax the muscle spasm of subscapularis, accompanied by gentle downwards traction, whilst an assistant applies counter traction in the axilla. The elbow is then adducted on to the chest and internally rotated to lay the arm across the chest during which the humeral head has usually popped rather noticeably back into place. The arm is then placed in a polypropylene sling for 3 weeks before gentle mobilization is allowed. If this procedure is performed under general anaesthetic, the operator will normally be pleasantly surprised that the shoulder reduces virtually instantaneously once the anaesthetist's muscle relaxants get to work – otherwise direct manipulation into the socket is easily performed.

What would you check and document before and after reduction?

The circumflex axillary nerve winds around the surgical neck of the humerus and may be damaged during dislocation *and* reduction. It gives motor supply to the deltoid muscle but testing this before reduction is somewhat cruel; fortunately, it also supplies sensation to an area over the anterolateral curve of the muscle. This should be examined both before and after reduction to ensure the nerve is uninjured, and this should be assiduously documented. I would also perform an x-ray to ensure reduction was adequate and that no bony damage had occurred during reduction.

Theodor Kocher (1841–1917). Swiss surgeon who was the student of both Billroth and Langenbeck. His work on thyroid physiology and pathology won him the Nobel Prize for Medicine in 1909. He had a personal series of over 2000 thyroidectomies, with an overall mortality rate of just 4.5 per cent.

13. PILONIDAL DISEASE

A young man presents with a pilonidal abscess in his natal cleft. What is your preferred treatment option?

See Figure 4.7. The immediate aim is to relieve the pain from his abscess. Incision and drainage of the abscess is required under general anaesthetic. No attempt is made to do anything more than that. The incision is made away from the midline.

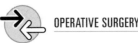

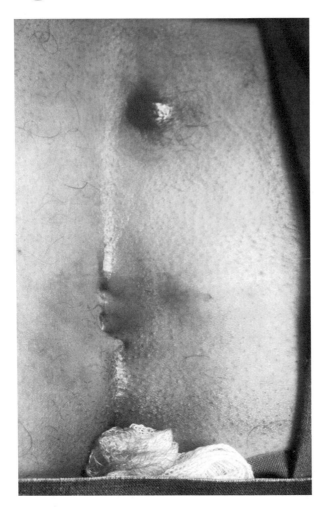

Figure 4.7 Pilonidal disease. Both midline pits and a lateral abscess are evident.

He returns to see you in clinic 3 months later with a healed scar but continuing symptoms from his pilonidal disease. What are the options and what is your treatment plan?

In clinic, he should be examined to look specifically for midline pits and lateral tracks. If he has midline pit disease and his symptoms are not too bad, conservative measures are continued, such as regular depilation of the area and exemplary personal hygiene. If he had symptomatic lateral tracks, excision should be offered. The decision has to be made whether the wound is laid open and left to granulate or whether the wound is clean enough to allow direct primary closure. In most non-infected cases, primary closure may be attempted but the patient warned that it may not be successful. Other approaches, such as those of Bascom, Karydakis and Limberg, aim to flatten the natal cleft and all have good success rates.

How does pilonidal disease develop and where else can it occur?

Opposing camps describe different aetiologies. One theory holds that it is a congenital nest of hairs that becomes enclosed as the skin closes over it; however, this does not explain why the hairs found in the bottom of the abscess in the natal cleft are demonstrably head hairs. The acquired theory suggests that chronic trauma allows a hair tip to penetrate the skin and the rolling motion of the buttocks causes the hairs to burrow in. It is also seen in the finger webs of people in certain occupations, notably hairdressers and sheepshearers.

Describe the steps of the Karydakis procedure

The patient is positioned prone under general anaesthesia with the buttocks taped apart. The area of the natal cleft is prepared and draped. An asymmetric ellipse is drawn on the skin of the natal cleft encompassing the lateral tracks in the wider half of the ellipse. The skin is incised according to the marked pattern and the tissue removed down to the level of the pre-sacral fascia. The tissue beneath the narrow flap is undermined until it can be approximated to the other side. The restraining tapes on the buttocks are freed and the skin closed with interrupted nylon sutures over a mini-vacuumed drain. The drain is removed at 24 hours and the patient allowed home. Stitches are removed between 2 and 3 weeks.

14. MASTECTOMY

What are the surgical options for a 42-year-old female patient with a 3 cm tumour in the lower inner quadrant of a small breast?

Initial surgical therapy for this woman would consist of either a wide local excision (WLE) or simple mastectomy; in both cases with or without axillary node clearance or sampling. Given that the lesion is under 4 cm and located peripherally, WLE should be considered. Potential problems with WLE are her young age, as she may be better served by mastectomy, and the cosmetic effect of WLE in a small breast. The surgical options are explained to her and she may decide, particularly with regard to the cosmesis of WLE in a small breast. It should be explained that, with a WLE, there is around a 10 per cent chance that an insufficient margin will be obtained at operation, requiring either a further WLE or mastectomy.

The treatment of the clinically uninvolved axilla is more problematical. The options are as follows.

→ *Blind radiotherapy to the axilla*. This provides local control but no prognostic information and will overtreat an uninvolved axilla. It is now rarely used owing to the significant morbidity of restricted shoulder mobility following radiotherapy.

→ *Axillary clearance to Level III.* This offers local control plus prognostic information but again risks overtreatment in an uninvolved axilla and increases the risk of side effects, such as lymphoedema.

→ *Axillary node sampling and later surgery/radiotherapy*, depending on the results. This sounds more precise, but needs two sittings and has all the problems associated with 'sampling', such as sampling error. It is not free of the risks of restricted shoulder movement and lymphoedema.

→ *Sentinel node biopsy.* Identification and operative frozen section of the sentinel node allows axillary clearance, if necessary. It has not been proven to be sufficiently accurate yet and, although it is a promising technique, the results of randomized trials, such as ALMANAC, are awaited before it becomes routine practice.

The patient should be made aware that the chance of having axillary involvement is around 30 per cent, but that an involved axilla should be treated with either radical radiotherapy or Level III clearance – but not both, as the morbidity rises sharply.

Describe a simple mastectomy. What are the limits of the dissection?

An elliptical skin incision is placed in skin crease lines, if possible, to encompass the nipple and the skin overlying the tumour. The flaps are raised and undermined up to the clavicle and down to the upper edge of rectus sheath and from the edge of sternum to the border of latissimus dorsi. The breast tissue is elevated from the pectoral fascia, which is left intact and dissected from the sternum laterally. The skin wound can be extended into the axilla to allow clearance or a separate incision can be made. The breast dissection is continued to include the axillary tail. All macroscopically obvious breast tissue has now been removed. Scrupulous haemostasis is undertaken and the skin flaps closed without tension or dog-ears, over a vacuum drain. The skin is closed by subcuticular absorbable suture. The drain is left until it drains less than 30 ml per day or until day 5, when it is removed regardless. The drain need not detain the patient in hospital, as many centres have arrangements with the district nursing service for drain removal in the community.

Which nerves should be seen at axillary dissection? What are the consequences of dividing them?

→ *The median pectoral nerve*, which runs upwards to enter the underside of pectoralis minor before passing into and supplying pectoralis major, is seen and preserved. Division results in minor weakness of the pectoral muscles, predominantly the lower costal fibres. Concomitant damage to the lateral pectoral nerve, however, will paralyse the entire pectoralis major.

→ *The intercostobrachial nerve* emerges from the chest wall just behind the origin of pectoralis minor, and supplies sensation to the medial upper arm and the axilla. Division of the intercostobrachial nerve is not unusual during axillary clearance, and gives a minor sensory loss on the lateral chest wall and medial upper arm.

→ *The thoracodorsal nerve* runs down the posterior axillary wall to enter the deep surface of latissimus dorsi; it should be easily identified and preserved but, if inadvertently divided or deliberately sacrificed, there is minimal deficit. It must be preserved with the vessels if a latissimus dorsi flap is considered for reconstruction.

→ *The long thoracic nerve* passes down the lateral thoracic wall just posterior to the mid-axillary line. It must be preserved, as division of the nerve produces winging of the scapula because of paralysis of serratus anterior.

Prior to surgery the patient wishes to discuss the reconstructive options. What are they?

There are several topics to discuss in this setting, the first of which is timing. Some women are suitable for immediate reconstruction at the time of mastectomy, which is less time consuming for the patient, although not necessarily so for the surgeon involved. Care must be taken to ensure that the oncological operation is not compromised because of cosmetic considerations. Alternatively, reconstruction can take place at a later date after all adjuvant therapy has occurred and the woman has recovered from the tribulations of mastectomy.

In terms of replacing lost tissue volume, the alternatives are placement of a prosthesis or transposition of a myocutaneous flap – or a combination of the two to achieve larger volumes. Subpectoral placement of a prosthesis alone is a simple procedure but tends to produce a rather unnatural looking breast mound. Myocutaneous flaps achieve a more natural appearance than a prosthesis but are limited by the volumes they can achieve. If circumstances dictate, the need for a large volume reconstruction to match the other side, consideration should be given to contralateral reduction surgery to achieve potentially better overall results. The commonest flaps in use are the pedicled latissimus dorsi flap or the TRAM flap (transverse rectus abdominis myocutaneous flap), which can either be pedicled or free grafted. The TRAM flap tends to provide a larger volume reconstruction. Nipple replacement can be achieved by synthetic 'stick on' placement after surgery, by tattoo and, occasionally, by nipple transplantation to a healthy site with later re-grafting to the reconstructed breast.

15. THYROID DISEASE

What forms of treatment are available to a young woman with symptomatic Graves' disease?

Graves' disease is an autoimmune cause of hyperthyroidism often characterized by striking eye signs of exophthalmos and lid lag. It is ten times more common in women than men and is particularly prevalent in women under the age of 40. The available treatments are medical, radioiodine therapy or surgery. None is ideal and all have drawbacks.

Medical treatment with drugs, such as carbimazole, does not treat the underlying condition but merely palliates the symptoms, which may be sufficient as 25 per cent of Graves' disease cases will resolve spontaneously. Treatment is for a set period – normally 12 months – and, if relapse occurs after stopping therapy, then a further long-term course of medical therapy is not usually indicated. However, it is used to render the patient euthyroid again before further treatment.

Radioiodine may be given as a single oral dose according to the estimated weight of the gland. Effects take 6–10 weeks to become evident and hyperthyroidism must be controlled in the mean time. Benefits include low cost and ease, combined with efficacy. Unfortunately, it is not suitable for women in the child-bearing years, as some evidence of transplacental effects exists, nor can parents hold their children for 2 weeks after treatment. Its major disadvantage, however, is late-onset hypothyroidism, which can occur up to 10 years after treatment. Radioiodine is contraindicated in patients with Graves' eye disease, since their eye signs will worsen by one grade with radioiodine therapy.

Surgery is an excellent treatment and is particularly suitable for certain patient groups:

→ those under 30 years of age
→ patients with ophthalmic Graves' disease
→ women wishing to get pregnant within the next 4 years
→ patients who do not wish to have radioiodine treatment
→ patients with large goitres at risk of extrinsic compression.

What are the drawbacks of medical therapy?

As already noted, it is a palliative rather than curative treatment. Like all medical therapies, it has side effects: dyspepsia, headache and sensitivity rashes are the commonest, but the most important is agranulocytosis, which occurs at an incidence of 4 per 1000. All patients started on carbimazole should be warned of the possibility of agranulocytosis and warned to seek medical help if they develop sore throats, excessive bruising or bleeding. Patients should have a baseline FBC taken at the start of therapy and this should be checked at clinic visits.

If surgery is indicated, what operation would you perform?

The choice lies between total or subtotal thyroidectomy. If total thyroidectomy is performed to prevent recurrence, thyroxine replacement is required. Subsequent surgery in those who develop recurrent Graves' disease in a hypertrophied thyroid remnant is difficult with increased risks of all complications. If a subtotal thyroidectomy is performed, approximately 10 g of thyroid tissue are left behind to avoid postoperative hypothyroidism.

How would you prepare the patient preoperatively and what would you tell her when gaining informed consent?

Preoperatively she needs her thyrotoxicosis controlling. A 2-week course of carbimazole often complemented with a β-blocker may be used to achieve this. Currently most centres use a block and replace regime of carbimazole and replacement thyroxine. Biochemical evidence of euthyroid status should be obtained before surgery. Additionally, treatment with Lugol's Iodine for the last pre-operative week is said to reduce the vascularity of the gland, although this is not universally accepted or practised. Similarly, in some centres, indirect laryngoscopy is performed before all thyroidectomies, but in others, only before recurrent neck surgery. It should be noted that 3 per cent of the population have some degree of vocal cord paralysis, which may be asymptomatic.

Informed consent should include reference to the scar and the inability to predict the quality of it. She should be warned about the risks of postoperative hyperthyroid storm. She should be told about the consequence (not a risk) of postoperative hypothyroidism and the need for treatment. She must also be warned of the risks of hypoparathyroidism, both permanent (1 per cent) and transient (~3 per cent), which is usually due to ischaemia of the parathyroids, rather than inadvertent removal. She must also be warned of the risk of laryngeal nerve palsy, which again may be permanent (1 per cent) or transient (~3 per cent). There is also a small risk of postoperative bleeding in the neck which can lead to respiratory embarrassment. This is due to laryngeal venous occlusion and oedema rather than laryngeal compression *per se*.

Describe the major steps of a total thyroidectomy

The patient is positioned supine with a slight head up tilt, the head supported on a ring with the neck extended and a sandbag between the shoulder blades. General anaesthesia and an endotracheal tube is usual. A transverse 'collar' skin crease incision is made symmetrically about the midline 3 cm above the sternal notch with the sternocleidomastoid as the lateral limits. Platysma is divided and the skin flaps are mobilized up to the superior thyroid notch and down to the sternal notch before a Joll's retractor is used to separate them. The deep cervical fascia is incised and the strap muscles retracted laterally. Each lobe is then mobilized by ligation in continuity and division of the middle thyroid vein branches on the gland itself. The superior thyroid artery and vein are dissected at the upper pole of the gland, being careful to avoid the external laryngeal nerve. The recurrent laryngeal nerve should be identified entering the operative field from below, lying obliquely to the oesophagus and trachea, passing forwards in the region of the inferior thyroid artery. Once safely identified and protected, the inferior thyroid vessels can be secured and divided on the gland to avoid devitalizing the parathyroids, which again should be identified and protected. The gland is now dissected free of its posterior attachments and removed. Absolute haemostasis is achieved by ligation of individual vessels and diathermy is avoided, if possible, to minimize damage to the parathyroids and the laryngeal nerves. The wound is closed in layers. In the event of any intraoperative bleeding, a small vacuum drain may be used, but is not required in an uncomplicated case. The patient is returned to the ward, accompanied by the necessary equipment to open all layers of the closure.

Robert Graves (1797–1853). Irish physician and painting companion of J.M.W. Turner. He published his account of exophthalmic goitre in 1835; he also described angioneurotic oedema and scleroderma.

16. LAPAROSCOPIC SURGERY

Describe a method of safely establishing a pneumoperitoneum

A 2 cm vertical incision is made just below and extending slightly into the umbilicus. The subcutaneous tissues are spread widely, and the umbilical stalk is cleared and grasped with Littlewood's forceps. A small hole is then incised in the base of the stalk and a pair of closed long artery forceps inserted into the hole. A 'give' will be felt as the peritoneum is punctured, after which the clip will move freely from side to side. The artery clip is withdrawn and used to enlarge the hole slightly, and the laparoscopic port inserted with a blunt trocar. After connection to the insufflator, gas flow can be turned up to high immediately. This is a variation of the Hassan open technique. Many gynaecological surgeons, and some general surgeons, use a closed technique, with blind insertion of a Veress needle into the subumbilical area and cautious insufflation. After establishment of the pneumoperitoneum, the sub-umbilical port is inserted blindly using a sharp trocar. This technique is considered to be less safe by the surgical Royal Colleges.

Where would you place the ports for a laparoscopic cholecystectomy?

There should be a 10 mm subumbilical port and a second 10 mm port in the epigastrium just to the right of the midline over the gallbladder itself. Two 5 mm ports are placed subcostally in the midclavicular line and anterior axillary lines.

What is Calot's triangle and why is it important?

It is the triangle bounded above by the liver edge, medially by the common hepatic duct and the cystic duct below. It is important because the cystic artery crosses through Calot's triangle to reach the gallbladder. The triangle should be dissected thoroughly to ensure the anatomy is clearly displayed. The cystic duct and artery should both be clearly seen before division. The myriad of anatomical variation should be remembered.

What additional procedure might you perform if there was a suspicion of a ductal stone?

You should perform an on-table cholangiogram. Cannulation of the cystic duct stump and injection of radio-opaque contrast will outline the biliary tree during fluoroscopy and demonstrate any filling defects within the biliary tree. Any stone thus outlined can be retrieved through a choledochotomy and the duct closed over a T-tube, which is then exteriorized. Alternatively, if there is suspicion of a ductal stone before surgery, a preoperative ERCP can clear the duct from below.

Outline the steps of a laparoscopic inguinal hernia repair

A pneumoperitoneum is safely established and three ports are inserted; a 10 mm umbilical port and a 5 mm working port in both iliac fossae. Using the inferior epigastric vessels as the principal landmark, the hernial orifices of both sides are examined. It is not unusual to discover other small hernias, not detected on clinical examination, as well as the one planned for repair. Any indirect sac is reduced from within or simply amputated, safe in the knowledge from direct vision that it is empty. The peritoneum lying between the pubic tubercle and the deep ring is stripped off, and a sheet of mesh is then stapled over the hernial orifices and the peritoneum replaced.

Alternatively, a balloon dissector can be introduced into the pre-peritoneal space to create a working space. The mechanism of repair is similar to the trans-peritoneal approach.

17. ABDOMINAL AORTIC ANEURYSM

What is an aneurysm?

It is defined as a localized dilatation of a blood vessel to more than twice the normal diameter; lesser increases are referred to as ectatic vessels. A generalized dilatation of the whole arterial system is known as arteriomegaly.

What is the single most important factor in deciding when to operate on an abdominal aortic aneurysm (AAA)?

The most critical factor is size. Although all other surgical criteria are assessed, including fitness for surgery and concomitant illness, the decision to offer surgery is usually made only after the aneurysm has reached an appropriate size. The size criterion for surgery currently rests at 5.5 cm diameter, although some surgeons advocate using a criterion of 6 cm in women as female aneurysms seem less prone to rupture. Smaller aneurysms that are symptomatic because of distal embolization or back pain, and aneurysms with a rate of growth greater than 1 cm in 1 year also merit repair. Studies have shown that repair below diameters of 5.5 cm is of no benefit, as the operative mortality outweighs the risk of rupture if left untreated. Patients with aneurysms smaller than 5.5 cm should be enrolled on an annual ultrasound screening programme and called for surgery when they attain the requisite size.

How would you image a patient with an aneurysm pre-operatively and what structures are you looking to identify?

As well as all their 'standard' surgical work-up, AAA patients need detailed imaging of the aneurysm itself. In particular, its exact relationship to the renal arteries must be determined, as suprarenal clamping should be avoided, if possible. The distal extent of aneurysmal vessels should also be determined as this directs whether a bifurcated graft will be needed if one or both iliac arteries are involved. Rarely, the aneurysm may extend above the diaphragm and require a combined thoracoabdominal approach. Aberrant anatomy, such as horseshoe kidneys, are best identified preoperatively so that due consideration may be given to any problems that they may cause. This information is best provided by arteriography or contrast CT scanning. In some centres three-dimensional CT reconstructions allow detailed morphological information to be gained without resort to angiography (Figure 4.8).

Is screening for AAAs effective?

It is effective in certain groups. Two large-scale studies have recently reported a definite survival benefit after screening for AAA in men over the age of 65. Below this age, the data are less clear for men. There is also clear evidence that screening in women is not effective.

Outline the principal steps in an elective AAA repair

Approaches to the aorta vary and either a transverse or long midline incision is acceptable. The small bowel is packed to one side and the fourth part of the

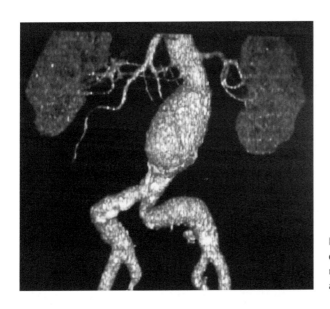

Figure 4.8 Three-dimensional computed tomography reconstruction of an infrarenal abdominal aortic aneurysm.

duodenum mobilized to the right. The posterior peritoneum overlying the aorta is incised. The neck of the aneurysm is cleared and controlled before attention is turned to the lower end. The distal extent of the aneurysm is identified and normal vasculature distal to the aneurysm is defined and controlled. A bolus of intravenous heparin is given and the vessels clamped achieving proximal and distal control. The sac is opened and clot, debris and arteriosclerosis cleared. Back bleeding from inferior mesenteric, lumbar or median sacral arteries is controlled by oversewing. A prosthesis suitable for the task, i.e. tube or bifurcated, is inserted after measuring for size. The proximal end is managed first and is sutured in place using a continuous double-ended synthetic monofilament suture. When the proximal join is secure and has been satisfactorily tested the distal end, or ends in the case of a bifurcated graft, is sutured in place and similarly tested. If at this point the distal colon is looking dusky, then the inferior mesenteric artery will need to be re-implanted. The aneurysm sac is closed over the graft to decrease the risk of aorto-enteric fistula. The peritoneum is reconstituted and the abdomen closed.

How do vascular and gut anastomoses differ?

Vascular anastomoses are invariably performed with a non-absorbable suture, prolene being the most popular, as opposed to gut anastomoses in which an absorbable suture is preferred. Whilst bowel may be joined by either a continuous or interrupted suture technique, vascular joins are performed continuously to ensure equal distribution of tension around the suture line. A bowel anastomosis aims to achieve inversion of the mucosa, whereas the vascular anastomosis is an everting technique.

18. VARICOSE VEINS

Detail how you would assess a patient with varicose veins

Specific points of interest in the history include:

→ duration and nature of symptoms
→ interference with daily life
→ whether a female patient has finished having her family
→ family history of varicose veins
→ occupation including amount of standing
→ past history of lower limb injury/plaster or surgery
→ history of deep venous thrombosis
→ use of the oral contraceptive pill.

The patient is examined standing upright with both lower limbs bare. Skin discoloration, thread veins and ankle flare are noted. The groin is examined to exclude the presence of a varix. The veins are examined to discern whether they represent the long or short saphenous distribution. If it is not clinically apparent, then a hand-held Doppler machine is used to ascertain reflux in the groin or at the saphenopopliteal junction. In uncomplicated, long saphenous primary varicose veins, no further investigations are needed. In the case of recurrent veins, complicated cases or those involving saphenopopliteal reflux, a venous duplex scan is ordered before offering surgery. This should also be performed in cases where there was a clear history or suspicion of DVT.

What is a saphena varix?

A saphena varix is a dilatation of the long saphenous vein just before the junction with the femoral vein. The valve here is incompetent, and it is often associated with descending varicose veins. It may present as a lump in the groin or be noticed during the examination of varicose veins. It empties on minimal pressure and refills on release, and it demonstrates a fluid thrill on percussion. At operation, a varix arises as a bluish swelling from within the cribriform fascia; often thin walled, care must be taken when dissecting around it otherwise a significant venous haemorrhage can occur obscuring the operative field.

What operation would you perform for a case of saphenofemoral incompetence? Briefly describe it

A saphenofemoral disconnection is performed with stripping of the long saphenous vein and multiple avulsions as necessary.

The patient is re-examined in the standing position before surgery and all varicosities marked with an indelible skin marker. The patient is positioned supine under general anaesthesia with 20° of head down tilt. A groin crease incision over the site of the saphenofemoral junction (SFJ) medial to the femoral pulse is made. The junction is identified, and all tributary branches are isolated and divided leaving the SFJ clear. The femoral vein is cleared for 2 cm above and below the junction to exclude any other branches, and the SFJ is then doubly ligated and divided, leaving a cuff of less than 1 cm on the femoral vein. A disposable plastic stripper is passed down the long saphenous vein to just below the knee and the end retrieved through a stab incision. The vein is then stripped. Multiple avulsions of the veins are performed as necessary through tiny stab wounds – these may be stitched or steri-stripped and the wound in the groin closed. Firm elasticated bandaging is applied.

What is the recurrence rate?

This varies tremendously depending on which studies are read but historically it has ranged between 7 and 65 per cent. Certainly approximately 20 per cent of varicose vein surgery is for recurrence.

How would you differentiate between the femoral and long saphenous veins at surgery?

At surgery, the differentiation may not be straightforward as the saphenous vein may be an incredibly robust vessel. The long saphenous vein (LSV) will have at least 3–4 tributaries joining it in its last 5 cm. The femoral vein receives only one branch in the groin and that is the LSV.

What are the tributaries of the long saphenous vein in the groin?

In spite of the oft-displayed textbook arrangement, they can be highly variable. In general, they consist of the lateral and medial thigh veins, superficial and deep external pudendal veins, the superficial circumflex iliac vein and superficial inferior epigastric vein.

19. BLEEDING DUODENAL ULCER

A 72-year-old man presents with frank haematemesis, hypotension and tachycardia. What is your management strategy?

This patient needs simultaneous assessment and resuscitation. Maintenance of a clear airway, supplemental oxygen and prevention of aspiration take priority.

Large-bore intravenous access, withdrawal of blood for FBC, clotting, U&E, LFT and crossmatch of 6 units are sent immediately, and an intravenous saline infusion started. Points of relevance in his history, which may be obtained from either the patient or other sources, such as his family or old hospital notes, would be:

→ similar previous episodes
→ history of ingestion of non-steroidal anti-inflammatory or steroid drugs
→ smoking and drinking habits
→ a history of indigestion and/or acid reflux
→ passage of melaena
→ recent weight loss
→ change of appetite
→ dysphagia.

→ **I would pass a urinary catheter to monitor his urine output, as this is the most sensitive measure of tissue perfusion**; if he required large volumes of fluid for resuscitation, I would consider placing a central venous line for pressure monitoring.

The next investigation would be an upper gastrointestinal endoscopy by an experienced therapeutic endoscopist using a double-channel gastroscope.

At OGD a large bleeding ulcer in the duodenum is found. How can you stop it bleeding?

A wide variety of means are available but each hospital may not have every method available. Laser coagulation of the ulcer base has been shown to be very effective, as has the use of a special heater probe. Injection of sclerosant solutions into the mucosa around the bleeding point have also been shown to be effective – ethanol is a typical sclerosant in common use; many people now also inject adrenaline, which acts as a vasoconstrictor. Direct diathermy can also be effective, although generally less so than these other forms of treatment.

If the haemorrhage is controlled, what would be the subsequent management?

After endoscopic haemostasis, the patient needs to be monitored closely in hospital. He should be started on high-dose proton pump inhibitor and many surgeons would prescribe eradication therapy on an empirical basis. Certain endoscopic and clinic stigmata are recognized as being predictive of further bleeding:

→ an actively bleeding vessel
→ clot adherent to the ulcer base   } OGD appearances
→ a visible vessel
→ age over 60 years
→ requirement for > 6 units of blood within 24 hours of admission.

This gentleman is at high risk of re-bleeding and his attending doctors should have a very low threshold for further gastroscopy if he shows signs of haemodynamic instability or continued blood loss.

If the haemorrhage cannot be controlled by endoscopic means, how should the patient be managed?

In a patient in whom endoscopy is unable to stop bleeding, I would proceed to emergency surgery. Through an upper midline laparotomy incision, a gastroduodenotomy is performed to reveal the bleeding ulcer at the back of the duodenum. This is under-run with a non-absorbable or long-lasting absorbable suture. Once haemostasis is assured, the bowel is closed as a pyloroplasty and the abdomen closed. In cases of bleeding from a gastric ulcer, the choice lies between performing a partial gastrectomy, if the patient is fit enough, or if not, exclusion of the ulcer by large PDS sutures or local ulcer excision may be life saving.

In what part of the duodenum is a bleeding ulcer likely to be and which vessel involved?

It is likely to be a posterior ulcer in the second part of the duodenum where it overlies the gastroduodenal artery; thus, as the ulcer erodes, it does so through the artery, which explains the often catastrophic haemorrhage. The gastroduodenal artery is a branch of the hepatic artery, which comes from the coeliac axis.

Draw the coeliac axis and its branches

See Figure 4.9.

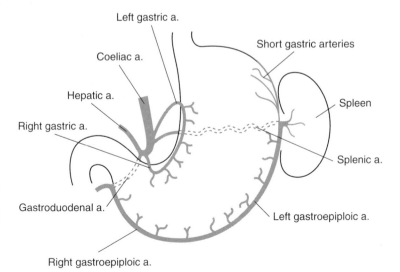

Figure 4.9 The coeliac axis.

20. FEMORAL EMBOLECTOMY

Define an embolus and give some examples

An embolus may be defined as an abnormal mass of undissolved material carried from one place to another in the bloodstream. Typical examples are as follows:

→ thrombus/clot – by far the commonest
→ tumour – cells from a malignant neoplasm may embolize; tumours, such as renal cell carcinoma, which have invaded along the renal vein or IVC, are particularly prone to embolization
→ fat – often following long bone fracture or orthopaedic procedures, although it can happen from soft tissue procedures alone
→ atheroma – from ruptured plaques
→ gas – air may embolize from opened neck veins during head and neck surgery or CVP line insertion
→ amniotic fluid – can enter the bloodstream during labour and leads to DIC, which may be fatal
→ foreign body – catheter tips from cannulae or talcum powder used to 'cut' heroin for intravenous abuse.

What are the sextet of symptoms that occur in acute peripheral ischaemia?

Peripheral embolization is characterized by the sudden onset of: pain, pallor, pulselessness, parasthesia, perishing cold and paralysis.

A 63-year-old female with atrial fibrillation suddenly develops a painful, cold right leg. What is the likely diagnosis and what are you going to do about it, giving details of any operation you might be considering?

The likely diagnosis is a femoral embolus, almost certainly related to her atrial fibrillation. She needs immediate heparinization and preparation for theatre after shaving of both groins and marking of the affected side for a femoral embolectomy.

This operation is preferably performed under general anaesthesia but can be done under local anaesthetic. A longitudinal skin incision over the common femoral artery is made and the common, superficial and profunda femoral arteries are exposed and controlled above and below with silastic slings, i.e. **gaining proximal and distal control**. An arteriotomy is made in the femoral artery at the level of the ostia of the profunda artery. Inflow is restored by passage of a Fogarty catheter proximally (Figure 4.10), inflation of the balloon and withdrawal. If clot is recovered and excellent flow produced, then the inflow is clamped, otherwise the procedure is repeated until satisfactory flow is generated. Using a slightly smaller catheter, the procedure is repeated down both distal arteries, retrieving all clot until acceptable back bleeding is produced; both vessels are then clamped. After irrigation of all three vessels with heparinized saline, if the patient is not already systemically heparinized, the arteriotomy is closed directly or with a vein patch, if necessary.

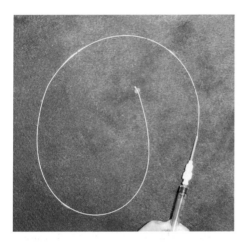

Figure 4.10 A Fogarty embolectomy catheter. The balloon is kept inflated by judicious finger pressure on the syringe during withdrawal through the vessel.

What are the common predisposing conditions?

The predisposing conditions are generally related to the list of common causes outlined above, e.g. femoral nailing will predispose a patient to fat embolism. The cardiological causes not described are atheroma, any cardiac arrhythmia – especially atrial fibrillation – and following a myocardial infarction, when mural thrombus may develop, which can easily embolize.

Thomas Fogarty (1934 –). Surgeon of the University of Oregon Medical School. As a junior resident in the early 1960s, he invented the embolectomy catheter that bears his name. He began inventing while a schoolboy, designing a new centrifugal clutch for a motor scooter, which is still in use today. He holds more than 60 US patents for medical devices. He also owns an award-winning vineyard in California.

21. FLEXOR TENDONS

A young man falls on to some broken glass and suffers a penetrating injury to the base of his right ring finger. Describe how you would assess this injury

Assessment of the injury includes details, such as hand dominance, occupation, mechanism of injury and time since injury. I would examine the hand thoroughly to look for any other injuries. The nature of the penetrating injury is noted, as is the condition of the tissues. Both active and passive movement of each finger joint is individually tested to identify deep or superficial tendon injury. Sensation to light touch is tested along both borders of all digits; this can be added to by using two-point discrimination testing, if necessary. Arterial supply and capillary refill over the whole hand are assessed. Given the mechanism of injury, an x-ray is mandatory to look for foreign bodies and any associated bony injury.

On examination the patient has altered sensation and inability to flex the PIPJ. What is the most likely nature of the injury?

He has probably cut the flexor digitorum superficialis tendon, and either cut or bruised the digital nerve to the ring finger on that side.

Where would you make the skin incisions in order to explore this injury?

The original entry wound should be excised and included in the incision. At the base of the finger, a 'Z' incision across the crease of the metacarpophalangeal joint would be appropriate. This can then be easily extended by zigzagging it in either direction; elevation of the flaps gives ample access to the tendons anteriorly and the digital nerves laterally.

Draw one method of suture to repair a flexor tendon

Many methods are described including those of Bunnell and Kessler. A modified Kessler suture is shown in Figure 4.11.

Stage I uses a 4/0 non-absorbable suture, and can use two sutures as shown here or a single suture for both sides. The second stage uses 6/0 nylon to oversew the paratenon.

What types of splints are available? Which could be used in this case?

In general, splints may be resting, static or dynamic. A resting splint aims to achieve immobilization, typically of inflamed tissues, such as painful rheumatoid joints. A static splint can be worn continuously until a fracture has healed, for example, or intermittently, such as the wearing of a night splint to relieve

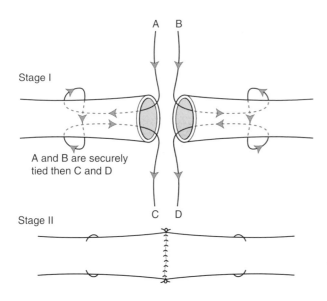

Stage I

A and B are securely
tied then C and D

Stage II

Figure 4.11 A modified Kessler suture. In Stage I, A and B are securely tied, then C and D, if a two-suture method is being used.

the symptoms of carpal tunnel syndrome. Dynamic splintage is usually employed after a tendon injury or repair, and allows movement of the joints and active use of the antagonists of those tendons that have been repaired but only passive movement of the injured tendons. Many modern rehabilitation regimes entail early mobilization using a dynamic splint, such as a modified Kleinert regime, but many hand surgeons will still immobilize a flexor tendon repair for 4 weeks before beginning physiotherapy. The wrist is flexed as are the MCPJs. The interphalangeal joints are kept extended. In this position of immobility, the collateral ligaments are held fully extended, and cannot fibrose and shrink; thus, when mobilization is resumed, a full range of joint movement is still possible.

22. AMPUTATIONS

What are the indications for lower limb amputation?

Amputation is necessary if the lower limb is dead or dying because of unreconstructable vascular disease, or if the leg is endangering the rest of the body because of infection, gangrene or tumour. Severe trauma or a disease, such as polio, which has left a useless limb, is also an indication for amputation.

At what level should the amputation be performed?

The level of resection should be sufficiently high to remove all unwanted tissue and allow healthy, viable tissues to heal. In general, effort should be made to remove the minimum amount of tissue, but careful thought must be given to eventual rehabilitation and some distal amputations, the Syme's forefoot amputation for example, are very difficult to rehabilitate. The below knee is an amputation that usually heals well with a good prosthesis-bearing stump for an artificial limb; rehabilitation potential is excellent. The below-knee and above-knee amputations are the commonest sites.

Describe the principal steps taken during a below-knee amputation

Two different patterns of skin flap are in common use: the Robinson skew flap or the long posterior flap. Both are equally acceptable and the long posterior flap technique is described here.

With the patient laid supine under general, spinal or epidural anaesthesia, the flaps are marked. A line transversely across the front of the leg sited 15 cm below the tibial tuberosity from mid-lateral point on either side of the leg is marked. This is then extended down the axial borders to a level just above the origin of the achilles tendon and completed across the posterior leg. The skin is incised, following the markings and the anterior compartment muscles are divided at the level of the skin incision and the vessels ligated. Elevation of the tibial periosteum is followed by division with a saw. The front of the tibia is cut at an angle to prevent the sharp leading edge traumatizing overlying tissues. The fibula is divided at least 1 cm higher. With both bones divided, the leg is hinged open to visualize the posterior compartment muscles. These are divided in an oblique fashion and finally divided at the level of the posterior skin flap. The remaining vessels are ligated and the sciatic nerve, or its two component nerves, sectioned by knife under tension, allowing retraction. The two bones ends are filed to achieve smooth bevelled surfaces. The posterior flap can now be filleted and trimmed to allow a generous but not too bulky stump to be fashioned. Immaculate haemostasis is achieved and then closure over a suction drain. The deep fascia is approximated and the skin closed with interrupted non-absorbable sutures avoiding 'dog-earing'. It is then firmly wrapped in wool and crepe.

What are the specific contraindications to a below-knee amputation?

The specific contraindications to a below-knee amputation (BKA) are:

→ a specific indication for a higher amputation
→ a fixed flexion deformity of the knee
→ inability to leave a tibial stump of at least 7.5 cm
→ insufficient tissue for adequate healing.

What are the complications of a below-knee amputation?

Complications can be those related to any operation and those specific to this one. Haematoma, infection and necrosis, or poor healing may all result from poor technique or an inappropriate level of amputation. A poor stump scar, osteophytes and stump ulceration may all require minor refashioning of the stump.

Stump neuroma causes an incredible shooting pain when compressed – more proximal section of the nerve may help. Phantom limb is a strange problem but one that definitely exists; it tends to settle gradually and does so in a distal to proximal fashion, i.e. the toes disappear from the phantom limb first then the ankle, etc. Two further neurogenic pains are causalgia, which is probably a sympathetic response, giving rise to a terrible burning sensation, and jacitation, which is a sudden jumping of the leg; it is often caused by a neuroma.

23. MORE HIPS

An unfortunate 26-year-old soldier falls off a 12-foot wall on an assault course and sustains an intracapsular fracture of the femoral neck. What procedure should he undergo?

He should have a dynamic hip screw (DHS). A DHS is performed in preference to a hemiarthroplasty, as would be performed in the elderly, for two reasons. Firstly, as a young man, the blood supply to the femoral head may well not be compromised by the fracture, allowing fixation and, secondly, a prosthetic joint in a young man would be disastrous, as it would inevitably wear out, leaving him to face a series of revisional procedures over the coming years. Whilst a DHS is an ideal solution to the acute injury, it should be noted that, if the metal work should need removal at a later date, it is extremely problematical, as DHS removal sets do not exist!

Is there any urgency or can he wait till tomorrow's trauma list?

An intracapsular femoral neck fracture in a young patient constitutes an orthopaedic emergency. Studies have shown that fixation within 6 hours greatly improves outcome – and the sooner the better. He cannot wait until tomorrow's trauma list.

Describe how you would perform a DHS

The patient is positioned supine on an orthopaedic traction table under either a general, or occasionally spinal, anaesthetic. The fracture is reduced by traction, abduction and internal rotation, and the reduction checked by fluoroscopy and held by the traction table. The good leg is widely abducted to allow the image intensifier access during the procedure. The area is prepared and draped with a transparent polythene sheet. Commencing just behind the greater trochanters, the skin is incised longitudinally for 15–20 cm down the thigh. Fascia lata and then vastus lateralis are divided in line to expose the upper lateral femur. The guide wires are passed across the fracture into the femoral head using a jig to ensure an angle of 135° to the femoral shaft and, when the wire position is satisfactory in two planes on fluoroscopy, the path is measured and drilled over the guide wire. The drill hole is then tapped before the screw is inserted over the wire until the image intensifier shows a satisfactory position in the femoral head, with the tip of the screw just abutting the subchondral bone. The wire is then removed. The periosteum is lifted and cleared on the lateral femur before applying a five-hole buttress plate over the end of the hip screw and the plate secured with screws through both cortices. The muscle layers are replaced and the wound closed over a suction drain.

24. TESTICULAR TORSION

> A 12-year-old boy presents with terrible pain in his right testicle. It came on suddenly about 5 hours ago and has been there ever since; there is no history of trauma. What would you expect to find on examination and what is the differential diagnosis?

I would expect to find a boy, obviously in pain, who is unwilling to let me examine his genitalia. The right testicle would be excruciatingly tender to examine, swollen and occasionally red. The 'normal' testis may lie in a high transverse (bell clapper) position.

The differential diagnosis includes:

→ testicular torsion – the most likely diagnosis
→ torsion of an appendage – such as a hydatid of Morgagni
→ orchitis/epidydymo-orchitis – there may be evidence of a concurrent UTI; mumps should be considered
→ idiopathic scrotal oedema – a rare condition occurring mainly in very young children; the pain is usually mild and swelling is the predominant feature.

> Would you perform any investigations and what is your treatment plan?

Given that I think this is testicular torsion, no investigation is appropriate as he needs urgent scrotal exploration. Colour duplex ultrasound has been advocated by some, but is neither sensitive nor specific for testicular torsion, so should not be used.

Outline the steps of any operative procedure you might be contemplating

The patient is positioned supine under general anaesthesia, and the external genitalia prepared with aqueous solution and draped. The affected testicle is grasped and pressed against the scrotal skin so that the tissues are tense, and a midline raphe incision is made. The many layers of tissue are incised with a knife and any minor bleeding stopped with bipolar diathermy. Once the final layer of the tunica vaginalis is opened, any reactive hydrocele empties and the testicle is viewed. If it is torted, the cord is untwisted and the testicle wrapped in warm wet packs for 10 minutes before viability is assessed. An obviously infarcted testis should be removed without untwisting. If the cord is not twisted, the appendages are examined. If one of those is twisted, it is excised. Whatever the course of events, a viable testicle is returned to the scrotum, a dead one is removed. Debate rages as to when a testicle should be fixed in the scrotum in a situation such as this. It is the practice of one of the authors (JPG) to fix both sides whenever he has operated on a truly torted testis, but to fix neither side if no torsion were present. It should be noted though that many surgeons will routinely fix both sides of any exploration to ensure recurrent testicular pain cannot be attributed to torsion.

What eventuality will you remember to warn him and his parents of when obtaining consent?

As detailed above, an infarcted testis must be removed to prevent the development of anti-sperm antibodies that would render an adult with a single testis infertile. All patients undergoing scrotal exploration for torsion must give consent for possible orchidectomy.

A 22-year-old male presents with a hard craggy mass in his right testicle. What investigations are you going to perform and what operation are you going to schedule him for urgently?

This young man has almost certainly got a testicular tumour. He needs an orchidectomy via an inguinal approach. This is both diagnostic, in that it safely yields tissue for histology and is therapeutic, being the only treatment required in many instances. Before his operation he should undergo imaging, either by CT or USS of his primary tumour, of his para-aortic lymph nodes and his liver. He should also have a chest x-ray, or preferably CT thorax. He requires serum α-fetoprotein, β-HCG and liver function tests performing. These tests are used to stage the disease and identify metastases. Only very rarely will preoperative imaging of the mass so conclusively exclude a malignant tumour as the diagnosis that the surgery is not performed.

How you would perform this man's surgery with particular reference to your approach?

The patient gives informed consent for an inguinal-approach orchidectomy. A groin incision is used as testicular tumours spread via the lymphatics of the spermatic cord to the para-aortic nodes on the posterior abdominal wall, reflecting the embryological development of the testes. If surgery were via a scrotal approach, any dissemination of tumour cells would then involve a further lymphatic field, as the scrotum drains locally to the inguinal nodes. Early high clamping of the cord in the inguinal canal obviates this risk.

The patient is positioned supine under general anaesthesia, and prepared and draped to expose the appropriate groin and the external genitalia. Using a groin skin crease incision, the external oblique aponeurosis is identified and divided in its line to reveal the spermatic cord. The cord is mobilized and, as early as possible, the cord is cross-clamped at a level close to the deep ring. The rest of the cord and the testicle are now dissected free, mainly by blunt dissection, and the tumour is delivered from the scrotum. The cord is divided and transfixed. The specimen is removed and sent for histology. After haemostasis, the groin is closed in layers and a scrotal support given for comfort.

What is this mass likely to be and describe a staging system? If he had Stage I disease, what is the prognosis?

Seminomas predominate in the fourth decade with teratomas being more common in the preceding decade; only 10 per cent of testicular tumours are non-germ cell origin, so this could conceivably be lymphoma, or a Leydig or Sertoli cell tumour. Given his age, it is most likely to be a testicular teratoma.

He is staged using the Royal Marsden Hospital staging system (see Table 4.1).

Table 4.1 Royal Marsden Hospital staging system for testicular tumours

Stage I	Tumour confined to one testicle
Stage II	Abdominal lymphadenopathy
A	<2 cm
B	2–5 cm
Stage III	Lymphadenopathy above diaphragm
O	No abdominal disease
ABC	Node size as stage II
Stage IV	Extralymphatic metastases
C	>5 cm

In stage I disease, the 5-year survival is of the order of 95 per cent.

Giovanni Morgagni (1682–1771). Professor of Anatomy in Padua, Italy. He is generally accepted as the 'father' of pathological anatomy. He was amongst the first to describe gallstones and provided the original description of haemopericardium after penetrating injury.

25. MINOR OPERATIONS

A young soldier has had several attempts to cure his ingrowing toenail (IGTN). He wants it 'sorted out once and for all'. What procedure will you offer him?

Assuming that he has already had several wedge resections without success and he is adamant he wants the problem sorting out definitively, he should be offered a Zadik's procedure on the affected side, bearing in mind the two contraindications to that procedure of active infection of the nail and peripheral vascular disease.

Explain how you would establish anaesthesia?

Although this procedure can be done under general anaesthetic, it can be easily performed under digital nerve block. Using 1 per cent lignocaine without adrenaline, infiltrate about 2–3 ml on either side of the base of his great toe to block the digital nerves as they enter the toe. This gives excellent anaesthesia.

Describe the procedure

Having achieved satisfactory anaesthesia, I would prepare the foot liberally with antiseptic, giving the toes as thorough a clean as possible and draping to expose the relevant toe. A tourniquet in the form of a thin rubber catheter is applied around the base of the toe to achieve a bloodless field and prevent dissipation of the lignocaine. The toenail is removed and two small 1 cm incisions are made sloping away from the corners of the nail bed. The overlying skin is elevated to reveal the germinal matrix. In the classical description, this is excised and the whole of the nail bed curetted down to periosteum. A modern variation is the addition of phenolization after excision of the germinal matrix, using 80 per cent phenol applied to the matrix for 3 minutes, taking care to protect healthy tissues from any spillage. After the allotted time, the phenol is washed out using surgical spirit and the tourniquet released. The two skin incisions are sutured, often on to the underlying periosteum to close the space left by the nail, and the toe dressed with a non-adherent dressing and soft gauze, leaving the tip of the toe visible. This procedure has a success rate of greater than 90 per cent.

You are asked by the doctors on call to perform a temporal artery biopsy. What disease is suspected and what are the sequelae if left untreated?

It is used to diagnose temporal arteritis, a giant cell arteritis, characterized by unilateral headache and temporal and jaw claudication, owing to involvement of the facial artery – this symptom is almost diagnostic. Transient diplopia from ocular muscle ischaemia is a precursor of the most feared complication – occlusion of the terminal branches of the ophthalmic artery giving sudden, irreversible unilateral blindness. It should be treated with high-dose steroids on suspicion of the diagnosis and therapy reviewed in the light of the biopsy results.

Describe how you would perform a temporal artery biopsy

The temporal artery in question is normally located just behind the hairline and is often easily palpable, particularly if it is inflamed, and should be marked prior to anaesthesia. The area is infiltrated with local anaesthetic and a small transverse skin incision made. The artery is freed from the surrounding tissue by sharp dissection and a 2 cm portion is excised between clips. The two ends are ligated and the skin wound closed.

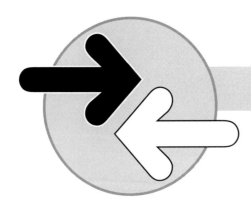

SECTION FIVE

SURGICAL ANATOMY

1. BREAST

Describe the structure of the adult female breast

The base of the adult female breast is fairly fixed, but the overall dimension and the position of the nipple is variable in the extreme. The base lies from the lateral sternal edge to the mid-axillary line, and extends from the second to the sixth ribs and overlies pectoralis major for the most part with small extensions over serratus anterior, the upper rectus sheath and external oblique muscles of the anterior abdominal wall. An extension of mammary tissue often extends into the axilla as the tail. The mature female breast is composed of many terminal duct lobular units that drain into branched ducts, eventually coalescing into a dozen or so major ducts opening on to the nipple. It should be noted that the distribution of ducts and tissue is not always congruous, i.e. breast tissue at the 6 o'clock position does not necessarily drain through the 6 o'clock nipple duct. The nipple is surrounded by a pigmented areola, itself ringed by elevated sebaceous glands known as tubercles of Montgomery. The ductolobular tissue of the breast is relatively sparse in the non-lactating breast, the majority of the breast volume is due to the interposed fatty tissue and it is the variations in the amount of adipose tissue that gives rise to the variations in size of the female breast. The breast is supported by a series of fibrous bands passing from the deep chest wall to the dermis – the ligaments of Astley Cooper.

What is the blood supply of the breast and describe its lymphatic drainage?

The breast's arterial supply is derived from perforating branches of the internal mammary artery, and branches from the lateral thoracic and thoracoacromial arteries. In general, lymph from the breast flows from superficial to deep and then passes either into the internal mammary nodes tracking alongside that artery or into the chain of axillary nodes, passing sequentially from one group to the next. In cases of lymphatic occlusion, lymph will flow across the midline into the nodes of the other breast, down into abdominal nodes or into nodes following the posterior intercostal vessels into paravertebral nodes. The lymph nodes of the axilla are arranged in five groups, which are listed below, although they do not always lie in strictly demarcated groups and the pattern may vary:

→ *Anterior nodes* lie in the medial axillary wall alongside the lateral thoracic artery. They receive the major part of the breast's lymphatic drainage as well as the anterior upper trunk.
→ *Posterior nodes* lie in the medial axillary wall behind the anterior group, with the subscapular artery, and drain the axillary tail and posterior upper trunk.
→ *Lateral nodes* lie on the medial side of the axillary vein, draining the upper limb.

→ *Central nodes* lie in the fatty tissue that fills the axilla and receive the drainage from the first three groups of nodes.

→ *Apical nodes* lie in the axillary apex and receive lymph from all the above four groups. This group drains to the supraclavicular nodes and thence to the thoracic duct or right lymphatic trunk.

What is the surgical relevance of the lymphatic supply?

Carcinoma of the breast spreads via the lymphatics. Potentially involved nodes should be examined and occasionally an occult carcinoma will present purely as axillary lymphadenopathy. The status of the axillary lymph nodes has been shown to be the single most important prognostic factor in dealing with carcinoma of the breast, and several techniques are in use to obtain this information, ranging from clearance of all accessible axillary nodes to sampling and sentinel node biopsy. At surgery, the nodes are said to be in one of three levels dependent on their relationship to the pectoralis minor muscle:

→ Level I – nodes lying beneath the lower border of pectoralis minor
→ Level II – nodes lying underneath the muscle itself
→ Level III – nodes lie medial and above the upper border of pectoralis minor.

To perform a satisfactory Level III clearance, the insertion of pectoralis minor on to the ribs may be divided.

What is peau d'orange?

It is the stippled, pitted appearance of the skin overlying an advanced breast cancer. Infiltration of the ligaments of Astley Cooper cause them to shorten and pull on the skin causing the dimpled appearance.

Sir Astley Paston Cooper (1768–1841) was the most famous surgeon of his generation. His first attempt to ligate the abdominal aorta above an aneurysm in 1817 laid the foundations for modern arterial surgery. He published widely on the anatomy of the breast, thymus, testes and hernia, naming the transversalis fascia. He was also the first surgeon to perform disarticulation at the hip joint successfully in 1824. He received his baronetcy, and 1000 guineas, in 1821 for removing an infected sebaceous cyst from the head of King George IV.

2. PERICARDIA

Describe the pericardia

The pericardia are the two layers of connective tissue that invest the heart, and are termed fibrous and serous pericardia respectively. The fibrous pericardium is a tough fibrous sac enclosing the heart and the roots of the great vessels, with which it fuses superiorly, whilst its base blends with the central tendon of the diaphragm. The serous pericardium is a layer of serosa that lines the fibrous pericardium and is then reflected over the entire surface of the heart as the parietal and visceral serous pericardia, respectively. The potential space between the two layers of serous pericardia forms a slippery sac within which the heart beats.

What are the surface markings of the fibrous pericardium?

See Figure 5.1. The right border extends from third right costal cartilage to the lower border of the sixth, just beyond the right lateral edge of the sternum. The inferior border extends from here to the apex, at the mid-axillary line in the fifth left intercostal space. The left border extends from here to the lower border of the left second costal cartilage, about 2 cm from the left sternal edge.

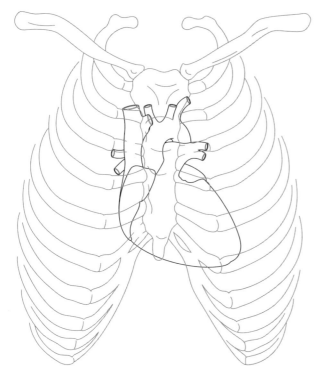

Figure 5.1 Surface markings of the pericardium.

What is the innervation of the pericardia?

The fibrous and parietal serous pericardia are supplied by branches of the phrenic nerve. The visceral serous pericardium receives no innervation.

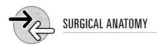

Describe the two prominent invaginations of the visceral serous pericardium

These are the oblique and transverse sinuses, where the serous pericardium is invaginated around vessels, leaving blind ending sacs. The oblique sinus lies between the left and right pulmonary veins and the inferior vena cava. The transverse sinus lies between the pericardium that cloaks the aorta and pulmonary trunk in a common invagination, and the pulmonary veins and superior vena cava.

How might a patient with a tense pericardial effusion present?

The presenting symptoms are those of left and right heart failure. If tense, an effusion will limit the pumping ability of the heart, giving rise to cardiac tamponade. Clinically, there is tachycardia, hypotension and pulsus paradoxus – an exaggeration of the normal inspiratory decrease in systolic blood pressure. The patient may also exhibit Kussmaul's sign – a raised JVP that rises with inspiration due to the impaired venous return. Beck's triad describes the features of a rising JVP, falling blood pressure and muffled heart sounds and is said to be indicative of cardiac tamponade.

How would you treat such a collection of fluid between the layers of pericardium?

Initially, pericardiocentesis is attempted by inserting a long large-bore pericardial needle into the angle between the xiphoid and the left seventh costal cartilage, directing it upwards and backwards, aiming for the tip of the left shoulder. Whilst advancing the needle, negative pressure is maintained on the syringe. Ideally, the patient should have ECG monitoring, as a ventricular arrhythmia indicates that the needle has advanced too far. Even aspiration of as little as 20 ml of fluid is sufficient to restore a reasonable cardiac output; however, if the fluid is blood, it is often clotted and aspiration is ineffective. In such cases, a small subxiphoid window can be made under local anaesthetic and a track made to the pericardium, which is incised – the technique of a 'pericardial window'.

Adolf Kussmaul (1822–1902). German physiologist who introduced pleural aspiration and gastric lavage, and described polyarteritis nodosa and mesenteric embolism, as well as recording his observations of the jugular venous pressure and the respiration in diabetic ketoacidosis.

3. HIPS AND PELVIS

What ligaments are attached to the pelvis?

On the posterior aspect of the pelvis lie the posterior sacroiliac ligaments, which are essentially continuous with the iliolumbar ligaments above and the sacrococygeal ligaments below. The sacrospinous ligament closes the greater sciatic notch and the sacrotuberous ligament closes the lesser sciatic notch turning them into their respective foramina. Anteriorly, the anterior sacroiliac ligaments and anterior longitudinal ligament lie at the back of the pelvis, whilst the obturator membrane closes off the majority of its foramen. The inguinal ligament attaches to the anterior superior iliac spine, and the pubic tubercle and the lacunar and pectineal ligaments lie on the adjacent bone. Within the bony pelvis, the puboprostatic ligaments, or pubovesical ligaments in the female, fill the 'U'-shaped gap between the muscular bands of each side of levator prostatae/pubovaginalis. The condensations of connective tissue around the middle rectal vessels attached to the pelvic side walls are known as the lateral ligaments of the rectum, although they are not true ligaments.

In women, the broad ligaments are the folds of peritoneum lying lateral to the uterus and attaching to the lateral pelvic walls in condensations known as the suspensory ligaments of the ovary. The round ligament of the uterus joins the tubo-uterine junction to the deep inguinal ring, and the lateral ligaments extend from the cervix to the lateral pelvic wall. The uterosacral ligaments extend backwards from the cervix to the pelvic fascia overlying piriformis.

The ligaments surrounding the hip joint are described below.

What passes through the greater sciatic foramen?

The piriformis muscle fills much of the foramen. The other structures are the superior gluteal nerve and vessels, inferior gluteal nerve and vessels, pudendal nerve, the internal pudendal vessels, nerve to obturator internus, sciatic nerve, posterior femoral cutaneous nerve, and nerve to quadratus femoris.

What is the surface marking of the sciatic nerve from the pelvis to the knee?

From the midpoint between the ischial tuberosity and greater trochanter downwards on the posterior thigh to the apex of the popliteal fossa.

Describe the factors maintaining the stability of the hip joint

Stability is maintained by a combination of three factors: bony, ligamentous and muscular. The femoral head is a snug fit inside the acetabulum, which is deepened further by the acetabular labrum and this is the primary factor maintaining stability. Three ligaments further stabilize the joint. The iliofemoral ligament is an inverted 'V', attaching above to the anterior inferior iliac spine and adjacent acetabular brim, and below to the upper and lower limits of the intertrochanteric line. The pubofemoral ligament passes from the iliopubic eminence and obturator crest on to the inferior joint capsule, and the ischiofemoral ligament winds around the joint from the inferior acetabulum to insert primarily into the capsule.

Muscular stabilization is provided by the short gluteal muscles, such as quadratus femoris and piriformis, whilst the two lesser glutei are important stabilizers during weight bearing on one leg – such as when walking – when they act to prevent adduction rather than as pure abductors.

Which ligament is of primary importance?

The ileofemoral ligament is the strongest and most important followed by the pubofemoral ligament. The ischiofemoral ligament contributes little, as very few of its fibres actually insert on to the femur itself.

Describe the capsular attachments of the hip joint

The capsule is attached circumferentially around the labrum and transverse ligament, from where it passes laterally to attach to the neck of the femur. It attaches anteriorly to the intertrochanteric line of the femur, but posteriorly it attaches more proximally, approximately half way up the femoral neck.

Classify fractures of the femoral neck. How does this relate to management?

Femoral neck fractures can be broadly divided into intracapsular or extracapsular fractures. Intracapsular fractures tend to disrupt the blood supply to the femoral head and have an increased risk of avascular necrosis of the head. Intracapsular fractures may be classified by the Garden classification, which describes the degree of displacement at the fracture site:

→ Garden Type I – incomplete fracture
→ Garden Type II – complete but undisplaced fracture
→ Garden Type III – complete fracture with partial displacement
→ Garden Type IV – complete fracture with complete displacement.

Undisplaced fractures may be treated with cannulated screws or a dynamic hip screw in the young, but patients over the age of retirement should normally be treated with hemiarthroplasty. Extracapsular fractures do not impair the blood supply of the femoral head and are usually treated using a dynamic hip screw.

What is the prognosis for patients with a fractured neck of femur?

Because of the co-morbidity of the elderly group of patients who sustain femoral neck fractures, the overall survival rate at 6 months is only around 50 per cent.

R.S. Garden, orthopaedic surgeon in Preston. He described his classification in the Journal of Bone and Joint Surgery *in 1961.*

4. CRANIAL BLOOD SUPPLY

What is the pterion and which bones meet there?

The pterion describes an area of the skull where the frontal, parietal, temporal and sphenoidal bones meet. It is at the outermost edges of the respective ossification centres where the ossifying bones fuse last. The pterion may have its own separate central ossification centre where the sutures meet, known as the pterion ossicle.

What is its surface marking, and why is the landmark and its surface marking so clinically important?

Its surface marking is two fingerbreadths above the zygomatic arch and a thumb's breadth behind the frontal process of the zygomatic bone. The pterion is the weakest part of the skull and is often fractured in head injuries; it overlies the anterior branch of the middle meningeal artery, which is disrupted in cases of overlying fracture and gives rise to an extradural haematoma. It is the site for an emergency temporal burr hole.

Describe the origin and distributions of the middle meningeal artery

The middle meningeal artery (MMA) is a branch of the maxillary artery, itself a terminal division of the external carotid artery. The MMA only supplies the bone of the skull and does not give supply to any intracranial contents.

What are the branches of the external carotid artery?

See Figure 5.2 on page 170.

Disruption of the MMA classically gives rise to an extradural haematoma. Describe the classic clinical presentation

An extradural haematoma usually occurs following a blow to the head. The classic presentation is of initial depression of Glasgow Coma Score, often to the point of unconsciousness, followed by a lucid interval, which may last for several hours. Thereafter, there is a rapid deterioration in conscious level and coma ensues. This deterioration is accompanied by signs of rising intracranial pressure and lateralizing signs, such as an ipsilateral dilated unresponsive pupil. Untreated, the rising ICP leads to coning, with loss of all reflexes bilaterally, bilateral pupillary dilatation and progressive brainstem compression.

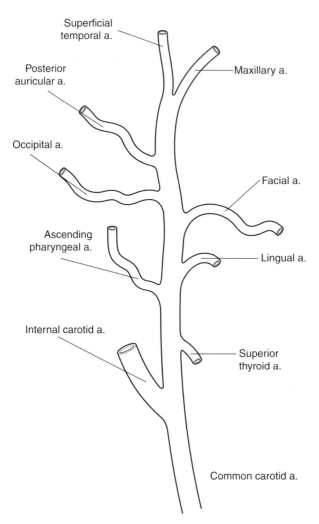

Figure 5.2 Branches of the external carotid artery.

What are the territories supplied by the three main cerebral arteries?

The cerebrum is supplied by the anterior, middle and posterior cerebral arteries, with the first two being branches of the internal carotid artery, and the latter a branch of the vertebral arteries via the basilar artery.

→ *Anterior cerebral artery* – supplies the whole of the medial surface of the hemisphere down to the corpus callosum and as far back as the parieto-occipital sulcus. It spills over on to the lateral surface to meet the distribution of the middle cerebral artery. It includes the superior frontal gyrus, and the motor and sensory areas for the contralateral leg and perineum.

→ *Middle cerebral artery* – supplies the bulk of the hemisphere and covers the entire lateral surface bar an area of the width of a single gyrus around the periphery. It supplies cortex that controls the contralateral half of the body excepting that detailed above.

→ *Posterior cerebral artery* – supplies the lower cortex below the parieto-occipital gyrus on the inferior, medial and lateral aspects. It includes the visual area of the opposite side.

What is the circle of Willis? Draw it

It is the anastomosis at the base of the brain of the ascending arteries that supply the brain. The optic chiasm and the pituitary stalk lie in the middle of the circle (see Figure 5.3).

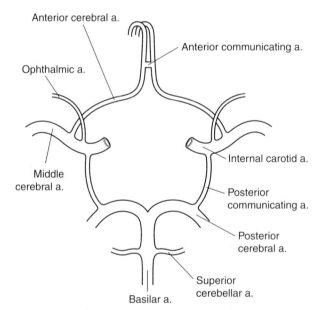

Figure 5.3 The circle of Willis.

Thomas Willis (1621–75). Acclaimed as one of the greatest physicians of the 17th century, he was not the first to describe the vascular anastomosis at the base of the brain, it having been partially described by Fallopius amongst others over 100 years previously. Willis also described typhoid, whooping cough and narcolepsy, as well as writing the first textbook of pharmacology, and differentiating between diabetes mellitus and insipidus by virtue of the taste of the urine.

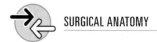

5. COMPARTMENTS

The bones, interosseous membrane and fascia divide the lower limb below the knee into several well-delineated compartments. Describe them and their contents

→ *The extensor compartment* lies between the deep fascia and the interosseous membrane, with the tibia lying medially and the fibula laterally. It contains tibialis anterior, extensor hallucis longus, extensor digitorum longus and peroneus tertius, along with the deep peroneal nerve and anterior tibial vessels.

→ *The lateral compartment* lies between the peroneal surface of the fibula and the deep fascia of the leg. In front and behind lie the anterior and posterior intermuscular septa. The lateral compartment contains peroneus longus and brevis, and the superficial peroneal nerve.

→ *The posterior compartment* is the calf. This is bounded posteriorly by the continuation of the deep fascia from the popliteal fossa, posterolaterally by the posterior intermuscular septum and anteriorly by the tibia, fibula and interosseous membrane. The posterior compartment contains tibialis posterior, flexor hallucis longus, flexor digitorum longus, soleus and gastrocnemius. It also contains the peroneal and posterior tibial arteries, the tibial and sural nerves and the short saphenous vein.

What is compartment syndrome?

Compartment syndrome occurs when there is a raised pressure in an osseofascial compartment. A raised compartment pressure leads to reduced capillary flow and decreased venous return, establishing a vicious cycle of oedema and worsening venous congestion until the pressure is such that the arterial supply to the compartment is compromised. This results in muscle and nerve ischaemia, which themselves compound the oedema and raise the pressure even further. Prolonged, raised intracompartmental pressure leads to irreversible ischaemia and cell death. Trauma and bleeding are two of the commonest causes and it should be remembered that no compartment is immune to its effects.

Which compartment is commonly affected and what is the resultant deficit?

The most commonly affected compartment is the extensor compartment of the leg. Loss of tibialis anterior and the long extensors results in loss of extension of the foot and hallux.

How do you diagnose compartment syndrome?

See Figure 5.4. The diagnosis is usually made clinically and requires a high degree of suspicion. The history may disclose previous trauma or injury. On examination, the affected compartment is swollen, firm and exquisitely tender to touch. Passive stretch of the involved muscle groups produces severe pain and is almost pathognomonic. A peripheral neuropathy may be present and usually develops before the motor signs, which are a late development. Superficial veins may become engorged but the distal arterial pulse is maintained until very late in the condition. Intracompartmental pressures can be measured using a transducer or a needle attached to a manometer. Indications for immediate open fasciotomy include single readings greater than 40 mmHg, a reading more than 20 mmHg greater than the contralateral (normal) compartment, or pressures greater than 30 mmHg for more than 4 hours.

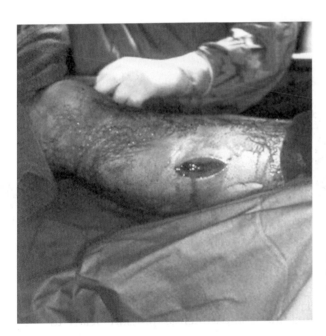

Figure 5.4 Compartment syndrome. The leg is tensely swollen – a previous inadequate fasciotomy wound is evident.

6. SCAPULA

What is the bone shown in Figure 5.5 and what are the prominent bony features?

This is a right scapula and can be orientated by the prominent spine that runs across the posterior surface, the laterally facing glenoid and the inferior angle. It has

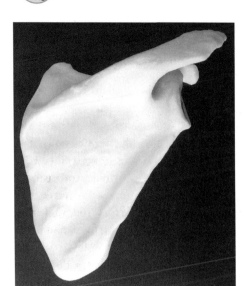

Figure 5.5

a concave costal surface with lateral and medial edges, a dorsal surface and an inferior angle. On the dorsal surface lies the spine, which separates it into supraspinous and infraspinous areas. Laterally, the spine expands into the acromion process with a facet for the clavicular articulation anteromedially. At the lateral angle, the scapula broadens out to form the scapular neck and thence the glenoid cavity, for articulation with the humeral head. The upper part of the glenoid projects forward as the base of the coracoid process. The superior border has a suprascapular notch just medial to the base of the coracoid process.

What muscles are attached to the scapula?

The muscular attachments are best considered by systematically working one's way around its bony outline and features.

→ *Dorsal surface.* Supraspinatus and infraspinatus either side of the dorsal spine. From just below the glenoid downwards along the lateral border attach the long head of triceps, teres minor, teres major and, finally, latissimus dorsi from the tip of the angle. Ascending the medial border, rhomboid major, rhomboid minor and levator scapulae take attachment. The inferior belly of omohyoid lies immediately medial to the suprascapular notch and overflows on to the costal surface and the adjacent transverse scapular ligament.

→ *Costal surface.* Subscapularis occupying the majority of the whole costal surface with serratus anterior attached in a rim around its outside along the medial and inferior borders.

→ *Spine.* Trapezius attaches all along the superior border, with deltoid along the inferior border.

→ *Coracoid process*. Pectoralis minor attaches medially, with the short head of biceps and coracobrachialis attaching together at the tip.

→ *Glenoid*. Long head of triceps attaches to the infraglenoid tubercle with the long head of biceps above the glenoid.

What ligaments are attached to the scapula?

The transverse scapular ligament bridges the suprascapular notch with the suprascapular artery above it and the nerve below. The coracoacromial ligament is a broad triangular ligament attaching from a point just anterior to the clavicular facet on the acromion to the lateral aspect of the coracoid process. The coracoclavicular ligament is in two parts; the conoid part from the knuckle of the coracoid fanning upwards to the underside of the clavicle, whilst the trapezoid part passes almost horizontally from the undersurface of the clavicle to the trapezoid ridge on the upper coracoid. They are extremely strong ligaments and maintain the integrity of the acromioclavicular joint. The coracohumeral ligament runs from beneath the coracoid to the greater tuberosity of the humerus blending with the joint capsule as it does so.

What factors maintain the stability of the glenohumeral joint?

In marked contrast to the hip joint, whose stability is primarily anatomical and ligamentous, the glenohumeral joint is stabilized in the main by its muscles. The glenoid is deepened by the glenoid labrum, which adds stability, but it is the muscular stabilization that is much more important. The muscles stabilizing the shoulder – subscapularis, supraspinatus, infraspinatus and teres minor – are collectively known as the rotator cuff, and all attached near to the joint and fuse with it. The long head of biceps sinks into the superior capsule providing additional strength above, whilst the long head of triceps supports the inferior joint surface when the arm is abducted, giving stability in this position. Stability is further increased by the coracoacromial arch, which by arching over the top of the glenohumeral joint acts to increase the area on which the humeral head can articulate.

7. TRIANGLES OF THE NECK

Describe the boundaries of the anterior and posterior triangles of the neck

The anterior triangle is bordered by the midline, the mandible and the medial border of sternomastoid; and the posterior triangle by the posterior border of sternocleidomastoid, the anterior border of trapezius and the clavicle. The anterior triangle may be further subdivided into submental, digastric, carotid and muscular triangles.

What is the differential diagnosis of a lump in the neck?

The differential diagnosis depends in part as to where the lump is located. Whilst some causes, such as lymphadenopathy and skin lesions, are common to both triangles, many causes are specific to one:

→ posterior triangle lumps:
  - pharyngeal pouch
  - cystic hygroma – in children
  - cervical rib
  - subclavian artery aneurysm – often a post-stenotic dilatation in association with a cervical rib
→ anterior triangle lumps:
  - thyroid
  - thyroglossal cyst
  - submandibular gland
  - parotid gland
  - branchial cyst
  - chemodectoma (potato tumour)
  - aneurysmal carotid artery
  - tortuous carotid artery
  - laryngocoele
  - sternomastoid tumour.

What is a cystic hygroma?

A cystic hygroma is a congenital lymphatic malformation lying at the root of the neck. It consists of thin-walled interconnecting cysts formed from the coalescence of the early lymphatic elements during development. Most are present at birth and may be large enough to obstruct respiration and swallowing. They are brilliantly transilluminable. Aspiration with or without sclerosant instillation provides symptomatic relief, although surgical excision is the preferred method of treatment.

What is a branchial cyst?

A branchial cyst is a smooth cyst that presents from under the anterior border of sternocleidomastoid at the junction of the middle and upper thirds of the muscle. This is the site of a rare, true fistula from the second branchial cleft, but these cysts are unlikely to represent true branchial cleft remnants. They are lined by heterotopic squamous epithelium and have lymphoid tissue in the cyst wall. There is rarely a deep track leading from the cyst. Diagnosis is confirmed by aspiration of milky fluid rich in cholesterol crystals. Treatment is by excision.

List the causes of cervical lymphadenopathy

See Table 5.1.

Table 5.1 Causes of cervical lymphadenopathy

Cause	Type	Example
Infection	Acute bacterial	Oropharyngeal infections such as tonsillitis and scalp infections from infected skin lesions
	Acute viral	Any upper respiratory tract infection; Epstein–Barr virus infection tends to leave a marked lymphadenopathy, even after subclinical infections
	Chronic	HIV infection; tuberculosis, although the brawny mass of matted nodes of history is rare in modern times
	Atypical	Toxoplasmosis gives rise to a few tender nodes but often little else specific. It may be an opportunistic infection in AIDS patients. Cat scratch disease generates large, persistent, often purulent, nodes up to 7 weeks after the cat scratch
Malignancy	Primary	Lymphomas of both sorts commonly present with cervical nodes; leukaemias, particularly chronic lymphatic leukaemia
	Secondary	Head and neck tumours, particularly oral cavity, pharynx and larynx. Thyroid cancers will also spread to cervical nodes and were previously often given the misnomer 'lateral aberrant thyroid'. Breast and gastrointestinal tract will also spread to these nodes, notably Virchow's node in the supraclavicular fossa
Rarities		Sarcoidosis gives rise to palpable cervical nodes in 30 per cent of cases, more commonly in Afro-Caribbeans than Caucasians. Lymph node hyperplasia can occur in response to a variety of stimuli, including rheumatoid arthritis, phenytoin or as an immune response to distant tumour.

What are chemodectomas?

They are rare tumours of the carotid body, sitting at the carotid bifurcation and often splaying it open, which is evident on angiography. They can be familial or bilateral, and are associated with chronic hypoxia. Usually benign, they may occasionally be malignant and can metastasize; patients may have other head and neck paraganglionic cell tumours, such as glomus jugulare tumours. Generally slow growing, they present as a mass in the anterior triangle of the neck with transmitted pulsation, which moves laterally but not vertically. They are so vascular that they may be compressible and demonstrate a bruit or thrill. Investigation is by angiography or MRI, although duplex ultrasound or CT may give useful information. Treatment is preferably excision by an experienced vascular surgeon and mortality rates are of the order of 1–2 per cent, with a similar risk of hemiplegic stroke. Radiotherapy can be used in high-risk cases with slightly worse results.

Rudolf Virchow (1821–1902). After graduating from Berlin military medical school in 1843, he published his work on thrombosis in 1845 and 2 years later founded his own journal, Virchows Archiv, *as some of the journals of the day had refused to publish his articles. He was appointed Professor of Pathology in Berlin in 1856, and went on to describe neuroglia, subdural haematoma and meningitis. He entered politics and was a member of the Reichstag from 1880 to 1893 and, at one stage, was Leader of the Opposition. He died after fracturing his hip jumping from a tram.*

8. ANATOMY OF THE FEMORAL REGION

Describe the femoral sheath

It is a downwards continuation of the extraperitoneal areolar tissue enclosing the abdominal aorta and inferior vena cava, and forms a fascial envelope from the psoas fascia behind and the transversalis fascia in front. It passes beneath the inguinal ligament and there contains the femoral artery and vein with the femoral canal lying most medially within it. The femoral nerve lies outside of and lateral to the femoral sheath.

What is the femoral ring?

See Figure 5.6. It represents the superior end of the femoral canal. It is bounded anteriorly by the inguinal ligament and posteriorly by the pectineal ligament, pectineus and its overlying fascia. Medially lies the lacunar ligament and laterally the femoral vein. The canal contains only fat and some lymph nodes, including Cloquet's node, which drains the glans penis/clitoris. The canal represents a

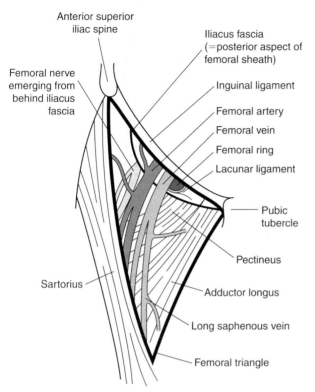

Anterior superior
iliac spine

Iliacus fascia
(=posterior aspect of
femoral sheath)

Femoral nerve
emerging from
behind iliacus
fascia

Inguinal ligament

Femoral artery

Femoral vein

Femoral ring

Lacunar ligament

Pubic
tubercle

Pectineus

Sartorius

Adductor longus

Long saphenous vein

Femoral triangle

Figure 5.6 The femoral ring
and triangle.

'dead space' into which the femoral vein can expand during times of increased venous return.

How do you differentiate between a femoral and an indirect inguinal hernia?

A femoral hernia emerges through the cribriform fascia of the sheath before turning upwards, thus its neck is below and lateral to the pubic tubercle. An indirect inguinal hernia emerges through the superficial inguinal ring, i.e. above and medial to the tubercle.

What structure may be at risk during a femoral hernia operation?

The femoral vein lies immediately lateral to the femoral canal, which must be occluded during the procedure to prevent recurrence, but the vein must be allowed room to expand with increased blood flow during lower limb activity. Over zealous suturing may directly damage the vein or compress it, leading to obstructed venous return and venous thrombosis. The accessory obturator artery is present in 50 per cent of people and usually passes along the lateral aspect of the femoral ring to the obturator foramen; however, in a significant proportion of people, it passes along the medial side of the ring. Division or digital stretch of the lacunar ligament, to open up the ring to allow delivery of the sac in difficult cases, risks damaging an aberrant vessel.

What is the femoral triangle?

It is an area of anterior thigh bounded by the inguinal ligament, the medial border of sartorius and the medial border of adductor longus. The femoral nerve and vessels lie at the base. At the apex of the triangle, the femoral artery and vein pass beneath the sartorius muscle into the adductor or Hunter's canal accompanied by the saphenous nerve and the nerve to vastus medialis. The femoral vessels pass from the canal through the adductor hiatus of the adductor magnus muscle and enter the popliteal fossa.

What are the branches of the femoral artery?

The common femoral artery gives rise to the inferior epigastric artery before it passes beneath the inguinal ligament. After passing beneath the ligament it gives off four branches in the groin, which are the superficial and deep external pudendal, superficial circumflex iliac and the superficial epigastric arteries. Thereafter, the vessel gives off the profunda femoris artery and continues itself as the superficial femoral artery and gives no further branches. The profunda femoris gives rise to lateral and medial circumflex arteries at the level of the greater trochanters, and subsequently a series of muscular perforating branches.

John Hunter (1728–93). The father of scientific surgery in this country; his contributions include the description of the descent of the testes, the demonstration of fat absorption by gut lymphatics, experiments on grafting and transplantation and the ligation of the superficial femoral artery in the subsartorial canal. He amassed an enormous collection of biological specimens, which now reside in the Royal College of Surgeons in London. His ischaemic heart disease was diagnosed by his student and later friend, Edward Jenner, and he died of an acute myocardial infarction at a particularly stormy board meeting at St George's Hospital.

9. VERTEBRAE

What type of vertebra is shown in Figure 5.7? How can you distinguish between cervical, thoracic and lumbar vertebrae?

This is a lumbar vertebra. It has a large, almost rectangular body without articular facets for ribs or transverse foramina. The transverse processes are long, slender

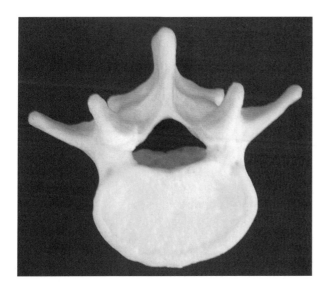

Figure 5.7

and well formed, and the spinous process large, oblong and horizontal. Thoracic vertebrae all have facets for articulation with ribs, the spinal foramina are circular and have spine-like spinous processes. The thoracic transverse processes point laterally, superiorly and posteriorly. Only cervical vertebrae possess foramina transversaria. They have triangular spinal foramina and bifid spinous processes.

What is the general structure of an intervertebral disc and what is its function?

The intervertebral disc is a secondary cartilaginous joint. The hyaline cartilage of two adjacent vertebrae are joined by a peripheral ring of fibrous tissue called the annulus fibrosus. This consists of strong concentric layers of fibres, which prevent movement in any direction. Contained within the annulus is the thick, jelly-like nucleus pulposus, lying nearer the back than the front. The nucleus pulposus accounts for about 15 per cent of the volume of the disc.

The intervertebral discs act to prevent lateral and anterior/posterior movement between vertebra, while allowing some flexibility for flexion and extension. They act as 'shock absorbers' between the vertebrae by allowing compression of the nucleus pulposus.

What pathological conditions can affect these discs?

The commonest pathological condition affecting intervertebral discs is a herniation of the nucleus pulposus through the annulus, commonly referred to as a 'slipped disc'. This usually occurs in adults and the herniation is commonly posteriorly or posterolaterally, reflecting the eccentric positioning of the nucleus pulposus. The herniated pulposus can compress the nerve roots as they exit the intervertebral foramina giving rise to neurological symptoms. More rarely, deep-seated infection can be harboured within the disc – discitis – causing severe back pain with minimal examination findings.

If the disc between L4 and L5 (L4 disc) herniates to the right, what will the patient or his astute examining clinician notice?

Backwards pressure of the disc causes back pain because of pressure on the posterior spinal ligaments. Lateral protrusion into the L4/5 foramen will compress the L_5 nerve root, producing neurological symptoms in that nerve's distribution, although a large prolapse may also compress adjacent roots. The patient complains of a shooting pain down the posterior right thigh exacerbated by coughing or sneezing, and describes a numbness or tingling down the lateral leg and on to the dorsum of the foot. On examination, there is typically weakness of the dorsiflexors of the foot and the extensors of the toes with wasting of the muscles if long-standing, which may be severe enough to produce a foot drop. There is a sensory disturbance over the lateral calf and dorsum of foot. There is little dysreflexia associated with an L_5 root compression.

If the C6 disc prolapses, what would he notice?

There will be a similar pattern of pain, muscle weakness, hyporeflexia and sensory loss as in lumbar disc prolapse, in the C7 distribution. There is neck pain and radiation down the arm into scapula, triceps and forearm extensors. There is tingling and numbness along the middle of the dorsal surface of the forearm and over the palmar surface of the middle three fingers. Weakness occurs in the triceps and finger extensors and, in time, wasting in these muscles occurs. The triceps reflex is diminished or absent.

10. INGUINAL CANAL

Describe the inguinal canal?

It is an oblique muscular canal in the abdominal wall connecting the intra-abdominal preperitoneal space at the deep inguinal ring to the superficial inguinal ring beneath the skin of the pubis.

What are its boundaries?

The deep ring, at the mid-point of the inguinal ligament, marks its commencement. Its floor is the rolled edge of the inguinal ligament and transversalis fascia laterally. The anterior wall is the external oblique muscle and aponeurosis with fibres of internal oblique laterally. The posterior wall is the conjoint tendon medially and the transversalis fascia alone in the lateral part. The roof is the lower edges of the internal oblique and transversus muscles as they arch over the canal, from in front of the lateral canal to insert into the pubic bone as the conjoint tendon behind the medial canal.

What traverses the canal?

It transmits the spermatic cord or round ligament of uterus and the ilioinguinal nerve. The spermatic cord is generally described as having three coverings and three groups of three constituents. The ilioinguinal nerve is usually included in this list for ease of recollection but it is not strictly a content of the cord.

Coverings
→ External spermatic fascia
→ cremaster muscle
→ internal spermatic fascia.

Arteries
→ Cremasteric
→ testicular
→ artery to the vas deferens.

Tubes
→ Pampiniform plexus
→ lymphatics
→ vas deferens.

Others
→ Genital branch of genitofemoral nerve
→ ilioinguinal nerve
→ processus vaginalis.

Where does a direct hernia occur?

A direct hernia occurs through a weakness in the transversalis fascia medial to the inferior epigastric artery and deep ring, whereas an indirect hernia passes through the deep ring and, therefore, lateral to the inferior epigastric vessels. These vessels are an important landmark during a transabdominal laparoscopic hernia repair.

What methods do you know to repair an inguinal hernia?

→ *Bassini repair* – now largely historical, it opposes the conjoint tendon and inguinal ligament. This is a repair under tension and often had a releasing incision performed in addition.

→ *Darn repair* – again uncommon in modern practice, it reinforces the posterior wall of the inguinal canal with a darn of non-absorbable sutures between the conjoint tendon and the inguinal ligament.

→ *Mesh repair* – originally called the Lichtenstein repair. Placement of a prolene mesh reinforces the posterior wall of the canal. It is the recommended technique of the Royal College of Surgeons working party on groin hernia repair.

→ *Mesh plug repair* – simply occludes the deep ring with a prolene mesh.

→ *Shouldice repair* – a highly effective double breasting technique.

→ *Laparoscopic repair* – may be done as a preperitoneal or intraperitoneal procedure.

How does the inguinal canal differ in children and why is that surgically relevant?

The obliquity of the canal only develops as the child grows, so in children, the canal is shortened and the superficial and deep rings overlie each other. In addition, childhood inguinal hernias are always due to a patent processus vaginalis. When operating on a child's hernia, the incision should be over the superficial ring. The procedure should be a herniotomy – division of the patent processus vaginalis – rather than formal posterior wall repair (herniorrhaphy).

How did Dr Shouldice repair hernias?

The Shouldice repair lays open the whole inguinal canal and double breasts the transversalis fascia using non-absorbable suture to strengthen the posterior wall. Edward Shouldice almost invariably performed the operation under local anaesthetic and used stainless steel wire as the suture of choice. The enviable recurrence rates (<1 per cent) from the Shouldice Clinic in Toronto are due to a combination of meticulous reproduction of this technique, and the superspecialization of the surgeons who perform nothing but groin hernia repairs.

11. KNEE LIGAMENTS

Describe the attachments of the cruciate ligaments of the knee. What do they do?

The anterior cruciate ligament is attached to the tibial plateau in front of the tibial spine, and passes upward and backwards to attach to a smooth area on the medial surface of the lateral femoral condyle. The anterior cruciate prevents backward movement of the femur on the tibia but also limits the extension of the lateral femoral condyle on the tibia, which is crucial to the 'screw home' mechanism that locks the extended knee.

The posterior cruciate ligament attaches from the posterior part of the tibial plateau behind the spine and the adjacent uppermost posterior tibial surface and passes upwards and forwards to insert into the smooth area on the lateral aspect of the medial femoral condyle. The posterior cruciate prevents the femur sliding forward off the tibia and is the only factor maintaining stability of the femur in a weight-bearing flexed knee. The cruciate ligaments are named from their tibial origins.

Which other ligaments attach around the knee joint?

The ligaments of the knee can be classified as extracapsular or intra-articular. The extracapsular ones are the patella retinacula, the patellar, tibial and fibular collateral and oblique popliteal ligaments. The intra-articular ligaments are the cruciate ligaments, the medial and lateral menisci, and their associated transverse and meniscofemoral ligaments. Although the cruciate ligaments are intra-articular, they are extrasynovial, as the synovial sheath clothes them anteriorly but leaves them bare posteriorly, as though they have been impressed into the synovium from behind. The joint capsule should also be included, as it is the capsular ligament of the knee joint.

Describe the medial and lateral menisci

The menisci are semilunar discs of fibrocartilage, which intervene between the articular surfaces of the femoral condyles and tibial plateau. They are avascular except where they attach. The medial meniscus is the larger of the two, attaching in front of the anterior cruciate ligament anteriorly and in front of the posterior cruciate posteriorly. It is also attached to the deep part of the medial collateral ligament. The lateral meniscus is more truly 'C'-shaped than its medial counterpart with the two horns attaching in front and behind the intercondylar spine of the tibia. It has no attachment to the lateral collateral ligament but receives a slip of insertion from the upper half of the popliteus muscle.

One meniscus is injured much more frequently than the other – which one and why?

Medial meniscus tears are more common because of the mechanics of the injury. The injury is caused by the femur being internally rotated on the tibia, a common movement in sport, whereas the lateral meniscus is damaged by external rotation of the femur on the tibia, a far less common movement pattern. It is also said that medial meniscal injuries are more common because the attachment of the meniscus to the collateral ligament means it is relatively fixed and cannot slide out from twisting compression injuries; in comparison, the lateral meniscus is able to move more freely.

What factors prevent the knee from dislocating?

The bony anatomy aids anteroposterior stability little, but the spine of the tibia prevents sideways movement of the femur on tibia. Stability of the knee joint is maintained primarily by the ligaments, with some help from the muscles. The cruciate ligaments are responsible for anteroposterior stability in flexion, whilst lateral stability and stability in extension are provided by both the collateral ligaments and the oblique popliteal ligament. The expansions of the vasti muscles aid stability, with vastus medialis in particular stabilizing the patella. The iliotibial tract stabilizes the partly flexed knee.

What is peculiar about the tendon of popliteus?

The tendon of popliteus is intra-articular but extrasynovial. It lies between the knee joint capsule and the synovial membrane, adherent to the capsule. Occasionally, it may be attached to the lateral meniscus, which it grooves as the bare tendon overlies the bare meniscus.

12. THORAX

Describe the divisions of the mediastinum

The mediastinum can be divided into four areas, described as superior, anterior, middle and posterior. Alternatively, the anterior, middle and posterior divisions may be collectively referred to as the inferior mediastinum, the two sections divided by a horizontal plane passing from the sternal angle to the lower border of T4. The three subdivisions of the inferior mediastinum are all bounded inferiorly by the domes of the diaphragm.

→ *The superior mediastinum* is bounded anteriorly by the manubrium, and posteriorly by the vertebral bodies of T1–4. The inferior limit is the horizontal plane described above and superiorly it is continuous with the root of the neck. It contains the great vessels, trachea, oesophagus and phrenic and vagus nerves. The great vessels are arranged asymmetrically such that the arteries lie on the left side and the veins on the right.

→ *The anterior mediastinum* is a very narrow, almost potential, space lying between the pericardium and the sternum. It is continuous with the superior mediastinum and contains only the thymus.

→ *The middle mediastinum* contains the pericardium and heart, the roots of the great vessels, the lung roots and the phrenic nerves. It lies between the posterior and anterior mediastina.

→ *The posterior mediastinum* lies between the posterior aspect of the pericardium and T4–12. It is open above with the superior mediastinum. It contains the descending aorta, the oesophagus, thoracic duct, azygous veins and thoracic sympathetic trunk.

What are the structures evident in this lung hilum?

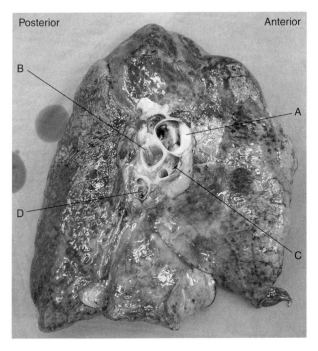

Figure 5.8 Left lung root.

See Figure 5.8. The left and right lung roots are arranged similarly. The pulmonary artery (A) lies superiorly, the main bronchus posteriorly (B) and the two pulmonary veins lie anteriorly (C) and inferiorly (D). On the right side the eparterial bronchus to the upper lobe (and the accompanying artery) branch off outside the lung and sit uppermost in the right lung root. The pulmonary ligament hangs down below.

What is the inferior pulmonary ligament?

The pulmonary ligament is a cuff of pleura, which hangs down from the lung root like a sleeve that is too big, allowing expansion of the structures of the lung hilum as required. It is not a ligament and has nothing to do with the lung!

What are the surface markings of the lungs and the pleura?

The pleural markings follow the lateral thoracic cage and extend superiorly 3 cm above the middle third of the clavicle. Anteriorly, the marking is the lateral edge of the sternum. On the left, the pleura deviates from the fourth costal cartilage and arches out to a point midway to the cardiac apex, while on the right the sternal margin is followed. On both sides, at the sixth costal cartilage, the marking turns laterally and runs obliquely around the chest to the level of the eighth rib at the mid-clavicular line, the 10th rib at the mid-axillary line and the 12th rib at the lateral border of erector spinae, crossing the 12th thoracic vertebra.

The lung markings are identical both laterally and superiorly, but the lower markings lie two rib spaces above those of the pleura. The lung hila lie behind the third and fourth costal cartilages at the sternal margin, level with T5, 6 and 7.

13. PANCREAS

What are the anatomical parts and topographical relations of the pancreas?

The pancreas is divided into head, neck, body and tail. The head is the widest part of the gland and lies within the 'C'-shaped concavity of the duodenum retroperitoneally. It overlies the inferior vena cava and the renal veins and is at the level of L2. It has a wedge-shaped lower extension, which lies anteriorly and to the left, known as the uncinate process. The neck is the narrow strip of gland that overlies the superior mesenteric and portal veins. The superior mesenteric vein is 'clasped' between the neck above and the uncinate process below. The body of the gland extends upwards toward the left upper quadrant and lies over the left renal vein, the aorta, the left diaphragmatic crus, the left psoas muscle and the left adrenal gland. The splenic artery runs just behind the upper border of the gland and the splenic vein lies behind, where it joins with the inferior mesenteric vein. The tail passes from the level of the left renal hilum to the splenic hilum enclosed in the layers of the lienorenal ligament and accompanied by the splenic artery and vein.

How does the pancreas develop?

The pancreas develops as two outgrowths of endoderm at the junction of the foregut and midgut. The ventral bud and dorsal bud grow into the ventral and dorsal mesogastrium, respectively, and are brought into apposition by rotation of the duodenum, which then lies retroperitoneally. The two primitive pancreatic outgrowths then fuse into a single gland with anastomosis of the two duct systems.

How many ducts does it have and where do they open into?

There are two ducts. The major duct (of Wirschung), developed from the ventral duct embryologically, is joined by the common bile duct at the ampulla and opens into the second part of the duodenum. The accessory duct of Santorini develops from the dorsal duct and drains the lower part of the head, opening at the minor duodenal papilla approximately 2 cm above the ampulla.

From where does the pancreas gain its blood supply?

The main supply to the neck, body and tail is from branches of the splenic artery, which courses behind the superior margin of the gland. The head is supplied by the superior and inferior pancreaticoduodenal arteries. The superior artery is a branch of the gastroduodenal artery, and ultimately the coeliac axis, whilst the inferior artery is a branch from the superior mesenteric artery. The two blood supplies meet at the level of the major papilla, and this represents the division between foregut and midgut.

After a very difficult splenectomy, you leave a drain in the splenic bed. Over the next 3 days it drains over 2000 ml of fluid. How might you ascertain if you had damaged the pancreatic tail and how might you treat such a pancreatic fistula?

Testing the fluid for amylase content will ascertain whether this is a pancreatic fistula. Levels greater than ten times the serum amylase are indicative of a pancreatic fistula.

These fistulae are generally treated conservatively. Initiation of intravenous feeding and somatostatin analogue therapy, such as octreotide, help reduce pancreatic secretions. In time, most of these fistulae will close spontaneously.

14. THE CHEST X-RAY (CXR)

Describe the mediastinal outline and its constituents on this CXR (Figure 5.9)

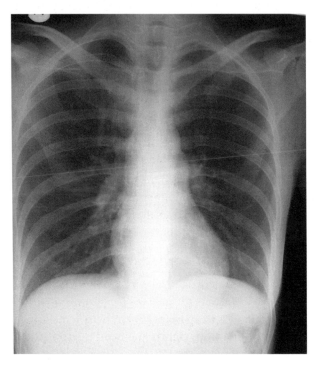

Figure 5.9

This is a standard posteroanterior film. The right mediastinal outline consists of the superior vena cava and the right atrium from above down. The left border is formed by the aortic arch, the pulmonary trunk, the left auricle, which is generally not very prominent, and the left ventricle, again from above down. The inferior margins are usually indistinct from those of the diaphragmatic domes, but represent the right ventricle and a small part of the left ventricle.

Describe the CXR of a tension pneumothorax. What would you do whilst waiting for the CXR to be developed?

If a tension pneumothorax is suspected, it should be treated presumptively rather than waiting for a CXR to confirm the diagnosis. A CXR, if taken, would demonstrate tracheal deviation and mediastinal shift away from the affected side. There would be loss of lung markings and a 'lung edge' on the collapsed side. There may be surgical emphysema. As soon as the diagnosis is suspected, either clinically or radiologically, then the tension should be relieved by insertion of a large bore (12 or 14G) cannula into the second intercostal space in the mid-clavicular line. A hiss of escaping air confirms the diagnosis. Decompression should be promptly followed by definitive management, by placing a chest drain in the fifth intercostal space just anterior to the mid-axillary line.

A shocked patient with a rigid belly and epigastric pain has all the clinical appearances of a perforated viscus, but his CXR shows no free gas. Is your diagnosis wrong?

Not necessarily, as the diagnosis may be correct because free gas is seen on the erect CXR in only 70 per cent of patients. The gas can be further sought on lateral decubitus films, abdominal ultrasound or CT. Absence of free gas should, however, prompt consideration of the other causes of an acute abdomen, so an abdominal CT may be the most appropriate next investigation.

Another patient has free gas under his diaphragm on CXR – must he have perforated?

Not necessarily. The commonest reason for free gas under the diaphragm is following abdominal surgery and this gas takes around a week to be absorbed. Laparoscopy, on the other hand, uses CO_2 for insufflation, which is much more rapidly absorbed. Care should be taken before ascribing free subdiaphragmatic gas to a laparoscopy more than 1 day before. Other 'non-surgical' causes of free gas are:

→ escape of air from the tracheobronchial tree in patients with obstructive airways disease, or ventilated patients
→ gynaecological causes – tubal insufflation, douching or vaginal examinations
→ pneumatoides cystoides intestinalis – a rare abnormality with multiple gas-filled sacs in the wall of the gastrointestinal tract
→ idiopathic.

In addition, a gas-filled viscus, such as the transverse colon, may interpose between the liver and diaphragm mimicking the appearance of free gas; this is known as Chilaiditi's sign.

Demetrius Chilaiditi (b. 1883). A native of Vienna, from whence he graduated in 1908, he practised as a radiologist in a variety of countries, describing his classical x-ray findings in 1910.

15. FEMUR

What is this (Figure 5.10)? Describe the principal bony features

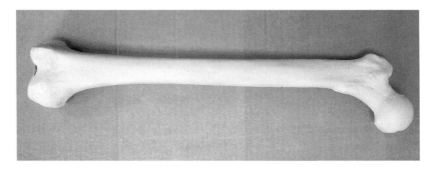

Figure 5.10

It is a right femur, which can be correctly orientated by noting the femoral neck, which angles upwards, backwards and medially, whilst the intercondylar notch faces posteriorly. The important parts are the femoral head with its central depression for the attachment of ligamentum teres. Below the head is a strong but narrow neck, which leads down to the greater trochanter. The lesser trochanter lies opposite and below, and the two are joined by the intertrochanteric line anteriorly and the intertrochanteric crest posteriorly. Running down the middle third of the posterior shaft of the femur is a bony ridge, known as the linea aspera, which flares out at the lower end into the medial and lateral supracondylar lines. The lower end of the bone is expanded into the medial and lateral femoral condyles with an intercondylar notch between.

What is the blood supply to the head of this bone? Which is most important?

The blood supply is by three routes. The most important is by the retinacular vessels from the trochanteric anastomosis, which travel within the joint capsule and are reflected back toward the head at the capsular attachment to the femur.

The central portion of the head receives supply from a small vessel in the ligamentum teres and there is also some supply to the head from the intraosseous vessels of the upper femur. It is said that the vessel to the head of the femur that travels within ligamentum teres obliterates as the patient ages and, by middle age, contributes nothing to the blood supply; division of the ligament at hip arthroplasty, however, is often followed by a considerable haemorrhage.

The posterior aspect of the shaft of this bone gives attachment to many muscles. Describe them

The upper posterior shaft receives, from medial to lateral, the insertions of iliopsoas, pectineus, adductor brevis, adductor magnus and gluteus maximus; each except iliopsoas attaches to a thin line along the linea aspera. The middle posterior shaft receives insertions into the linea aspera of adductor longus and the continued tendon of adductor magnus. Vastus medialis arises from the whole length of the medial lip of the linea aspera, more medial than those insertions listed. The length of the lateral lip gives origin to vastus lateralis with the origin of the short head of biceps femoris just medial and the origin of vastus intermedius just lateral to it.

Describe the main features of the patella

The patella is the largest sesamoid bone of the body and lies within the tendon of the quadriceps complex. It is roughly triangular in outline with the apex lowermost and has a convex anterior surface and a smooth articular posterior surface. The articular surface is divided from top to bottom by a vertical ridge. The quadriceps tendon inserts into the upper part of the bone and a flat tendon from vastus medialis inserts horizontally into the medial aspect. The patella is attached below to the tibia via the patellar ligament and the expansions of the patellar retinacula, which extend from the lateral and medial edges of the bone, derived from their respective vastus muscle, and sweep downwards adjacent to the patellar ligament to the tibia. The lower border of the patella lies at the level of the tibial plateau.

16. JOINTS AND CARTILAGE

Give a general classification of joints

A joint is the union of two or more bones and may be fibrous, cartilaginous or synovial. A fibrous joint, as its name implies, unites the bones by fibrous tissue alone, which may or may not ossify. The skull sutures are fibrous joints that ossify, whereas the lower tibiofibular joint represents a fibrous joint that remains unossified.

What are the characteristics of primary and secondary cartilaginous joints?

A primary cartilaginous joint is one where bone and hyaline cartilage meet. All epiphyses are primary cartilaginous joints, as are costochondral junctions. They are completely immobile and very strong to the extent that the adjacent bone will fracture before the primary cartilaginous joint separates. A secondary cartilaginous joint, otherwise known as a symphysis, is the union between bones where the articular surfaces are covered with hyaline cartilage and united by fibrocartilage. Although the fibrocartilage may contain fluid, or even gel in the case of an intervertebral disc, which is part of a secondary cartilaginous joint, there is never a synovial membrane. The presence of small amounts of fibrocartilage allows some degree of movement in contrast to a primary cartilaginous joint.

Describe the features of a synovial joint

Synovial joints include all limb joints and have six specific characteristics. All synovial joints have:

→ bone ends covered by hyaline cartilage
→ an enclosing capsule
→ a joint cavity
→ a capsule reinforced by ligaments
→ a lining of synovial membrane
→ a range of movement.

The synovial membrane lines all non-articular surfaces within the joint and secretes the fluid that acts as lubrication. Anatomically, the joint capsule is actually the capsular ligament of the joint and should be included in any list of ligaments for a particular joint.

How do the different types of cartilage differ?

Cartilage is a dense connective tissue characterized by cells and fibres embedded in a ground substance. There are three different types as follows.

→ *Hyaline cartilage.* This is the commonest type, with a highly hydrated amorphous matrix of collagen and ground substance. It is avascular, obtaining its nutrient supply by diffusion from adjacent tissues and, although deformable, if injured, it regenerates by formation of fibrous tissue rather than new cartilage. It is found on all synovial joint surfaces, the epiphyseal growth plates of growing bones, tracheobronchial tree and larynx.
→ *Fibrocartilage.* This has many similarities to ligaments and tendons and has a matrix with obvious bands of thick collagen. Cells within it are grouped longitudinally. It is resistant to both pressure and shear forces, and has a normal but scant blood supply, reflecting its low metabolic demands. This type of cartilage is found in intervertebral discs, the menisci of the knee, intra-articular joint discs, such as the temporomandibular joint, and in the symphysis pubis.
→ *Elastic cartilage.* This has a matrix with a combination of many elastic fibres and some collagen fibres. It is easily deformable, but springs back into place. It is avascular and never calcifies or ossifies, as both hyaline and fibrocartilage are apt to do with increasing age. It forms the elastic framework of the pinna, epiglottis and eustachian tube.

17. UPPER LIMB NERVES I

Draw the brachial plexus

See Figure 5.11.

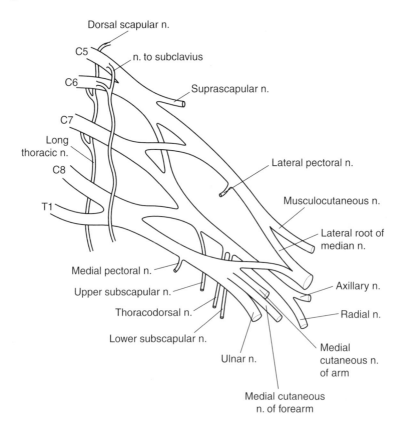

Figure 5.11 The left brachial plexus showing roots, cords, trunks and branches.

Describe the cords and their anatomical positions

The cords are named lateral, medial and posterior, which represents their relationship to the second part of the axillary artery, which they surround.

Describe the two common patterns of trauma to the brachial plexus giving rise to recognizable deformities

The commonest brachial plexus injury is a downward traction injury, especially from childbirth or a fall on the shoulder, as in high-speed motorcycle accidents.

It injures the upper cord ($C_{5/6}$) and is known as Erb–Duchenne paralysis. The affected muscles are deltoid, supraspinatus, infraspinatus, biceps, brachialis, brachioradialis and supinator brevis. The arm hangs internally rotated due to an unopposed subscapularis, with the forearm extended and pronated and is generally referred to as the 'waiter's tip' position. Sensory loss does not occur from isolated C_5 lesions but, with C_6 lesions, there is sensory loss over the outer surface of the arm.

In a lower plexus injury resulting from forced abduction of the arm, usually at birth, the C_8T_1 roots are affected. There is paralysis, and later wasting, of the small muscles of the hand and sensory loss on the medial 3½ fingers and inner forearm. It is known as Klumpke's palsy. If the T_1 root is affected, Horner's syndrome will also occur.

Describe the course of the radial nerve. How is it commonly injured?

The radial nerve is a direct continuation of the posterior cord of the brachial plexus and receives contributions from $C_{5-8}T_1$ – it is the nerve of the extensor compartment of the forearm. It exits the axilla by passing beyond its posterior wall, lying on the tendon of latissimus dorsi and traverses the triangular space of the arm. It descends the arm behind the fibres of the medial head of triceps, only occupying its position in the radial groove in the lowest part, deep to the lateral head of triceps. Here, it pierces the lateral intermuscular septum and lies between brachialis and brachioradialis, and passes through the cubital fossa beneath brachioradialis. It gives off the major posterior interosseus branch and continues downwards, sequentially lying on supinator, the tendon of pronator teres, the flexor digitorum superficialis, and flexor pollicis longus. It winds round the lower end of the radius to reach the back of the hand.

The radial nerve is prone to injury at two sites throughout its course, namely, in the axilla itself, and as it lies against the periosteum of the humerus in the lower radial groove. In the axilla, it is susceptible to compression injuries from poorly fitted crutches, although this is less common due to the introduction of 'elbow' crutches. More commonly, compression of the radial nerve in the axilla is due to a 'Saturday night palsy', whereby the patient falls into a deep slumber, usually alcohol assisted, with the arm hung over the back of a chair. Injury in the spiral groove occurs in cases of fracture of the humerus and, in this instance, the nerve may be divided, crushed or bruised.

What is the resultant deficit from an injury to the radial nerve at the level of: (1) the axilla, (2) the mid-shaft of the humerus and (3) the wrist?

1   When injured in the axilla, the characteristic deficit is a loss of elbow extension and the triceps reflex, and a wrist drop because of the loss of wrist and metacarpophalangeal extension. The interphalangeal joints can still extend

by virtue of the lumbricals. Sensory loss is a surprisingly small area over the first dorsal interosseus.

2 A mid-shaft of humerus fracture injures the nerve in the radial groove. By this stage, it has given off the nerves to triceps and so elbow extension is intact, but with this exception, the resulting motor and sensory losses are identical to those resulting from an axillary injury.

3 Lower injury, below the level of the supinator muscle, demonstrates weakness of finger extension but the wrist drop is minor, as brachioradialis is competent via its intact posterior interosseous nerve supply. The closer to the wrist joint the injury occurs, the more minor the extensor weakness becomes as the radial nerve typically gives off its branches much more proximal than the muscles it supplies.

Wilhelm Erb (1840–1921). A German neurologist who popularized the use of electrodiagnosis in neurology; he was also the first clinician to use the tendon hammer routinely.

Guillaume Duchenne (1807–75). French neurologist who never held a hospital appointment but merely practised privately throughout his career. He discovered that external electrical stimulation could cause muscles to move, and introduced this as a diagnostic tool. He performed the first biopsy on a live patient.

Augusta Klumpke (1859–1927). Although American, she studied medicine in Switzerland and Paris. She described the birth palsy that bears her name whilst still a student.

18. CEREBROSPINAL FLUID

Discuss the formation of cerebrospinal fluid

Cerebrospinal fluid is mainly produced by the choroid plexuses, which line the third, fourth and lateral ventricles with some being generated from the other cerebral capillaries. Although the total volume of CSF is only 130 ml or so, about 500 ml per day is produced, reflecting a constant circulation and resorption of fluid. It can exchange substances with the extracellular fluid, but this is regulated by the tight junctions of the blood–brain barrier; the overall composition of CSF is determined by the secretory role of the choroid plexus.

Describe the pathways by which CSF flows and is resorbed

See Figure 5.12. The CSF flows in a caudal direction from the lateral ventricles into the third ventricle via the interventricular foramen of Monro, and then

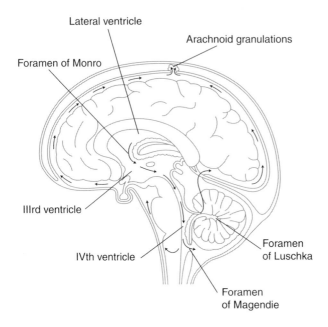

Lateral ventricle

Arachnoid granulations

Foramen of Monro

IIIrd ventricle

IVth ventricle

Foramen of Luschka

Foramen of Magendie

Figure 5.12 The normal pathway of cerebrospinal fluid flow. Reprinted from *Neurology and Neurosurgery Illustrated* 3/e, Lindsay KW et al, © 1997 Elsevier Ltd, with permission from Elsevier.

through the Sylvian aqueduct of the midbrain into the fourth ventricle. From here, CSF then reaches the subarachnoid space via the foramina of Luschka and Magendie, passing into the pontine cistern and cerebromedullary cistern, respectively. Once within the subarachnoid space, it circulates around the surface of the brain and spinal cord before being resorbed into the venous circulation by the arachnoid villi. These herniate through the arachnoid mater and lie within the major venous sinuses, especially the superior sagittal sinus, and thus lie in the subdural space. Over time, the discrete arachnoid villi coalesce into clumps known as arachnoid granulations.

What is hydrocephalus? How is it classified and how is it caused?

Hydrocephalus is defined as an increase in the volume of CSF within the cerebral ventricles. It is usually, although not always, caused by impaired absorption rather than excessive secretion. It may be classified as an obstructive or communicating hydrocephalus, depending on the site of obstruction to flow. In the obstructive type, there is a blockage to CSF flow within the ventricular system itself, compared to the communicating type, whereby the blockage is outside the ventricular system. Hydrocephalus may also be described as congenital or acquired. The causes of hydrocephalus are shown in Table 5.2.

How would you obtain a sample of CSF for analysis?

By performing a lumbar puncture. The patient is placed on their left side with knees drawn up and the back flexed. The preferred level is at L3/4, as this level

Table 5.2 Causes of hydrocephalus

Type	Pathology	Cause
Acquired obstructive	Aqueductal stenosis	Infection Haemorrhage
	Mass effect/compression	Tentorial herniation Tumours Abscess Granulomata
	Obstructing lesion	Intraventricular haematoma Arachnoid colloid cyst
Congenital obstructive	Structural anomalies	Chiari II malformation Dandy–Walker Syndrome – atresia of the IVth ventricle outlet foramina Aqueductal stenosis
Communicating	Leptomeningeal thickening	Infection Haemorrhage Carcinomatous deposits
	Increased CSF production	Choroid plexus papilloma
	Hyperviscosity of CSF	

Reprinted from *Neurology and Neurosurgery Illustrated* 3/e, Lindsay KW et al, © 1997 Elsevier Ltd, with permission from Elsevier.

is easily identified as being level with the iliac crests. It can be checked by counting up from the lumbosacral junction, and is marked. It is essential that lumbar puncture is a sterile procedure. The skin is prepared with antiseptic solution. Hand scrubbing, masking and gowning are as for any other sterile procedure. Up to 5 ml of 1 per cent lignocaine are injected into the skin and paravertebral muscles as local anaesthetic. A spinal needle is advanced forward, aiming for the previously identified vertebral space. A 'give' is felt as the needle pierces the tough ligamentum flavum and then passes through dura and arachnoid layers to enter the spinal canal. The stylet is withdrawn from the needle and the CSF specimen(s) collected, noting its colour and turbidity. The needle can now be connected to a manometer, if required to measure the pressure within the cerebrospinal system.

Alexander Monro (1773–1817). Scottish anatomist who succeeded his father as Professor of Anatomy in Edinburgh. He was in turn succeeded by his own son; there was an Alexander Monro as Professor from 1720 to 1846.

Hubert von Luschka (1820–75). German anatomist and Professor in Tubingen, where he described the foramen in 1859. He also was the first to describe polyposis of the colon in 1861.

François Magendie (1783–1855). An experimental physiologist who only later turned to anatomy, he demonstrated that anterior spinal roots were motor, whereas the posterior roots were sensory, independently of Charles Bell in Scotland.

19. SPACES AND FOSSAE

Describe the boundaries and contents of the triangular and quadrangular spaces of the upper limb

See Figure 5.13. Both these named spaces are spaces of the upper limb. The triangular space lies below teres major, and between the humerus and long head of triceps. It transmits the radial nerve and profunda brachii vessels. The quadrangular space is bounded laterally by the humerus and medially by the long head of triceps. Superiorly lies subscapularis with teres major inferiorly, although, when viewed from behind, the upper border is the teres minor muscle. Through this space pass the axillary nerve, and the posterior circumflex humeral artery and vein. The quadrangular space lies above the triangular one with the teres major muscle as the shared boundary.

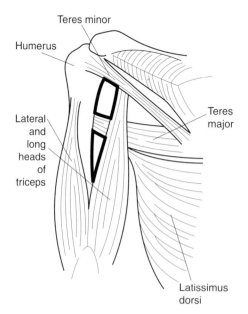

Figure 5.13 The quadrangular and triangular spaces viewed from behind.

Describe the boundaries and contents of the axilla

The axilla is the space between the side of the chest wall and the arm; it disappears during full abduction of the arm. It has an anterior wall, which consists of pectoralis major, pectoralis minor, subclavius and the clavipectoral fascia. The posterior wall is formed by subscapularis and teres major, and extends more inferiorly than does the anterior axillary fold. The tendon of latissimus dorsi winds round the lower edge of teres major in the posterior axillary fold. The medial wall is the upper part of serratus anterior, with the lower limit being defined as the level of the fourth rib. The anterior and posterior walls converge laterally to the humerus. The apex is bounded by the clavicle, scapula and first rib, and is the continuity between the axilla and the posterior triangle of the neck.

The cords of the brachial plexus enter the axilla from above and surround the second part of the axillary artery – the relationship of cords to artery being responsible for the naming of the medial, lateral and posterior cords. The axillary vein traverses the axilla, lying medial to the artery the whole way. Within the fatty tissue that fills the remainder of the axilla lie several groups of lymph nodes and the branches of the axillary vessels demanding care when dissecting in this region.

Describe the boundaries and contents of the popliteal fossa

The popliteal fossa is a diamond-shaped depression lying behind the knee joint. The upper borders are the tendon of biceps femoris laterally and those of semimembranosus and semitendinosus medially. The lower borders are the two heads of gastrocnemius. The roof is the popliteal fascia, a downwards continuation of the fascia lata of the thigh. The floor is formed by the popliteal surface of the femur, capsule of knee joint and popliteus muscle. It contains the popliteal artery and vein, the tibial and common peroneal nerves and a small group of lymph nodes. The short saphenous vein enters the fossa to join the popliteal vein at a variable level about the knee joint.

Describe the boundaries and contents of the antecubital fossa

The antecubital fossa of the arm is triangular in shape and is bounded by pronator teres, brachioradialis and a line joining the humeral epicondyles. It is roofed by the deep fascia of the forearm, with the bicipital aponeurosis, in addition, medially. The median basilic vein, median cutaneous nerve of the forearm, median cephalic vein and the lateral cutaneous nerve of forearm all lie on the bicipital aponeurosis, from medial to lateral. Below the aponeurosis, the fossa itself contains the median nerve, brachial artery and tendon of biceps, with the nerve lying most medial of the three. If brachioradialis is retracted laterally, the radial and posterior interosseous nerves are seen to lie in the lateral extremity of the antecubital fossa.

20. BASE OF SKULL AND CERVICAL SPINE

Label this photograph of the base of a human skull (Figure 5.14; 1–10) and
detail what traverses the major foramina (A–I)

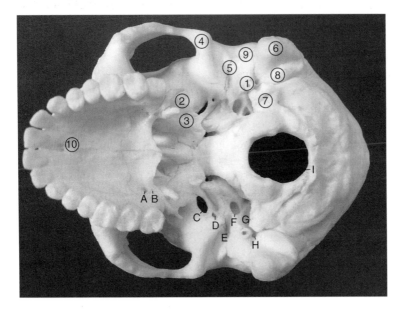

Figure 5.14

1	Styloid process	7	Jugular notch
2/3	Lateral and medial pterygoid plates	8	Digastric notch
4	Zygomatic process	9	External acoustic meatus
5	Squamotympanic fissure	10	Incisive fossa
6	Mastoid process		

A   Greater palatine foramen – greater palatine nerve
B   Lesser palatine foramen – lesser palatine nerves
C   Foramen ovale – mandibular nerve
D   Foramen spinosum – middle meningeal vessels
E   Foramen lacerum – closed by fibrous tissue
F   Carotid canal – internal carotid artery
G   Jugular foramen – vagus, accessory and glossopharyngeal nerves, internal jugular vein
H   Stylomastoid foramen – facial nerve and stylomastoid branch of posterior auricular artery
I   Foramen magnum – dura, lower medulla, spinal arteries, vertebral arteries, and the
    spinal roots of the accessory nerves

Describe the articulations of the base of the skull and the first two cervical vertebrae

The first cervical vertebra is named the 'atlas' and is atypical. It has a wide vertebral foramen divided into two by the transverse ligament; the spinal cord lies in the posterior segment, whilst the anterior part holds the dens of the second vertebra tightly. The second cervical vertebra – the 'axis' – is notable for the peg of bone that projects superiorly from the body of the vertebra, and this odontoid peg (or dens) articulates with the transverse ligament of the atlas, as well as the large articular facets. The horizontally disposed superior articular facets of the atlas articulate with the occipital condyles of the skull. This joint is supported by several ligaments. The alar ligament passes from the apex of the dens outward to the medial side of the occipital condyles on either side, whilst the superior longitudinal band blends with the transverse ligament of the atlas and attaches to the midline occiput. The whole joint is reinforced by the anterior and posterior atlanto-occipital and atlanto-axial membranes, as well as the anterior longitudinal ligament.

Describe how you would assess a lateral cervical spine film in a trauma situation

The film should first be assessed for adequacy. An adequate film should be well penetrated and demonstrate the whole of the cervical spine, including the top of the first thoracic vertebra. If the radiograph is insufficient, then it must be repeated with downwards traction on both arms, if possible; alternatively, a 'swimmer's view' through the axilla will demonstrate the lower vertebrae. The spinal column is checked for bony alignment by following the lines of the anterior vertebral bodies, anterior spinal canal, posterior spinal canal and the tips of the spinous processes. Each vertebra is examined sequentially, assessing the body, lateral masses, pedicles, facets, laminae, and transverse and spinous processes for fractures. The soft tissues of the pre-vertebral space and between spinous processes are assessed for widening, and any obliteration of the pre-vertebral fat stripe is noted. Any radio-opaque foreign bodies or bone fragments should be identified. After clearance of the cervical spine on clinical grounds in conjunction with the lateral neck radiograph, the patient should have anteroposterior and peg views taken to complete the radiographic assessment of the cervical spine.

21. WRIST FRACTURES

What fracture does the x-ray in Figure 5.15 show? Describe the relevant features

This x-ray of the left wrist shows a Colles' fracture. It is a transverse fracture of the distal radius and is the common result of a fall on an outstretched hand,

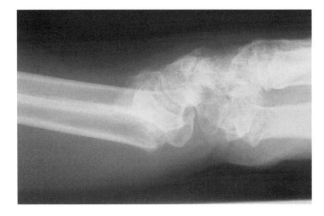

Figure 5.15

particularly in postmenopausal, osteoporotic women. The clinical appearance is said to be a 'dinner fork' deformity. The x-rays will show a transverse radial fracture within 2.5 cm of the radiocarpal joint, often with an associated fracture of the ulnar styloid process. The fracture is displaced with the distal radial fragment angulated dorsally and radially, with some degree of ulnar rotation and impaction.

What are the complications of a Colles' fracture?

Whilst malunion of a Colles' fracture is fairly common, the functional deficit from it rarely causes significant trouble in the elderly population, in whom it commonly occurs. In this population, greater degrees of residual angulation and deformity are generally acceptable than in the younger working population. There are exceptions to this, of course, and the elderly concert pianist will also require minimal residual deformity after reduction. The radioulnar joint may become subluxed after the fracture and displacement of the distal radius; the ulna head becomes prominent and may cause impingement in rotation after fracture healing. This may be treated by excision of the ulna head. The tendon of extensor pollicis longus may rupture, either acutely, or more commonly, after a delay of a few weeks, which may be due to the interruption of its blood supply by the injury or repeated abrasion against the roughness of the fracture site. The median nerve may be damaged acutely or from compression in an acute carpal tunnel syndrome. This type of fracture is susceptible to Sudeck's atrophy, a reflex sympathetic dystrophy, which leaves the hand painful, stiff and hypersensitive to all modalities of stimuli.

How would you manipulate a Colles' fracture?

After obtaining fully informed consent and after the administration of an appropriate anaesthetic, such as haematoma block, Biers block or a short general anaesthetic, the fracture is manipulated aiming to reverse the pattern of the injury. The distal fragment is disimpacted by placing traction on the hand, whilst an assistant applies counter-traction by holding the arm above a flexed elbow. The surgeon's thumbs are placed over the dorsal aspect of the distal fragment, encircling the wrist with the fingers and the fragment pushed ventrally and to the ulnar side. Maintaining slight traction, a plaster is applied in full pronation and ulnar deviation at the wrist with slight palmar flexion and this position maintained until the plaster is solid. A check x-ray is required unless performed in theatre with an image intensifier.

What are Smith's and Barton's fractures?

A Smith's fracture is sometimes referred to as a reverse Colles', as the characteristic radiographic appearance is of a distal radial fracture with volar angulation and proximal displacement. Barton's fracture is actually a fracture dislocation of the wrist with an intra-articular radial fracture and displacement of the whole carpus in either a dorsal or volar direction.

Abraham Colles (1773–1843) became Professor of Surgery and Anatomy in Dublin in 1804, and described his fracture 10 years later. He originally did not recommend any treatment for it, as he felt that adequate pain-free function could be achieved without manipulation. J.R. Barton described his fracture–dislocation in 1838, and Robert Smith his in 1847.

22. STOMACH

What is the blood supply to the stomach? How is this knowledge utilized when performing an oesophagectomy?

The stomach derives its blood supply from the coeliac axis, the first non-paired major branch of the abdominal aorta. The lesser curvature is supplied by branches of the left gastric artery in the upper part and right gastric artery, a branch of the common hepatic artery, in the lower part. The greater curve is supplied by the left and right gastroepiploic arteries. The left is a part of the short gastric series arising from the splenic artery and the right arises from the gastroduodenal artery, again a branch of the common hepatic artery. Both sets of arteries anastomose with each other on their respective gastric curves and then anastomose again with the supply of the other curve, approximately two-thirds of the way from the greater to the lesser curve.

During oesophagectomy, the short gastric, left gastroepiploic and left gastric arteries are divided to mobilize the upper portion of the stomach so that it can be pulled up to form the neo-oesophagus. The stomach then derives its blood supply wholly from the right gastric and gastroepiploic arteries and their anastomoses.

What sorts of partial gastrectomy do you know?

The variations are less about the gastrectomy than about the method of restoring gastrointestinal continuity. The Billroth I partial gastrectomy excises the distal stomach and directly re-anastomoses the free duodenal end to the partially closed gastric remnant. A Billroth II reconstruction forms a gastroenterostomy between a loop of small bowel that is brought up and the gastric remnant. The proximal free end of the duodenum is closed and left as a blind end. In a roux-en-Y reconstruction the duodenal stump is closed and the small bowel divided at the upper jejunum. The distal end is anastomosed to the stomach and the duodenal 'stem' is anastomosed to the small bowel some 50 cm downstream (Figure 5.16).

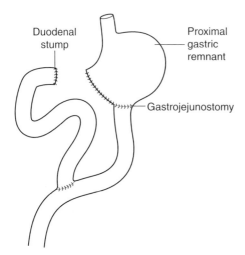

Duodenal stump

Proximal gastric remnant

Gastrojejunostomy

Figure 5.16 Roux-en-Y reconstruction following distal gastrectomy.

What is the gastric innervation? What are the results of denervation of the stomach? Does it vary according to the level of nerve section?

In common with the rest of the gut, the stomach receives a sympathetic vaso-motor supply, which travels with the arterial branches to the organ accompanied by afferent pain fibres. The stomach's major supply is parasympathetic via the vagi, which principally control motility and secretion. The anterior vagus runs down from the oesophageal plexus within the lesser omentum, close to the lesser curve in the company of the left gastric artery – at this level, it is often called the anterior nerve of Latarget. It gives branches to the anterior stomach and a large hepatic branch to the pyloric antrum. The posterior vagal trunk runs down the back of the lesser omentum, behind the anterior trunk, as the posterior nerve of Latarget. It gives off a coeliac branch that follows the left gastric artery backwards and numerous other branches that supply the posterior stomach.

Truncal vagotomy with section of both trunks over the lower oesophagus has been the traditional operation for the treatment of complicated ulcer disease as it radically reduces gastric secretory function; however, it also paralyses the pyloric antrum and must be coupled with a drainage procedure, such as pyloroplasty or gastrojejunostomy to avoid gastric stasis. Highly selective vagotomy divides the individual nerves as they supply the acid producing body and antrum, leaving pyloric function intact, and is the procedure of choice in the surgical treatment of refractory peptic ulcer disease, which these days is most uncommon. A variation of this theme is a posterior truncal vagotomy, which leaves the anterior pyloric nerves intact, coupled with an anterior seromyotomy. This may be performed via a laparoscope. Since the introduction of proton-pump inhibitors, the incidence of vagotomy of any description has fallen dramatically.

What is dumping?

Dumping is a term first described by Andrews in 1920 to describe the symptoms that can occur after gastric resections. It is now known that there are two sorts of dumping as follows.

→ *Early or vasomotor dumping.* Rapid emptying of hyperosmolar chyme from the residual stomach into the intestine causes fluid shifts from the vascular compartment; this causes a fall in plasma volume and vasomotor symptoms, such as weakness, dizziness, fainting, headache, palpitations, sweating and dyspnoea.
→ *Late dumping or reactive hypoglycaemia.* This is less common than early dumping. Rapid transit of high carbohydrate load into small intestine causes excessive insulin release and a later reactive hypoglycaemia 1–3 hours after eating.

Theodor Billroth (1829–94). Professor of Surgery in Zurich at the age of 31 and latterly in Vienna. He performed the first successful partial gastrectomy in 1881, the first laryngectomy for cancer and did pioneering work with colonic resection and anastomosis. He was also an early proponent of audit, publishing his 5-year results for many operations.

23. BLADDER

What is the nerve supply to the urinary bladder?

The bladder receives both sympathetic and parasympathetic nerve supplies. The primary innervation, including motor supply, is parasympathetic via the pelvic splanchnic nerves. The sympathetic supply is largely vasomotor and inhibitory to the detrusor muscle and is derived from the $L_{1,2}$ outflow, arriving via the superior hypogastric and pelvic plexuses. The sensation of bladder distension reaches the spinal cord through the parasympathetics, but true pain, as felt with a bladder stone, reaches the cord in both sympathetic and parasympathetic fibres.

Describe the pathways involved in micturition

Micturition reflexes begin to appear and get progressively stronger after the bladder volume has reached approximately 200 ml in most adults. Initially, as the volume increases, the bladder distends with minimal increase in intravesical pressure. As this level of accommodation is exceeded, the sensory stretch receptors in the bladder wall are stimulated, especially from the area of the posterior urethra. These afferent stretch impulses pass through the parasympathetic pelvic nerves to the sacral cord from where efferent signals pass back to the bladder wall to cause contraction of the bladder muscle. The micturition reflex is a completely autonomic spinal cord reflex, but can be facilitated or inhibited by higher cerebral centres after 'toilet training'. These centres lie in the pons of the brainstem with some mainly inhibitory ones in the cerebral cortex. The higher centres keep the micturition reflex partially inhibited, except when micturition is desired. They can prevent micturition, even when the micturition reflex is occurring by continual tonic contraction of the external urethral sphincter, until an appropriate time. When urination is desired, cortical centres facilitate the micturition reflex and inhibit the external urethral sphincter to allow urination.

When micturition begins, it is self-regenerating, i.e. the contraction of the bladder stimulates more stretch receptors, which leads to further reflex contractions. Thus, the micturition reflex consists of a progressive and rapid pressure increase, followed by a period of maintained pressure, before return of the pressure back to the basal tone of the bladder. If it occurs and the bladder is not emptied, then it remains inhibited for a few minutes to an hour.

Voluntary urination usually occurs by a person contracting the abdominal muscles, which raises the pressure in the bladder, forcing urine into the bladder neck and stretching it. This stimulates the micturition reflex and inhibits the external urethral sphincter.

In what operative procedures are the bladder nerves commonly endangered?

The bladder nerves are commonly endangered during pelvic dissection. The parasympathetic and sympathetic supply come together in the superior and inferior hypogastric plexuses, and continue as the pelvic nerves. They are particularly at risk during mesorectal excision for rectal cancers, since the plane of dissection is the plane of the pelvic nerves.

What bladder changes occur following complete transection of the spinal cord? How may these problems be managed?

Immediately following transection of the spinal cord, all vesical reflex activity is lost and gradual bladder distension is the norm for a period varying from 24 hours to several weeks. Thereafter, as long as the sacral cord itself is intact, then local reflexes will return and automatic bladder emptying will occur in response to distension. Transection of the cord means that all cortical input is lost and the bladder function again becomes purely reflex, as in a toddler. In the initial stages, an indwelling urethral catheter is to be avoided as the risks of urinary sepsis are high – the alternatives are the insertion of a fine-bore suprapubic catheter or intermittent catheterization. Although reflex micturition may return, this can often be accompanied by incoordination between the detrusor contraction and the relaxation of the voluntary sphincteric musculature. This can result in high bladder pressures. This detrusor-sphincter dyssynergia can be difficult to treat, and may require ablation of the urinary sphincters and permanent drainage arrangements.

24. THE NECK

What are the branchial arches, pouches and clefts?

The branchial arches are condensations of mesoderm that develop in the wall of the primitive pharynx and fuse ventrally to form horseshoes of tissue. The spaces between the arches on the external surface are known as the branchial clefts, whilst the branchial pouches are the internal grooves between adjacent arches. They are also referred to as pharyngeal arches and pouches. The subsequent differentiation of these arches is complex and not completely understood. In general, the first arch develops into the mandible and maxilla, the second into the hyoid bone along with part of the third arch. The remaining three arches form the cartilage of the larynx. Not only do the arches differentiate into bone and cartilage, but each develops associated musculature and has a dedicated cranial nerve and artery. The pouches lying between the arches each develop a dorsal and ventral diverticulum, which in turn develop into recognizable features. The eustachian tube, middle ear and mastoid antrum develop from the first pouch, whilst the second adds a contribution to the middle ear and develops into both the tonsillar apparatus and the tympanic cavity. The third pouch gives rise to the thymus and inferior parathyroids, whilst the superior parathyroids develop from the fourth pouch. The fifth pouch regresses as the ultimobranchial body, from which the parafollicular cells of the thyroid develop.

Outline the major anatomical features and relations of the thyroid gland

The thyroid gland has two lobes joined in the midline by an isthmus. The gland lies in the front of the neck behind the pretracheal fascia, with the isthmus at the level of the second to fourth tracheal rings. Each lateral lobe is narrower above than below. The gland receives its blood supply from the superior and inferior thyroid arteries. The superior artery, a branch of the external carotid, enters the gland at the apex of the lobe, and supplies the upper half by anterior and posterior branches. The inferior artery, from the thyrocervical trunk, divides into four or five branches that pierce the pretracheal fascia to supply the lower pole. An additional vessel, the thyroidea ima artery, supplies the lower isthmus in 3 per cent of people – it has a variable derivation. The venous drainage is by named vessels that accompany the arteries, and a middle thyroid vein that drains directly into the internal jugular vein. Behind the gland lie the parathyroid glands and the thyroid lobes overlie the common carotid artery within its sheath. The lateral aspects of the lobes are related to the strap muscles, under whose cover they reside. The medial lobar surfaces are related to the larynx, trachea, cricothyroid and inferior constrictor muscles. The recurrent laryngeal nerve approaches the medial surface of the gland from below, just anterior to the tracheoesophageal groove. The external branch of the superior laryngeal nerve passes to the medial upper pole, lying behind and medial to the superior thyroid artery.

What muscles attach to the hyoid bone?

The hyoid bone has no fixed skeletal attachment and thus is highly mobile. It lies in the front of the neck level with the C3 vertebral body. Seven of its attached muscles are divided into infrahyoid and suprahyoid groups. The suprahyoid muscles are digastric, attached to the base of the lesser horn, stylohyoid attaching to the base of the greater horn, and mylohyoid and geniohyoid both inserting into the body of the bone. The infrahyoid muscles are the sternohyoid and omohyoid, both of which arise from the lower border of the body of the hyoid and the thyrohyoid from the greater horn. These three infrahyoid muscles are often considered together with the sternothyroid muscle as the 'strap' muscles of the neck. In addition to these two groups of muscles, the hyoid is connected to the pharnyx and tongue by the middle constrictor and hyoglossus muscles respectively, both arising from the length of the greater horn.

List the various layers encountered in the surgical approach to the thyroid gland

After incision of the skin, platysma is divided. Thereafter the investing layer of the deep cervical fascia is encountered and divided. The strap muscles abut one another in the midline and should be separated, and on occasion division of sternohyoid and sternothyroid may be necessary for removal of a large goitre.

The next layer encountered is the pretracheal fascia, which should be opened; there may also be a false sheath of connective tissue overlying the thyroid itself.

25. UPPER LIMB NERVES II

Describe the origin and course of the ulnar nerve

The ulnar nerve is a continuation of the medial cord of the brachial plexus with contributions from the $C_{7,8}T_1$ nerve roots. It runs down the arm behind the brachial artery, angling backwards and passing through the medial intermuscular septum. It descends on triceps, and lies on the humeral shaft between the medial epicondyle and the olecranon. It passes between the two heads of flexor carpi ulnaris to enter the flexor compartment of the forearm. It passes downwards on the surface of flexor digitorum profundus beneath flexor carpi ulnaris. It emerges just above the wrist, accompanied by the ulnar artery, to cross the flexor retinaculum, alongside the pisiform bone, where it divides into its terminal superficial and deep branches. It supplies muscles on the ulnar side of the forearm but primarily is the nerve of supply to most of the intrinsic muscles of the hand. It gives sensory supply to the ulnar 1½ digits.

Where is the ulnar nerve vulnerable to injury?

The ulnar nerve is particularly vulnerable to injury at the elbow or the wrist. As it passes behind the olecranon, it is prone to compression injury and gives rise to a cubital tunnel syndrome. It may also be injured in association with elbow fractures, particularly if malunion then produces a marked cubitus valgus, which stretches the nerve around the medial epicondyle. Wrist injuries that produce ulnar nerve symptoms are generally compression types within Guyon's canal. This may be caused by a deep ganglion or occur in association with a carpal tunnel syndrome of whatever cause. The ulnar nerve, in common with the other ventral wrist structures, is vulnerable to penetrating injury from deliberate self-harm by slashing of the wrist.

Describe the lesion resulting from injury to the ulnar nerve: (1) at the wrist and (2) at the elbow

1 With a 'low' wrist injury, a claw hand develops. The little and ring fingers are flexed at the interphalangeal joints because of paralysis of the interossei and hyperextended at the metacarpophalangeal joints due to paralysis of the lumbricals. There is hypothenar wasting, weakness of finger abduction and thumb adduction. A sensory deficit occurs over the ulnar 1½ digits.

2 With an injury at the elbow, a 'high' lesion, there is a less pronounced claw, because the ulnar half of flexor digitorum profundus is also paralysed, leading to less flexion at the interphalangeal joints. The sensory deficit is identical to a low lesion. This is known as the ulnar paradox, i.e. the higher lesion gives rise to a less severe deformity.

Where is the median nerve most commonly injured?

The median nerve is most commonly injured at the wrist, owing to lacerations or entrapment syndromes in the carpal tunnel. Elbow dislocations and forearm fractures may lead to damage at the elbow. Isolated higher injuries are very rare. Penetrating injury from gunshot wounds or stabbings may injure any of the upper limb nerves at any level.

What lesions result from median nerve injury: (1) at the elbow and (2) at the wrist?

1 Injury at the elbow gives rise to a motor loss in the forearm pronators, long flexors of the thumb, index and ring fingers, i.e. the hand and wrist, except flexors, excepting the flexor carpi ulnaris and the ulnar side of flexor digitorum profundus. The hand deviates to the ulnar side, when flexing the wrist, and the index finger cannot be flexed. Flexion of the terminal phalanx of the thumb is lost, as is abduction and opposition; the thenar eminence wastes. Sensory loss is over the palmar surface of the thumb and radial 2½ fingers.
2 An injury at the wrist gives the same 'hand' signs as the higher injury but the long flexors are intact. The sensory loss is reduced, with 'thenar sparing', as the thenar cutaneous branch arises before the nerve passes beneath the flexor retinaculum.

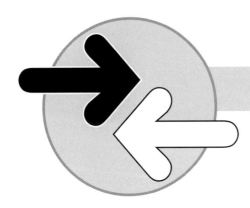

SECTION SIX

CLINICAL PATHOLOGY

1. FISTULAE AND SINUSES

Define fistulae and sinuses. Are they normal or abnormal?

A fistula is an abnormal communication between two epithelial lined surfaces. A sinus is a blind-ended track communicating with an epithelial surface. A fistula by definition is always abnormal. A sinus may be normal or abnormal, e.g. a cardiac sinus is normal, whereas a pilonidal sinus is abnormal.

Give an example of a common fistula

The commonest example of a fistula is the track following ear piercing! In medical practice, the commonest fistulae are entero-enteric fistulae but these are often clinically silent. The commonest presenting fistula is a fistula-in-ano.

What are the common causes of fistula-in-ano?

It is commonly associated with cryptoglandular sepsis in the anal glands, which may present as a fistula or abscess. Incision and drainage of such an abscess will of course convert it into a fistula. There is an increased incidence of fistula-in-ano associated with certain conditions, such as diabetes mellitus, Crohn's disease, tuberculosis and HIV infection. These conditions should always be considered when assessing a patient who presents with either a perianal abscess or fistula.

Classify fistula-in-ano

It is easiest to classify them according to their relationship to the anal sphincters, which can be represented diagrammatically (see Figure 6.1).

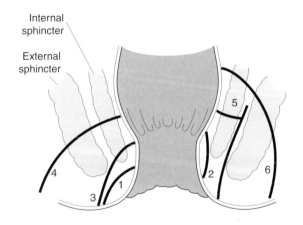

Figure 6.1 Types of fistula-in-ano in relation to the anal sphincters. 1, subcutaneous; 2, submucous; 3, low anal fistula; 4, high anal fistula; 5, intersphincteric fistula; 6, pelvirectal fistula.

Subcutaneous (1) and submucous (2) fistulae lie below the sphincters, while low anal fistulae (3) traverse the internal sphincter alone. High anal fistulae (4) traverse both internal and external sphincters, whilst intersphincteric fistulae (5) pass down between the two muscles, with the internal opening at a variable level. Pelvirectal (6) fistulae open internally above the anorectal ring.

Goodsall's rule describes the path taken by a fistulous track. With the patient in the lithotomy position, an external opening above a horizontal line through 3 and 9 o'clock will horseshoe round to enter the anal canal, whereas an opening below this line will tend to pass straight forward to enter in the posterior midline.

How can fistula-in-ano be treated?

Treatment depends on ascertaining the correct level of the fistula. Subcutaneous, submucous and low anal fistulae may safely be treated by laying open the fistula over a probe, after identifying the level of the internal sphincter, without comprising sphincter integrity. A similar approach to a high fistula may result in catastrophic division of the sphincters and result in faecal incontinence. This problem can be overcome by passing a seton through the fistula. If left loose, this will facilitate drainage of sepsis and when removed around 50 per cent will heal. If tied tightly as a cutting seton, then as this is progressively tightened every 2 weeks under anaesthetic, it will slowly 'cheese-wire' through the sphincter muscle, allowing fibrosis to take place behind and thus maintaining the integrity of the sphincter mechanism. Difficult or recurrent fistulae may be approached by excising the track as a core, known as core fistulectomy, with a local advancement flap to repair the internal opening. Complex fistulae may require a combination of a local procedure, such as fistulectomy, with a covering defunctioning stoma.

A 32-year-old man presents with a tense perianal abscess. How would you manage this?

In the first instance, he needs incision and drainage of his abscess to relieve his pain. Under general anaesthesia, in the lithotomy position, a digital rectal examination is performed to assess internal induration and the extent of the abscess. Rigid sigmoidoscopy and proctoscopy are then used to look for an internal opening and evidence of proctocolitis. After that the abscess is incised, sending a sample of pus for microscopy, culture and sensitivity. Thorough irrigation of the cavity and digitation to break down any loculations are necessary. The cavity should then be lightly packed. In addition to his operative management, other diseases, such as diabetes mellitus, should be excluded.

You arrange to see him in clinic 3 weeks later. Which results do you need to have at hand?

The most important result is that of the culture report from the pus swab you took. If it yielded skin commensal bacteria only, then the abscess is liable to be a boil on the perianal skin and requires no further treatment. If, however, the culture report yields enteric organisms, then the abscess is likely to be due to a fistula, which may require further management. Despite this, clinical examination is the most important investigation to assess whether anything further needs to be done at this point. This should include rectal examination, sigmoidoscopy and proctoscopy.

2. AMYLOID

What is amyloid? How can you identify it in tissues?

It is a proteinaceous material laid down extracellularly in a variety of forms and locations giving rise to a varied clinical picture. There is a typical β-pleated sheet molecular configuration that gives amyloid its affinity for certain dyes, e.g. Congo or Sirius red. It is always extracellular, being frequently present on basement membranes. The affected tissue tends to become waxy and hard. All amyloid deposits exhibit apple green birefringence on Congo red staining and have a characteristic β-pleated sheet structure on microscopy.

How can you classify it?

Amyloid deposition may be classified according to the specific protein involved. All consist of protein p plus another protein.

→ *AL*. This is myeloma-associated or primary amyloid. The L stands for light chain, as it has a direct immune origin from excess light chain fragments. There is a predilection for the connective tissues within the heart, liver, kidneys and spleen.
→ *AA*. Reactive or secondary amyloid. It is secondary to a chronic inflammatory stimulus, such as tuberculosis, rheumatoid arthritis, ulcerative colitis, Hodgkin's disease, hypernephroma or syphilis. The additional protein is serum amyloid A (SAA), an acute-phase reactant produced by interleukin stimulation of hepatocytes.
→ *AS*. Amyloid pre-albumin is the precursor protein and it is associated with Alzheimer's disease.
→ *AH*. Haemodialysis-associated amyloid. The H protein is β_2-microglobulin, which is too small to be filtered and, therefore, reappears in the serum and is deposited.
→ *AF*. Hereditary neuropathic and familial Mediterranean fever. The F protein is pre-albumin.

How does it cause problems clinically?

It may give rise to systemic or local amyloidosis. The symptoms obviously depend on the site of deposition. Systemic amyloidosis affects a wide range of organs.

Clinically, this produces diffuse generalized organ enlargement with hepatomegaly, splenomegaly, macroglossia and organ dysfunction, heart failure and proteinuria amongst others. Senile amyloidosis with minute deposits of pre-albumin in the heart and walls of blood vessels is common in the elderly. Localized amyloidosis may be found in the stroma of peptide-producing tumours, especially medullary carcinoma of the thyroid. Localized deposits may be found elsewhere with no apparent predisposing cause; the skin, lungs and urinary tract are most frequently affected. Amyloid deposition within organs is rarely asymptomatic. Cardiac deposition causes a constrictive cardiomyopathy, which is the commonest cause of death in systemic amyloidosis. Deposition in the kidney between the basement membranes gives rise to nephrotic syndrome, whilst an enlarged 'sago spleen' is the result of splenic deposits. Deposits in the ligaments of the wrist are a rare cause of carpal tunnel syndrome.

Amyloid was first identified by Rudolf Virchow in 1842 who gave it its name, which means 'starch-like', as it stains mahogany brown with iodine and blue–violet with acid, as does starch.

3. HELICOBACTER PYLORI

Draw and describe *H. pylori*

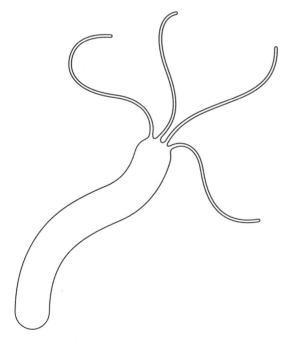

Figure 6.2 *Helicobacter pylori.*

See Figure 6.2. It is a spiral, flagellated mobile bacterium. It is approximately 4 μm in length, Gram negative and urease producing.

In what diseases is it implicated?

It is causally implicated in the pathogenesis of peptic ulcer disease. Its prevalence increases with age and is present in over half of the population over 60 years of age. Increased *H. pylori* infection rates correlate with low socioeconomic status and immigrant populations. It has a direct cytotoxic effect on gastric mucosa, producing an inflammatory response, and also induces hypergastrinaemia and hyperchlorhydria. Antral infection rates are greater than 90 per cent in duodenal ulcer and about 60 per cent in gastric ulcers. Eradication of the organism radically reduces recurrence rates for healed ulcers. Infection with *H. pylori* is associated with a chronic gastritis, typified by a lymphocyte and plasma cell infiltrate, which may progress to atrophic gastritis. Because of increased mucosal damage and inflammation, *H. pylori* is deemed a causative agent of duodenal and gastric ulceration and is a risk factor for the development of gastric cancer. The *H. pylori* antigens induce the appearance of mucosal-associated lymphoid follicles in the gastric submucosa and *H. pylori* infection is linked to a higher rate of MALT-type gastric lymphoma.

There is evidence that *H. pylori* may be associated with extradigestive disease. The proposed mechanism of injury is the immunological response to the *H. pylori* antigens, proinflammatory substance production, antigen mimicry and reduced folate and iron absorption. Diseases with this association are ischaemic heart disease, carotid artery stenosis, cholesterol gallstones, Raynaud's phenomenon and some immunological diseases, such as, Henoch–Schönlein purpura, Sjögren's syndrome and autoimmune thrombocytopenia, sideropenic anaemia and liver cirrhosis.

How can you diagnose *H. pylori* infection?

There are six methods of diagnosis:

→ rapid urease tests
→ culture
→ polymerase chain reaction
→ histology
→ C^{13} urea breath test
→ serology.

The commonest tests are the rapid urease tests (CLO, Pyloritec, etc.), which provide a result in 24 hours. The test utilizes the organism's ability to cleave urea; when positive for *H. pylori*, the action of urease turns an indicator compound from yellow to red in a commercially available test slide. They are approximately 90 per cent sensitive. Culture is performed in a microaerobic environment and is 98 per cent sensitive. The polymerase chain reaction test comes as a testing kit based on purified antigens and uses the enzyme-linked immunosorbent assay technique. Histology relies on the organism being visible under light microscopy on an antral biopsy and is also around 98 per cent sensitive.

The C^{13} urea breath test is based on *H. pylori*'s ability to hydrolyse the radio-labelled urea to produce labelled CO_2, which is subsequently exhaled and detected in the breath. It is the most accurate of the tests, being both 100 per cent sensitive and specific. Serology for *H. pylori* antibodies (IgG) is 98 per cent sensitive, but only 88 per cent specific, because unfortunately the test remains positive for many months after eradication.

It should be noted that therapy with a protein pump inhibitor at the time of endoscopy significantly decreases the sensitivity of both rapid urease tests and histology for *H. pylori* infection.

How would you manage someone with *H. pylori*-positive duodenal ulcer?

In simple *H. pylori*-positive cases, the aims are twofold. Firstly, ulcer healing, and, secondly, *H. pylori* eradication to reduce recurrence rates. There are many successful eradication regimens. One such is omeprazole 20 mg BD, metronidazole 400 mg TDS and clarithromycin 200 mg BD for 1 week followed by 3 weeks of omeprazole 20 mg OD.

H. pylori was first isolated by Barry Marshall and Robin Warren, two microbiologists from Perth, Western Australia, who initially classified it as a Campylobacter *because of its spiral shape – 'campylobacter' means 'curved bacteria'. Marshall also devised a method of detection, the CLO test, which is so named as an abbreviation of* 'Campylobacter-*like organisms'.*

4. MELANOMA

Define melanoma and discuss aetiology and epidemiology

Melanoma is a malignant neoplasm of epithelial melanocytes primarily arising in the skin, although it may also occur in the nasal cavities, on the retina and in gastrointestinal mucosa. It is most common in fair-skinned individuals living about the equator. Its incidence is rising rapidly owing to increased exposure to ultraviolet radiation – the main aetiological factor. An episode of severe sunburn appears to be more important than chronic exposure. It is twice as common in women; 70 per cent of melanomas arise *de novo*, with one-third arising out of previously present naevi. Enlargement, alteration of pigmentation, itching, bleeding and ulceration all arouse suspicion of malignant transformation. Benign melanoma does not exist.

What types of melanoma are there?

The four common types of melanoma are as follows.

→ *Superficial spreading* – about 65 per cent of lesions, with better prognosis owing to an initial horizontal growth phase.
→ *Nodular* – about 28 per cent. They have a worse prognosis because there is no horizontal growth phase.
→ *Lentigo maligna melanoma* – about 7 per cent of lesions arising out of a Hutchinson freckle but only about 5 per cent of such freckles transform into melanoma. They generally have a good prognosis.
→ *Acral lentiginous* – about 1 per cent in Caucasians but commoner in dark-skinned races. They occur in the hairless skin of palms or soles.

What information would you look for on the histology report of an excised melanoma?

The following should be specifically checked:

→ confirmation of the patient's details
→ the diagnosis confirming melanoma
→ the type of melanoma
→ the growth phase – horizontal has a better prognosis than vertical
→ the depth of invasion – Breslow thickness
→ excision margins
→ degree of mitotic activity.

Describe Breslow thickness. Are there any other staging methods?

Breslow thickness is a system first published in 1970 that correlates depth of tumour with prognosis; it is specific for melanoma (see Table 6.1).

Table 6.1 Breslow thickness

Depth (mm)	5-year survival (per cent)	10-year survival (per cent)
<0.78	98	95
0.78–1.6	85	75
1.6–3.6	70	60
>3.6	40	30

Another staging method is Clarke's levels, which correlate depth of invasion through the layers of dermis with survival. Breslow thickness has been shown to be a better predictor of clinical outcome.

How would you treat a suspicious pigmented lesion beneath a great toenail?

The toenail should be removed under appropriate anaesthetic, and either the lesion excised, if possible, or otherwise an incisional biopsy performed. If the histology report confirmed malignant melanoma, then amputation of the digit giving at least 2 cm proximal clearance should be arranged.

A 31-year-old female presents with an irregularly pigmented naevus on her back that has recently become itchy. She is very keen not to have too big a scar – how would you deal with this woman?

A thorough history is taken and examination is performed, looking for other naevi, lymphadenopathy and scars of previous operations, which may indicate removal of other lesions. In the first instance, possible diagnoses should be discussed, including malignant melanoma, and arrangements made to remove the lesion under local anaesthetic. A 2 mm margin is sufficient initially but the patient should be warned that, if it was reported as melanoma, further excision would be necessary.

The pathology report comes back showing malignant melanoma of a superficial spreading type with a Breslow depth of 2.6 mm with tumour up to one resection margin. What do you now tell her and arrange to do?

After explanation of the histology report, she should undergo further excision of the scar with a 2–3 cm margin all round. If this left a defect that could not be closed directly, then referral to a plastic surgeon should be considered for excision and subsequent flap closure of the defect, or proceed and use a split skin graft.

What is the long-term prognosis for this patient?

The 5-year survival from this depth of tumour, if node negative, is 70 per cent. Most recurrences are within the first 2 years, and virtually all by 5 years. The 10-year survival rate falls to 60 per cent.

What is sentinel node biopsy and explain how it might usefully be applied here?

Injection of a radioisotope into the area of the primary tumour will drain via the same lymph nodes as the tumour. A hand-held gamma detector can then identify which group of nodes are actually draining the tumour bed, which in a lesion situated in the mid-back may not be entirely obvious at first presentation. By removing the first draining node identified by the gamma detector, i.e. the one with the highest count, for histology, it can be ascertained if the tumour has metastasized. The assumption is that, if the sentinel node is clear, then the other nodes are also clear and lymphadenectomy is unnecessary.

Sentinel node detection can also be performed using methylene blue injection of the tumour itself and looking for the first node to turn blue, if the pathway of lymph drainage is known. Unfortunately, after a primary excision, sentinel node biopsy may not be completely accurate because local lymphatic drainage will have been disturbed by the initial procedure. Sentinel node biopsy is not yet in routine clinical practice but still the subject of controlled trials.

5. REFERRAL TO THE CORONER/NCEPOD

When would you refer a patient to the coroner?

The role of the coroner is to investigate deaths to ensure that no suspicious circumstances are attached to them. There are certain circumstances, listed below, in which referral to the coroner is mandatory. There are other cases in which one should voluntarily seek guidance from the coroner or his officer. Incidentally, the coroner is also the proper officer to investigate the finding of treasure troves. Coroners in the UK are either medically or legally trained and often both, but a background in medicine is not obligatory.

The circumstances requiring mandatory referral to the coroner are as follows.

→ When the cause of death is unknown.
→ Where a doctor has not attended the deceased in the terminal illness or when the patient's normal medical practitioner did not attend within 14 days of the death.
→ When the death is associated with any medical treatment. This includes any death within 24 hours of an operation or anaesthetic.
→ Sudden death – including all deaths within 24 hours of admission to hospital.
→ When death may be due to industrial accident or disease, road traffic accident, domestic accident or violence. Deaths from poisoning (which include alcohol), abortion, suicide or neglect must also be reported.
→ Deaths in which there may or will be claims of negligence against medical or nursing staff.
→ Deaths in custody.

If there is any doubt as to the cause of death or the circumstances surrounding death, or simply to check whether a cause of death is acceptable on the certificate, it is advisable to discuss the matter with the coroner or, more commonly, his officer.

What is NCEPOD?

NCEPOD is the National Confidential Enquiry into Perioperative Deaths. In 1987, regional CEPOD was performed in three health regions run by an association of surgeons and anaesthetists; following the first report, it was immediately expanded to a national survey and became NCEPOD. This is a national body that considers the factors involved in perioperative deaths in order to try to identify areas in which practice could be improved. It looks for potentially remedial factors in anaesthesia, surgery and other invasive medical procedures. The data collected are not research, and do not compare units or clinicians. The data are subject to 'crown privilege', which means the data cannot be sub-poenaed. All data are shredded after use.

NCEPOD reports annually with recommendations for practice. Each year, the report focuses on a particular facet of surgical practice, such as out-of-hours operating, care of the elderly surgical patient or cancer surgery. The first NCEPOD report was published in 1989 and looked at deaths in children under 10 years old. In 1990, NCEPOD surveyed 10 per cent of all deaths within 30 days of surgery and this standard remains today. Recent recommendations include that surgeons and anaesthetists should be involved in multidisciplinary audit, patients with aortic stenosis should have pre-operative echocardiography and every effort should be made to refer emergency cancer presentations to a multidisciplinary oncological team.

In 2003, the name changed to National Confidential Enquiry into Patient Outcome and Deaths (still NCEPOD) to reflect its expansion. Additionally, in 2003, NCEPOD became separate from the Association of Surgeons, and became an independent body. In 2002–3, the survey included patients under the care of physicians, general practitioners and 'near-miss' occurrences. In 2003–4, there will be a 3-month survey of all endoscopic procedures by surgeons and physicians. Future reports will focus on intensive care of medical patients in 2004, ruptured abdominal aortic aneurysm in 2005 and emergency medical admissions in 2006.

What are the specific exclusions to the NCEPOD data collection?

So far, the report does not consider deaths related to obstetric care, of either the baby or mother. Hospital dental surgery is included but community practice is excluded.

It is interesting to note that several private hospital groups also participate fully in NCEPOD reporting and funding, as do the hospitals on the Channel Islands and the Isle of Man.

6. HAEMATURIA

How would you investigate haematuria?

A thorough history is taken, asking specifically about other urinary tract symptoms, foreign travel, associated pain, family history of renal disease or calculi and a full clinical examination.

A mid-stream urine specimen is taken for urinalysis and culture/sensitivities to confirm haematuria and exclude infection. A serum sample for urea and electrolytes is also taken to assess renal function. The patient is asked to perform a flow-meter test in the clinic. The patient needs their entire urinary tract imaging; if stone disease was a possibility, an IVP is requested and ultrasound of the kidneys, ureter and bladder, and arrangements to perform flexible cystoscopy under local anaesthetic to examine the bladder mucosa should be made.

What is in your differential diagnosis? How would this differ if you lived in Egypt?

The common differential diagnoses include urinary tract tumour, infection, calculi and interstitial renal disease. In Egypt, schistosomal infection is a predominant cause of bladder symptoms, as it causes a chronic inflammatory cystitis and increases the risk of developing squamous cell carcinoma, which is much more common in Egypt than elsewhere – even other places where schistosomiasis is endemic. If 'surgical' investigations draw a blank and haematuria persists, then referral to a nephrologist for further investigation should be considered.

What types of bladder cancer occur?

By far the most common type of bladder cancer is transitional cell carcinoma (Figure 6.3), which accounts for over 90 per cent of cases, followed by squamous cell carcinoma in a further 5 per cent. Adenocarcinoma constitutes only about 1 per cent of all cases, which may be in an urachal remnant, in an area of glandular metaplasia in the base of the bladder or be metastatic. These figures are generally true for most of the world but, as already mentioned, are not valid in areas of endemic schistosomiasis, particularly Egypt, where the rate of squamous cell carcinoma is much higher.

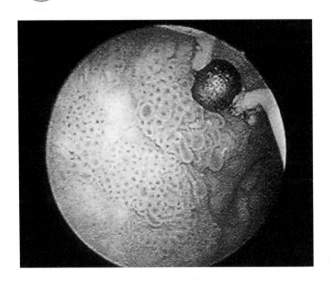

Figure 6.3 A transitional cell carcinoma of the bladder being treated by 'rollerball ablation'.

How is the extent of transitional cell carcinoma of the bladder usually described?

Transitional cell carcinoma is usually classified according to the TNM classification:

Tx	Primary tumour cannot be assessed
T0	No evidence of primary tumour
Tis	Carcinoma *in situ*
Ta	Non-invasive papillary tumour
T1	Tumour invades subepithelial tissue
T2	Tumour invades superficial muscle (inner half)
T3	Tumour invades outer half of deep muscle (T3a) or perivesical fat (T3b)
T4	Tumour invades prostate uterus, vagina, pelvic or abdominal wall

Discuss the various treatment modalities available to treat TCC

Superficial tumours may be managed in the first instance by endoscopic resection and follow-up cystoscopy, as between 50 and 80 per cent will recur at some stage. Recurrent tumours, or those of high pathological grade, although still superficial, require more intensive therapy with chemical instillations into the bladder – commonly used agents are mitomycin C, Adriamycin and BCG. The first two have a direct toxic effect on the urothelium, whilst BCG also stimulates a non-specific mononuclear infiltrate, which has been shown to be helpful.

Carcinoma *in situ* (CIS) is a difficult condition to treat. If it is localized and asymptomatic, conservative treatment may be adopted; however, widespread or symptomatic CIS requires instillational therapy with BCG and, if that fails, cystourethrectomy. This appears to be overly radical surgery for an *in situ* disease, but it is a 'field change' disease with a high risk of later urethral recurrence.

Invasive tumours require more aggressive therapy from the outset unless they are beyond the realms of curative treatment as many are at presentation. The options are radical cystectomy or radiotherapy, with neither being shown to have any particular advantage over the other. Primary radiotherapy, however, can be followed by salvage cystectomy, if necessary, later. In any event, the 5-year survival for patients with muscle invasive tumours at presentation is about 50 per cent irrespective of treatment modality.

7. DEEP VEIN THROMBOSIS

What is Virchow's triad?

Virchow's triad, first described in 1845, postulated that thrombosis is predisposed to by three general factors.

→ *Alterations in the vessel wall.* Conditions such as atheroma disturb the normal non-turbulent flow of blood and create stagnant areas of low flow in which thrombosis may develop. The exposure of subendothelial collagen to the circulation by even the smallest endothelial injury causes adherence of platelets and release of pro-aggregatory tissue factors.
→ *Alterations in the constituents of the blood.* These may be increased cell numbers as in polycythaemia, myeloma and thrombocythaemia, causing increased blood viscosity, or may be pro-thrombotic aberrations of the normal clotting mechanisms such as Factor V Leiden mutations or Protein C or S deficiencies.
→ *Alterations in blood flow.* Turbulent flow in aneurysms, at sites of bifurcation, through narrowed, atherosclerotic vessels or over damaged endothelium, disrupts the normal laminar flow of blood. In laminar flow, the cellular components of blood flow centrally are separated from the endothelium by plasma. Non-laminar flow brings the cellular elements in contact with the vascular endothelium, increasing the risks of platelet activation and adherence.

Outline the current guidelines for prevention of thromboembolic disease in surgical patients

These are guidelines formulated by the Thromboembolic Risk Factors (THRIFT) Consensus Group and originally published in 1992. They define high-, moderate- and low-risk surgery, and the recommendations for prophylaxis are based on the risks of deep vein thrombosis and fatal pulmonary embolus in each group.

High
The risk of DVT is 40–80 per cent and the risk of PE is between 1 and 10 per cent:

→ long bone fracture or major orthopaedic surgery
→ major pelvic or abdominal cancer surgery
→ major surgery lasting longer than 2 hours
→ trauma or illness in patients with previous DVT/PE/prothrombotic condition
→ acute lower limb paralysis.

High-risk groups should receive high-dose prophylaxis with either sub-cutaneous heparin or one of the newer low-molecular-weight heparins, which have the advantage of once-daily dosing. Compression stockings should be worn unless specifically contraindicated and pneumatic calf compression used intra-operatively, if available.

Moderate
The risk of DVT is 10–40 per cent and that of PE between 0.1 and 1 per cent.
  Major general, urological, gynaecological, cardiothoracic, vascular or neuro-logical surgery and any of the following:

→ age over 40 years
→ obesity
→ varicose veins
→ malignancy
→ infection
→ heart failure or recent myocardial infarction
→ paralysis of lower limbs
→ inflammatory bowel disease or nephrotic syndrome
→ polycythaemia
→ paraproteinaemia
→ paroxysmal nocturnal haemoglobinaemia
→ Behçet's syndrome or homocystinaemia.
→ major trauma (other than pelvis/lower limb) or burns
→ major immobilizing medical illness, e.g. heart or lung disease, cancer, inflam-matory bowel disease, septicaemia
→ minor surgery, trauma or illness in patients with previous DVT, PE or thrombophilia.

Moderate-risk patients should receive low-dose heparin prophylaxis and com-pression stockings.

Minor

The risk of DVT is less than 10 per cent and risk of PE less than 0.01 per cent.

→ minor surgery <30 minutes at any age with no other risk factors
→ major surgery >30 minutes at age <40 with no other risk factors
→ minor trauma or medical illness.

Low-risk patients should be mobilized immediately postoperatively.

What are the appearances of the post-DVT limb?

The post-thrombotic limb is characterized by chronic swelling with 'brawny' oedema and varicose veins owing to perforator incompetence. There is varicose eczema, with inflammation and discoloration owing to haemosiderin deposition above the medial malleolus. There may be signs of active or healed venous ulceration in the gaiter area, most typically just above the medial malleolus. There is lipodermatosclerosis around the ankle – the fibrotic response to chronic inflammation, which leads to a narrow atrophic ankle with oedema above – 'the beer-bottle leg'.

8. STAGING AND GRADING

What are the differences between staging and grading?

Grading is a solely histopathological assessment of a specimen and is generally on a scale of 1–3, with 1 representing a well-differentiated tumour in which recognizable patterns of the parent tissue are evident, whilst 3 is poorly differentiated with totally disorganized architecture and no relationship to parent tissue. Staging is the attempt to classify tumours into strata according to a variety of criteria, which gives an indication of prognosis. Initially purely clinical, it may now involve pathological data.

Give examples with regard to breast cancer

Breast cancer is graded histologically into well differentiated, moderately differentiated and poorly differentiated. Additional information usually supplied describes vascular and neural invasion.

Breast cancer is usually staged using a TNM system:

T_{is}	Carcinoma *in situ*
T_0	No evidence of primary tumour
T_1	Tumour <2 cm

(Continued)

T_2	Tumour 2–5 cm
T_3	Tumour >5 cm
T_4	Tumour of any size
a	Fixed to chest wall
b	Oedema, lymphocytic infiltration, skin ulceration or satellite nodes
c	Both a and b
N_0	No palpable nodes in ipsilateral axilla
N_1	Palpable nodes
N_2	Fixed ipsilateral axillary nodes
N_3	Clavicular nodes or arm oedema
M_0	No distant metastases
M_1	Distant metastases

Stage according to UICC is shown in Table 6.2. Locally advanced breast cancer (T_4) is shown in Figure 6.4.

Table 6.2 Stage according to UICC

Stage	TNM	Description	5-year survival
I	$T_1 N_0 M_0$	Early breast cancer	84 per cent
II	$T_1 N_1 M_0$; $T_2 N_{0-1} M_0$	Early breast cancer	71 per cent
III	Any T, $N_{2-3} M_0$; T_3, any N, M_0	Locally advanced breast cancer	48 per cent
IV	Any T, any N, M_1	Metastatic breast cancer	18 per cent

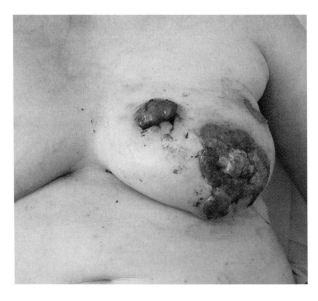

Figure 6.4 Locally advanced breast cancer (T4).

In the case of breast cancer, how can these be combined to give prognostic information?

The Nottingham Prognostic Index (NPI) is a pathological system that combines tumour grade, node status and tumour size, and has been validated as an accurate prognostic score:

Grade

Well differentiated	1 point
Moderately differentiated	2 points
Poorly differentiated	3 points

Positive lymph nodes

No nodes	1 point
1–3 nodes	2 points
>3 nodes	3 points

NPI = Grade + lymph node score + [size of tumour (cm) $\times$ 0.2]

A further point is added if vascular invasion is present.

Table 6.3 Nottingham Prognostic Index

NPI score	Prognosis	5-year survival
2.0–2.4	Excellent	93 per cent
2.4–3.4	Good	85 per cent
3.4–5.4	Moderate	70 per cent
>5.4	Poor	50 per cent

It can be seen from Table 6.3 that the 5-year survival figures for the good, moderate and poor grades of the NPI coincide closely with stages I–III of the TNM/UICC figures.

9. INFLAMMATION

What are the characteristics of inflammation?

These were described in around AD 30 by Celsus as rubor, tumour, calor and dolor, which in English equate to redness, swelling, heat and pain. Galen added loss of function (*functio laesa*) over a century later.

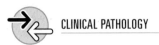

Which cells are commonly involved

Initially, the first cells involved are neutrophils, which exit the capillaries owing to the increased permeability afforded by the release of histamine and related substances from damaged endothelium; via the release of interleukins, these cells then control recruitment of other cell types and metabolic activity. Neutrophils are later followed by the arrival of activated macrophages. Between them, these two cell types are responsible for the demolition phase after injury, ridding the body of the debris of injury, and protecting against the ingress of bacteria and foreign matter. As the wound moves into the remodelling phase, these cells become less important, and fibroblasts and myofibroblasts assume primacy, although the macrophage is still important as a source of angiogenic stimuli for the formation of granulation tissue.

How is inflammation mediated?

Mediation of the inflammatory response is a complex interaction of many chemical messengers, some derived from the tissues, others released by activated cells. In addition, they may be preformed and stored, only being released when needed, such as histamine or serotonin, or they may be manufactured during the acute inflammatory event and released directly, such as prostaglandins, leukotrienes and cytokines.

What are interleukins? Outline the action of the common interleukins

Interleukins (ILs) are one class of substances under the general heading of cytokines that are responsible for modulation of the function of other cell types. They, along with the other cytokines, such as tumour necrosis factors and interferons, are polypeptides principally derived from activated lymphocytes and macrophages (see Table 6.4).

What is the complement cascade?

Complement is a series of proteins, numbered C1–9, synthesized in the liver and excreted into the plasma in an inactive form. When activated the complement compounds are chemotactic for phagocytes, promote opsonization and increase capillary permeability as part of the generalized inflammatory response. Once activated, the cascade allows other complement compounds to be activated in turn to allow continued opsonization of bacteria.

What defects of the complement system may be important clinically?

The pro-inflammatory role of complement can lead to host damage. This may be manifest by either inadequate activation of the system, resulting in susceptibility

Table 6.4 Interleukins

Interleukin	Source	Action
IL-1	Macrophages	Stimulates T cells and antigen presenting cells. Stimulates B cells, antibody production, and haematopoiesis. Potent pyrogen
IL-2	Activated T cells	Causes T-cell proliferation
IL-3	T lymphocytes	Promotes growth of blood cell precursors
IL-4	T cells/mast cells	Promotes B-cell proliferation and IgE production
IL-5	T cells/mast cells	Causes eosinophil growth
IL-6	Activated T cells	Synergistic with IL-1 or tumour necrosis factor α (TNFα)
IL-7	Thymus/bone marrow	Allows development of T- and B-cell precursors
IL-8	Macrophages	Chemotactic for neutrophils
IL-9	Activated T cells	Promotes T-cell and mast cell growth
IL-10	Activated T cells, B cells and monocytes	Inhibits inflammatory and immune responses
IL-11–IL-18		These have all been identified and are active in promoting haematopoiesis and cell proliferation and attraction

to infection, or it may be a hypersensitivity state because of excess complement activity. The best-known complement disorder is hereditary angioedema. Deficiency of C1 inhibitor leads to long-term activation of the system and minor traumatic stimuli can lead to frighteningly rapid mucosal oedema and airway occlusion. Another complement-associated disease is systemic lupus erythematosus (SLE), associated with increased release of complement responsible for microvascular injury. Other complement deficiencies lead to a susceptibility to pyogenic or neisserial infection.

Aurelius Celsus (25 BC–AD 50). A Roman gentleman, but not medically qualified, he wrote an eight-volume masterpiece called De Re Medicina, *in which he enunciated the cardinal signs of inflammation amongst other things.*

Galen (AD 131–201) was surgeon to the gladiators and Marcus Aurelius. He described operations for varicose veins, cleft lip, nasal polyps and the suturing of intestines, as well as naming the great vein within the skull that bears his name.

10. COLORECTAL CANCER

What does this radiological examination (Figure 6.5) show and what is the likely diagnosis?

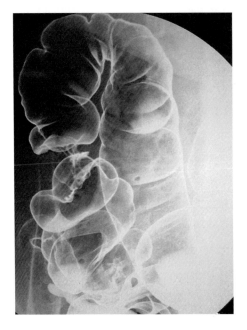

Figure 6.5

This is a double-contrast barium enema, which shows a colonic stricture. The stricture has a shouldered appearance, with loss of mucosal detail. This shouldered apple-core lesion would immediately make colonic carcinoma the most likely diagnosis.

How can the spread of colorectal cancer be assessed and staged?

It can spread by local extension, by lymphatic spread to local nodes, by portal spread to the liver and by systemic haematogenous spread either directly or via the liver to distant organs. Pre-operatively, this is assessed by a chest x-ray looking for evidence of pulmonary deposits, and an abdominal ultrasound or CT looking for evidence of liver disease. For rectal tumours, the extent of local extension is assessed by MRI scanning.

The pathological staging system attached to colorectal cancer (CRC) is that of Cuthbert Dukes, originally written in 1932 and classifying only rectal tumours (see Table 6.5). It is now used for all colorectal tumours and is the standard in the UK; other systems including TNM are widely used in addition to Dukes' staging.

Table 6.5 Dukes' staging system

Dukes' stage	Description	5-year survival rate
A	Tumour confined to the bowel wall. No lymph node involvement	90 per cent
B	Tumour outside of bowel wall. No lymph node involvement	70 per cent
C	Lymph node involvement. C_2 if the highest node is involved, otherwise C_1	C_1 – 60 per cent, C_2 – 35 per cent
D	Distant metastasis. This stage was added later	~15 per cent

What surgery would you perform for a CRC:

In the distal transverse colon?

An extended right hemicolectomy. The transverse colon at that point often has a variable blood supply and, to obtain oncological clearance, the entire colon supplied by the ileocolic and middle colic arteries is resected. In addition, the theoretical risk of poor marginal artery supply to the splenic flexure is avoided.

12 cm from the anal verge?

At this height, an anterior resection would be appropriate, with either a hand-sewn or a stapled anastomosis.

4 cm from the anal verge?

An abdomino-perineal resection. Although an ultralow, sphincter-saving anterior resection might be possible, you would need to think very carefully before doing so, particularly with regard to the patient's age, mobility and pre-operative sphincter control.

What could you do if the patient had liver metastases?

In virtually all circumstances, surgical intervention should be considered. In the vast majority of cases, patients present because of symptoms from their primary tumour, be it bleeding, faecal frequency, anaemia, tenesmus or impending obstruction. The liver should be fully assessed for resectability before operating. If potentially resectable, then a potentially curative colonic resection is performed, but if there were no chance of hepatic resection, then a palliative procedure should be considered. This may be a colorectal stenting procedure, a tumour bypass or a defunctioning stoma to alleviate symptoms. In the longer term, in those that survive their surgery, consideration should be given to chemotherapy, usually infusional 5-fluorouracil intravenously or sometimes given into the hepatic artery.

In a well patient with liver metastases, various forms of hepatectomy can be performed, depending upon the distribution of the lesions, removing up to 90 per cent of hepatic tissue with regeneration of the remaining liver. Currently, less than 25 per cent of patients are suitable for consideration of resection of hepatic metastases. In those that do undergo surgery, the current 5-year survival rate is around 40 per cent.

Describe the evidence supporting the colonic adenoma–carcinoma sequence

There is no definite but much circumstantial evidence for this sequence. In about 80 per cent of people with a colorectal cancer at least one other adenoma is found. The distribution of adenomas around the colon matches that of carcinomas and, in areas where anomalies of distribution of one exist, so the distribution of the other varies similarly. In excised carcinomas, there are often areas of adenoma and, similarly, adenomas may be excised endoscopically and found to contain some carcinomatous elements. The strongest circumstantial evidence comes from familial adenomatous polyposis (FAP). Here, the genetic defect carpets the colon in many hundreds of adenomas at an early age and, if untreated, all patients will have developed carcinoma by the age of 40.

Cuthbert Dukes (1890–1977). Consultant Pathologist at St Mark's Hospital, London. In 1932, he published 'Classification of cancer of the rectum' in the Journal of Pathology and Bacteriology. *Aside from this classical paper, he made significant contributions to other areas of colorectal pathology. He instituted a registry of familial polyposis-related cancers at St Mark's, which yielded much information about this disease. Most unusually for a pathologist, he also visited patients at home and published a paper in* The Lancet *in 1947 detailing the problems of living with a permanent colostomy.*

11. SCREENING FOR DISEASE

What is the purpose of a screening test?

To detect at an early treatable stage a serious disease in an asymptomatic population.

What are the requirements for a successful screening programme?

→ A disease that is an important problem, is treatable, or can be pre-empted, and it is known that early detection yields better outcomes.

→ An identifiable target population containing the majority of those at risk.

→ Resources available for a screening programme:
  ● programmed – patients are identified, then asked to be screened
  ● opportunistic – patients with risk factors are screened for associated diseases at presentation.
→ resources and facilities for treatment of newly diagnosed disease.

And what characteristics should the test have?

The test should be sensitive, specific and reproducible. It should be acceptable and safe to the screened population, and should generally be non-invasive. It must be cost effective.

Explain sensitivity and specificity

→ *Sensitivity* describes the ability of the test to detect all the people who actually have the disease, i.e. true positives. For example, a test that is 90 per cent sensitive will miss 10 per cent of the population who actually have the disease; these are the false negatives. A high sensitivity is required so that large numbers of people with the disease are not missed.
→ *Specificity* describes the ability of the test genuinely to exclude the disease in those who do not have it, i.e. few false positives. For example, a test that is 80 per cent specific will pick up 80 true cases and 20 false positives per 100 cases. A high specificity is desirable so as not to falsely diagnose or worry people who do not actually have the condition.

Describe the UK breast screening programme

Following the 1986 Forrest report, the UK introduced 3-yearly mammographic screening for women between the ages of 50 and 64 years. Women undergo two-view mammography at the first visit and single view thereafter. Suspicious films are followed up by further views and clinical examination. Imminent changes to the service include taking two views at each visit (by 2003) and raising the upper age limit to 70 years (by 2004).

What are the controversies surrounding breast cancer screening in UK?

Studies from around the world have shown definite reductions in mortality from breast cancer after introduction of breast screening. The two most famous trials were the Health Insurance Plan (HIP) of New York and the Swedish Two Counties studies, both of which used a screening interval shorter than the UK programme. The sequelae of using 3-yearly screens, as opposed to 2-yearly (Swedes) or even yearly (New York), is the incidence of interval cancers that present clinically with the rate roughly doubling for each interval year. It has been estimated that it costs in the region of £1 million for each breast cancer detected. The first reports of the UK programme failed to show any significant reduction in mortality, although later reports are showing benefits. There is no demonstrable benefit from screening women under the age of 50.

Describe an effective screening programme for a non-malignant disease

Screening the abdominal aortas of men over the age of 65 by a single abdominal ultrasound has been shown by several large randomized trials to reduce the mortality from abdominal aortic aneurysms. It has also been shown to be cost effective. Screening in women is not effective, presumably because of the lower rate of rupture of these aneurysms in women.

Describe an instance of targeted screening

Investigation of the siblings of an index case of a heritable disease would be classed as targeted screening. Good examples are colonoscopy for families of patients with familial adenomatous polyposis or hereditary non-polyposis colorectal cancer.

12. CALCULI

Define a calculus

A mass of precipitated solid material in a duct or organ.

What are the commonest types of calculi to develop?

The commonest types are: biliary; urinary; pancreatic; salivary and prostatic. Prostate calculi are probably the commonest with the majority of TURP specimens containing stones, although not necessarily the most clinically prevalent.

How may renal calculi cause symptoms and what are they made of?

Passage of the stone down the ureter gives rise to a most excruciating short-lived colicky pain, which recurs after only a few minutes. During an attack, the patient generally rolls from side to side in an attempt to relieve the agony. The diagnosis is in doubt if there is no blood on urinalysis, as this is an almost universal finding.

Two clinical presentations deserve special consideration in this setting. Beware the middle-aged patient presenting with their first attack of renal colic, as a leaking abdominal aortic aneurysm is a major differential diagnosis. The young patient with excruciating pain and no blood in the urine may be seeking opiate analgesia for personal gratification. If the stone obstructs the urinary system, the resultant hydronephrosis gives a dull loin ache with colicky exacerbations. It is easily infected, resulting in a pyonephrosis with concomitant systemic upset and may be the cause of septicaemia. It may result in complete destruction of the kidney. Infection both increases the risk of urinary stones and is increased by the presence of calculi. Virtually no stone passes through the urinary system without making the urothelium bleed. The haematuria may be microscopic on dipstick testing alone or may occasionally present as frank haematuria.

Renal stones may be classified as primary or secondary. Primary stones are made up of urate, oxalate, cystine or xanthine, owing to an excess of these metabolites in the urine as a result of metabolic abnormalities. Secondary stones are made up of calcium phosphate, calcium bicarbonate and the magnesium ammonium phosphate triple stone.

What factors predispose to renal calculi?

→ Anatomical abnormalities that might cause stasis in the system or reflux. Such conditions include a duplex system, urethral valves in newborns or horseshoe kidney.
→ Stasis for other reasons – pelviureteric junction obstruction is the commonest.
→ Infection – particularly by *Proteus* species, which are urea-splitting, thus causing an alkaline urine that causes precipitation and hence calculi formation.
→ Increased concentration of calcium ion. This will cause both nephrocalcinosis and calculi formation, and occurs in hyperparathyroidism.

How can renal stones be retrieved?

→ They may pass naturally. This is likely, if the stone is less than 5 mm in diameter on the KUB film, and becomes increasingly unlikely as size increases. Only 10 per cent of stones greater than 8 mm will pass spontaneously.
→ Ureteroscopy and graspers or a Dormier basket will be able to retrieve smaller stones in the lower third of the ureter.
→ Lithotripsy will allow larger stones to be broken down, thus allowing passage or removal by one of the other means.
→ Percutaneous nephrolithotomy – progressive dilation of a track into the kidney may sometimes allow percutaneous extraction of a large staghorn calculus.
→ Open nephrolithotomy is rarely required these days but was traditionally performed for large staghorn calculi of the renal pelvis (Figure 6.6).

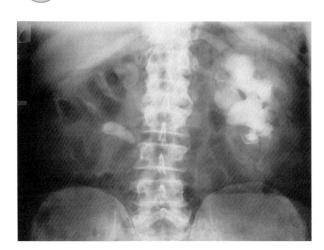

Figure 6.6 X-ray of staghorn calculi.

13. WOUND HEALING

Describe the processes involved in the healing of a skin wound

This is traditionally divided into healing by primary or secondary intention, although the underlying processes are essentially the same. Healing by primary intention occurs in cleanly incised wounds with closely opposed edges where there is minimal soft tissue loss, the surgical wound being a good example. The stages of healing are as follows.

→ *Haemostasis.* A combination of arteriolar constriction, fibrinogen and plate-let activation alongside the coagulation cascades promote haemostasis. The haematoma at the site of injury is rich in thrombin and platelet-derived growth factor, which stimulates fibroblast division.

→ *Inflammatory response.* Capillary dilatation gives rise to a fluid and cellular exudate. This is initially neutrophil rich and serves to remove the tissue debris and bacteria at the site of injury. One to two days after injury the cellular infiltrate is predominantly macrophages.

→ *Epidermal growth.* Within hours of injury, cell migration occurs to cover the raw area, aided by an increased mitotic proliferation of new epidermal cells from the basal layers a few cells remote from the cut edge. These cells grow under the surface of the fibrin/fibronectin clot and will also track down along suture lines; this is the reason epidermoid inclusion cysts sometimes occur.

→ *Dermal events.* Macrophage infiltration begins demolishing the inflamma-tory exudate. These macrophages also secrete the cytokines, which attract fibroblasts and increase the activity of local fibroblasts to secrete extracellular repair proteins. Tumour necrosis factor α secretion occurs, which is a potent stimulus to angiogenesis from the wound edges. Part of the process of new blood vessel formation is a degradation of the capillary wall of the existing vessels to allow budding to occur; this also makes the capillaries leaky, creating an exudative mass of fragile capillaries, which we see as granulation tissue.

→ *Collagen deposition.* Hydroxyapatite deposition begins within hours of injury, which is subsequently converted to collagen, polymerized and, over the course of many months, remodelled to gain its ultimate strength, which is always weaker than the original tissue.

It should be noted that the dermal and epidermal events take place simultaneously and are only separated here for ease for description.

Healing by secondary intention occurs in those wounds where there has been loss of epithelial and subepithelial tissue. It varies only quantitatively from healing by primary intention but does demonstrate wound contraction in addition. This is true contraction of the wound edges and may in some species be able to close a defect entirely. It is distinct from the epidermal ingrowth that occurs and from the contraction that occurs with the drying of the fibrin clot. The contraction is produced by the action of myofibroblast cells that appear at the wound edges.

Describe the classical stages in the healing of a long bone fracture

Fracture of a long bone results in haemorrhage from the torn ends of periosteum and from the disrupted marrow as well as the surrounding soft tissue. This fills the bone defect with a clot rich in plasma proteins – the stage of haematoma formation. It is the site of the subsequent inflammatory response with neutrophil and later macrophage invasion. The macrophages are particularly important for resorption of the necrotic bone and marrow, which occurs at the fracture site and for a little distance back from it. Subsequent resorption of the haematoma leads to formation of granulation tissue. Following this, there is formation of callus around the outside of the fracture site mediated by osteoprogenitor cells from the torn periosteal ends. Initially, this provisional callus traverses the outside of the bony defect and only later does medullary callus actually fill the gap. Conversion to woven bone occurs in most cases by gradual endochondral ossification of the provisional callus. By this stage, the fracture is immobile and healed, although it will take many months to regain full strength, as this woven bone is gradually resorbed and replaced by true lamellar bone.

Describe the complications of a bony fracture and its healing

The systemic complications of fractures are thankfully not common but are important.

Hypovolaemic shock may occur after long bone fracture; a femoral fracture may lose 2 L of blood into the surrounding soft tissues. Disruption of the marrow releases fat globules into the circulation, giving rise to fat embolism, a cause of ARDS in these patients. ARDS may occur in the absence of fat emboli as a result of a systemic inflammatory response to the injury and conversely fat emboli may be identified in the absence of bony fracture. The fracture may also be a portal for infection and subsequent septicaemia.

The local complications may be broadly divided into early or late complications.

Early local complications include infection of the bone or overlying soft tissues and neurovascular injury, especially at particular sites, such as a supracondylar humeral fracture, causing brachial artery injury. There may be associated joint injury or the fracture may cause additional soft tissue injuries, such as a pneumo-thorax associated with rib fracture. All long bone fractures must be carefully assessed to exclude the presence of a compartment syndrome, which may cause disability far in excess of the fracture itself.

Late local complications are generally complications of bone healing rather than the injury itself.

→ Delayed union or non-union may occur. These are separated only temporally. The dividing line between delayed healing and no healing is vague.

→ Although a fracture may heal, its position may be such as to be described as mal-union.

→ Elbow injuries are particularly prone to myositis ossificans, which is depos-ition of calcific material in the muscles and soft tissue around the joint. It occurs more severely after passive movement, so active mobilization is the key in rehabilitating elbow fractures.

→ All bone fractures may predispose to osteoarthritis, either by direct disruption of the joint or by imperfect healing causing altered patterns of wear on joints.

→ Bone injuries in children impinging on the growth plates may cause permanent disruption of growth leading to short limbs.

→ Certain bones are at particular risk of avascular necrosis following fracture owing to peculiarities of their vascular supply. Good examples are the necro-sis of the proximal pole of the scaphoid after a 'waist' fracture as the arterial supply is from distal to proximal and that of the femoral head after intra-capsular femoral neck fractures interfering with the retinacular supply.

→ Less common but potentially disabling complications include Volkmann's ischaemic contracture after a missed vascular injury or reflex sympathetic dystrophy, which may occur after a trivial injury.

14. THYROID

How would you assess a patient with an enlarged thyroid gland (Figure 6.7)?

By history, examination and special investigation. The history includes all rele-vant information about hypothyroid or hyperthyroid symptoms, area of

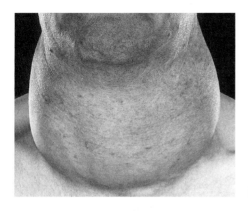

Figure 6.7 An enormous symmetrical goitre.

upbringing, exposure to radiation and duration of symptoms. The examination makes an assessment of the thyroid status by regard to the pulse, sweaty palms, tremor, and quality of the integument as well as the gland itself. The gland should be assessed for the following features:

→ degree of enlargement
→ nodular or diffusely enlarged
→ tenderness
→ retrosternal extension
→ lymphadenopathy
→ tracheal deviation
→ SVC compression
→ presence of eye signs; **although I would not look for eye signs, if the clinical findings were not those of Graves' disease**.

Blood should be sent for thyroid function tests, a description that varies from laboratory to laboratory but generally includes a thyroid-stimulating hormone (TSH) assay, and only goes on to include T4 and T3 testing if the TSH is abnormal. Thyroid autoantibodies are requested, but are non-specific for thyroid autoimmune disease, but the long-acting thyroid-stimulating hormone (LATS) of Graves' disease is not testable.

Fine-needle aspiration cytology (FNAC) of any lump is mandatory. It will reveal whether a nodule is cystic or solid, and provides a sample for cytological examination.

An ultrasound scan can give information about the morphology of the gland and the disposition of nodules, and whether areas are solid or cystic, but **it is neither sensitive nor specific for thyroid malignancy**, as the incidence of carcinoma in cysts, multinodular change and solitary lumps is similar.

What diagnoses can you confidently make on FNAC?

Possible results are:

→ benign
→ papillary carcinoma
→ follicular cells
→ thyroiditis
→ lymphoma
→ insufficient sample.

It is important to remember that FNAC looks at the cells themselves, not the way in which there are arranged, which in some instances is crucial. Thus, it can give a definite answer of benign thyroid tissue or papillary carcinoma, but can only tell you that there are follicular cells present, as the differentiation between follicular carcinoma and adenoma rests on the presence of an intact – or otherwise – capsule, which is not possible from cytology alone.

Discuss thyroid cancers, their treatment and prognosis

→ *Papillary carcinoma.* This is the commonest type accounting for >70 per cent of all thyroid cancers and occurs in the young, and women twice as often as men. It may be radiation induced. Papillary carcinomas are often multifocal and demonstrate early lymph node spread, with 40 per cent having nodal disease at presentation, and late haematogenous spread. Lymph node spread does not worsen prognosis. Treatment is by total thyroidectomy and resection of palpable local nodes. Postoperatively high-dose thyroxine is given to completely suppress TSH. Radio-iodine may be used to ablate any remaining thyroid tissue. Five-year survival approaches 100 per cent.
→ *Follicular carcinoma.* This has an incidence of about 15 per cent of thyroid malignancies and a mean age of onset of 50 years of age; it is increased in iodine-deficient areas. It is usually a solitary lesion with early haematogenous spread. Treatment is by total thyroidectomy with or without radio-iodine. The 5-year survival is between 50 and 100 per cent depending on the presence of metastases.
→ *Medullary carcinoma* presents as a hard lump with spread to cervical lymph nodes. Eighty per cent are sporadic, the rest familial, some as part of MEN syndromes. Treatment is by total thyroidectomy. Surgery is curative in the absence of metastases, but the 5-year survival falls to 50 per cent with metastases.
→ *Anaplastic carcinoma.* Typically presents in elderly patients with rapidly growing tumours and pressure symptoms. Treatment is by debulking and radiotherapy, but is generally palliative. Most patients are dead within 6 months.
→ *Lymphoma.* This accounts for less than 2 per cent of thyroid tumours and are usually B-cell tumours often arising in Hashimoto's thyroiditis. Treatment is with steroids, radiotherapy and, more rarely, thyroidectomy.

It is a peculiarity of thyroid cancers that males fare less well than females across all types except thyroid lymphomas. Increasing age is a further poor prognostic indicator, as is increasing grade and extra thyroidal spread in non-papillary tumours.

15. BONE DISEASE

Describe the causes of osteoporosis and osteomalacia?

Osteoporosis is a decrease in the bone density associated with an increased risk of fracture. The bone is fully mineralized, but the trabecular plates and spas are thinned and reduced. Predisposing conditions include old age and the post-menopausal state, which are known as idiopathic causes, and secondary causes such as:

→ immobilization
→ thyrotoxicosis
→ drug therapy from steroids, alcohol and heparin
→ Cushing's syndrome
→ rheumatoid arthritis, although this may be a disuse effect.

Diagnosis should not rely on plain radiographic evidence, as changes are only evident after one-third of the bone has been lost. Bone densitometry is accurate at an earlier stage. Serum calcium, alkaline phosphatase and vitamin D levels are normal. Treatment is aimed at the prevention of bone loss and, therefore, fractures. In post-menopausal women, hormone replacement therapy has been shown to decrease the rate of bone loss. Exercise, fluoridation and vitamin D also appear to help, although the effects on fracture reduction are less clear-cut.

Osteomalacia is characterized by deficient mineralization and an increase in the production of osteoid, unmineralized bone matrix. The causes include:

→ calcium/vitamin D deficiency, which may be nutritional, malabsorptive or metabolic
→ sunlight deprivation
→ renal tubular disease.

In children, it classically presents as rickets with the cardinal features of tibial bowing, bone pain, muscular weakness, failure to thrive and bossed forehead.

Blood tests are more useful in the diagnosis of osteomalacia than osteoporosis, as serum calcium and phosphate are reduced, as is urinary calcium. Serum alkaline phosphatase is increased. Plain x-rays show areas of thinning of the bone, known as Looser's zones. A bone biopsy will show widened seams of increased amounts of osteoid.

Osteoporosis is a common cause of pathological fractures. Give a definition of a pathological fracture and list other causes

A pathological fracture is one through a previously abnormal bone.

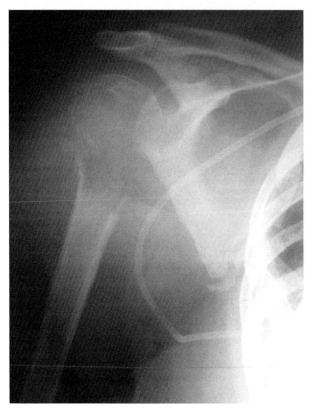

Figure 6.8 A pathological fracture through the surgical neck of humerus through a malignant deposit.

The causes are:

→ osteoporosis – the commonest cause
→ bony metastases
→ osteomalacia/rickets
→ primary bone tumour
→ congenital defects such as osteogenesis imperfecta. This is a defect of collagen manufacture resulting in weak bones, and in some types, blue sclera. Surviving patients suffer multiple fractures in the early years of life.

What tumours commonly metastasize to bone? Which are sclerotic and which are lytic?

Generally adenocarcinomas metastasize to bone. The two commonest are breast and prostate, with bronchus, thyroid and kidney making up the majority of the rest. All are porotic except prostate, which may be porotic, but is more commonly sclerotic.

Which primary malignancies affect bone?

→ *Osteogenic sarcoma.* A tumour of the young (10–30 years), with males slightly more commonly affected than females. A second peak occurs in the elderly in association with Paget's disease. It commonly occurs in the ends of long bones, typically around the knee. The typical radiographic appearances are sunray spicules of new bone formation and Codman's triangle of raised periosteum. The treatment is surgical resection in a specialist unit, where the chances of limb sparing surgery are increased, and chemotherapy. Five-year survival rates of about 60 per cent in those who present without metastases are achievable.

→ *Chondrosarcoma.* A malignant tumour of cartilage, particularly in the flat bones and vertebrae. Treatment is along similar lines to osteogenic sarcoma, but the 5-year survival is slightly worse.

→ *Multiple myeloma.* A tumour of the medullary plasma cells giving rise to abnormal protein production. The alkaline phosphatase is normal. The x-ray appearances are classical – multiple punched out lesions, typically in the skull producing a 'pepperpot skull'.

→ *Ewing's sarcoma.* A very aggressive malignant tumour usually presenting below the age of 20 years. It gives an onionskin appearance on x-ray. A raised ESR and fever are common presenting features. Treatment is by excision and chemoradiotherapy. Five-year survival is up to 60 per cent.

16. INFLAMMATORY BOWEL DISEASE

Describe the typical pathological features of Crohn's disease

Crohn's disease is a segmental, discontinuous, full-thickness inflammation of the bowel affecting the whole gastrointestinal tract from mouth to anus, which may have associated extraintestinal manifestations. Terminal ileitis is the commonest gastrointestinal lesion. The mucosa is reddened with small apthous ulcers that develop into superficial spreading ulcers with submucosal oedema and an increase in lymphoid tissue. This process may progress to deep narrow transmural ulcers and may result in fistulation – a common feature of Crohn's disease. Extensive fissuring may leave islands of raised mucosa – cobblestoning. In advanced disease, the bowel wall becomes fibrotic, giving rise to small bowel strictures or even longer 'hosepipe' segments. Although Crohn's is recognized as a chronic granulomatous condition, granulomata are only found in about 70 per cent of specimens.

What is a granuloma?

It is a collection of activated macrophages.

What surgical interventions are common in Crohn's disease?

As Crohn's is a disease of the whole gastrointestinal tract, no resectional procedure is likely to be reliably curative as compared to ulcerative colitis. Surgical intervention should, therefore, be kept to a minimum and the maximum length of bowel preserved. However, it should be noted that recurrence rates are independent of resection extent and are not increased if there is microscopic, but not macroscopic, Crohn's disease at the resection margins. Patients should be considered for surgery before advanced disease occurs, because mortality and morbidity are reduced and more conservative resections are possible with early surgical intervention. Localized terminal ileal disease may be treated by a limited ileocaecal resection, which in many cases turns out to be the only surgical intervention necessary. Small bowel strictures should ideally be treated by strictureplasty, as opposed to resection and anastomosis, as this will preserve intestinal length. Perianal sepsis with fistulation is a particular problem associated with Crohn's disease and surgical intervention should be weighed against the risk of perianal recurrence. It should be treated by clinicians with specialist interest in the condition. A presentation of multiple/recurrent fistula should always raise the question of Crohn's disease involvement.

What are the typical clinical features of ulcerative colitis?

The commonest presentation is with diarrhoea with marked faecal urgency. There is often blood present with the diarrhoea. This may be associated with abdominal pain, although pain is more often a feature of Crohn's disease. There is associated malaise, anorexia and weight loss. There are several well-recognized extraintestinal manifestations of the disease, some of which are related to disease activity, such as pyoderma gangrenosum, erythema nodosum, mucous apthous ulcers, iritis and large joint arthritis. Those not related to disease activity include sacroileitis/ankylosing spondylitis, chronic active hepatitis, cirrhosis, sclerosing cholangitis, primary biliary cirrhosis and clubbing.

How is it treated?

The treatment is primarily medical. In the acute attack, steroids are used to induce remission, which is then maintained by 5-aminosalicylic acid (5-ASA) derivatives, such as mesalazine. Localized proctitis may be treated by foam ene-mata of either steroids or 5-ASA, but widespread disease requires oral or IV therapy. Treatments including oral budesonide and azathioprine have been used to reduce the impact of standard steroid therapy.

What are the indications for surgery in ulcerative colitis?

This is generally for one of the following three reasons.

→ Failure of medical therapy. Signified by recurrent attacks, rapidly relapsing disease on maximal medical therapy, or where the disease is causing chronic disability or failure to thrive.
→ Acute complications of the disease, such as toxic dilatation, perforation or uncontrollable haemorrhage.
→ Prophylaxis. Ulcerative colitis increases the risk of colonic adenocarcinoma; the risk is calculated at 1 per cent per year after 10 years of disease.

What surgical options are available for the elective management of ulcerative colitis?

See Table 6.6.

Table 6.6 Elective surgical options for ulcerative colitis

Operation	Advantages	Disadvantages
Proctocolectomy and ileostomy	Single operation No surveillance needed	Permanent end stoma All disease removed
Colectomy and ileorectal anastomosis (if rectal sparing)	Single procedure No stoma	Residual rectum with recurrent disease and cancer risk needing surveillance
Proctocolectomy and pouch reconstruction	Usually continent All disease removed	Often >1 operation Complications are common (30%)

Burrill Bernard Crohn (1884–1983). Crohn was a practitioner at the Mount Sinai Hospital and presented his paper on the condition of regional ileitis in 1932 at the meeting of the American Gastroenterology Society (ASG). He was the most junior of the researchers who wrote the paper, but his name gained the primary position only because of alphabetical order and has remained attached to the disease ever since. Three years later he was elected President of the ASG. He went on to build up a hugely successful practice at Mount Sinai dealing with granulomatous enterocolitis and remained professionally active to the age of 88.

17. TISSUE SAMPLING

By what methods can you make a tissue diagnosis?

Tissue diagnosis can be made by obtaining cells for cytology, a biopsy for histology or complete excision of the lesion for histological examination.

What methods of collecting cytological material are there?

Cells for cytology may be obtained from surface lesions by scraping or brushing them, as in cervical smear cytology. Aspiration of fluid collections, such as ascites, can be examined cytologically, as can lavage specimens, as is commonly performed during bronchoscopy. These large volume aspirates are centrifuged to collect the cellular material, then examined microscopically. Solid lesions may yield cells for cytology by fine needle aspiration.

Describe how you would perform FNAC

The procedure is first explained to the patient. The equipment is set up, with an 18-gauge needle on a 10 ml syringe, with 2–3 ml of air in the syringe. The left hand is used to steady the lesion, the overlying skin swabbed with an alcohol wipe and the needle inserted at right angles to the skin and into the lesion. A note should be made of the texture of the lesion as it is entered, as this sometimes gives a clue to its origin. Once the needle tip is in the lesion, suction is applied to the syringe barrel and the needle passed through the lesion several times in different planes. The needle is withdrawn, releasing the negative pressure just before exiting the lesion and a dressing applied with firm pressure over the needle hole. The contents of the needle and syringe are expelled onto pre-labelled glass slides or into cytology fluid in its container. Slides can then be treated according to the preference of the local cytologist with regard to air or alcohol fixation. Slides or cytology fluid are sent to the cytologist with a request card detailing the relevant clinical information.

What are the limits of cytology?

Interpretation of the specimen relies on an experienced cytologist. The sample may be insufficient to give any clues. It should be remembered that it is a sample – a clinically malignant lump may give rise to a FNAC report of 'no malignant cells seen'; this does not exclude the diagnosis of malignancy. The greatest limitation is that it gives no information on the architectural arrangement of cells within the lesion, which may be important. FNAC, for example, cannot differentiate a thyroid follicular adenoma from a carcinoma.

FNAC of a breast lump will commonly be reported as C 1–5. What do those grades mean?

It is a reasonably reproducible grading system designed to minimize inter-observer discrepancy:

→ C1 – insufficient for diagnosis
→ C2 – benign
→ C3 – cellular atypia
→ C4 – suspicion of cancer
→ C5 – malignant.

Define biopsy

A biopsy is defined as a representative sample of tissue for histological diagnosis. It follows, therefore, that excisional biopsy is a misnomer. A biopsy may be incisional, wedge, punch or shave in type.

What is a 'core biopsy' and where do we see it used?

A core biopsy is performed to remove a representative piece of tissue for histological examination so that cell architecture can be assessed in addition to cytological features. It is performed under local anaesthetic under direct control for palpable lumps or radiological control for image-defined lesions. Local anaesthetic is injected into the skin overlying the lesion, which is punctured with a scalpel blade, allowing the larger core needle to be advanced to the lesion. When the core gun (see Figure 6.9) is fired, the hollow needle advances followed by its cover. When the needle is withdrawn, the covering part of the needle is drawn back enabling a core of tissue to be removed for histological examination. It is commonly used in diagnosis of breast lumps and in the assessment of intra-abdominal masses under radiological control.

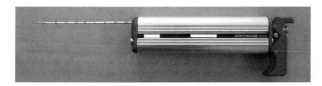

Figure 6.9 One of the variety of core biopsy guns available.

18. CARCINOGENESIS

How may viruses cause disease?

There are three basic mechanisms by which viruses cause disease.

→ *Direct cytopathic effect.* Virus particles damage the cells, and their membranes, in particular, resulting in an increased permeability and consequent dysfunction. This is the mechanism of effect of the hepatitis A virus in the liver, acute infection causing hepatic dysfunction from hepatocellular damage.

→ *Induction of the immune response.* Infected cells themselves are not harmed but the virus causes new antigen expression on the cell surface. These new antigens are not recognized, and evoke an immune response, which, if adequate, will destroy the infected cells. However, in an individual who mounts a poor immune response, the infected cells are not lysed, and the patient may become a symptomless carrier of the virus particles. An example is hepatitis B virus infection, which has both acute disease and carrier states.

→ *Incorporation of the viral genetic material into the host cell genome.* DNA viruses can be directly incorporated, whereas RNA viruses copy a DNA transcript into the host DNA. This occurs in RNA viruses that have the ability to cause reverse transcriptase enzyme activity, commonly known as retroviruses. An example of a viral-mediated neoplasm is Burkitt's lymphoma occurring in response to Epstein–Barr virus.

What are the main classes of carcinogens, and give an example of each?

The five main classes are as follows.

→ *Chemicals.* Exposure to different chemicals may give rise to certain tumours. Evidence for these effects has traditionally been epidemiological. The best-known example is tobacco and its combustion products. There are a number of associated tumours, but the commonest is carcinoma of the lung. The most important combustion products are the hydrocarbons, e.g. 3,4-benzpyrene.

→ *Viruses.* As discussed above, viruses can cause neoplastic transformation. A further example is hepatitis B virus and hepatocellular carcinoma, which are strongly associated.

→ *Radiation – both ionizing and non-ionizing.* Exposure to ultraviolet light, usually in sunlight, is a major factor in the development of skin cancers, particularly basal cell carcinomas and malignant melanomas. The radiation causes damage to the host skin cell's DNA, which leads to neoplastic growth.

→ *Biological agents.* Some tumours are related to other organisms, or even compounds produced by our own cells. Examples include tumorigenesis induced by oestrogens, and cholangiocarcinomas being induced in patients infected with the Chinese liver fluke *Clonorchis sinensis*.

→ *Miscellaneous*. This includes carcinogens where mechanisms are not understood, such as asbestos and mesotheliomas and lung tumours.

What are occupational cancers?

They are malignancies that occur as a direct result of exposure to a carcinogen in the course of a particular occupation. Traditionally, the evidence for such cancers has been epidemiological and is typified by the observation of Sir Percival Pott in 1775 of a greatly increased incidence of scrotal tumours in chimney sweeps exposed to hydrocarbons in soot. A further example of clustering of cancer cases by occupation was noted in 1895 when aniline was (wrongly) attributed to be the cause of bladder cancer in the chemical dye industry. Subsequent work has identified certain aromatic amines, such as β-naphthylamine as being the agent responsible. It is estimated that up to 20 per cent of bladder cancers in Europe and the USA are still occupationally related.

19. SKIN CANCER

Classify skin cancers

Malignant neoplasms of the skin may be primary or secondary. Secondary lesions may occur as cutaneous metastases from most tumours. Of the primary lesions, basal cell carcinoma (BCC) is commonest followed by squamous cell lesions and then malignant melanoma. Thereafter there are rarities: Merkel cell tumour, Paget's disease of skin, sebaceous carcinomas and sarcomas. Lymphoma has a cutaneous variant called mycosis fungoides.

Describe a classical BCC

See Figure 6.10. Also known as a rodent ulcer, they typically present in the hair-bearing skin of elderly people, commonly with a long history of sun exposure. Other predisposing factors include smoking, xeroderma pigmentosum and radiation/radiotherapy exposure. They appear as a small waxy nodule, which progresses into an ulcer with a pearly rolled edge and telangectasia, although several different macroscopic appearances are described. Although malignant, they rarely metastasize, but can be locally invasive and potentially disfiguring.

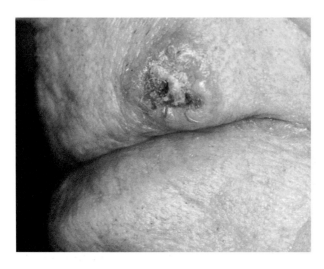

Figure 6.10 A typical BCC on the face. Note the rolled edge and the classical location.

Where are they commonest?

They are commonest on the face above a line drawn from the angle of the mouth to the external auditory meatus, although they can appear anywhere except the palms of the hands and soles of the feet.

How can BCCs be treated?

Treatment is usually by local excision with margins of less than 0.5 cm for discrete lesions; this allows histological confirmation of tumour type and completeness of excision. Small lesions can be treated by cryotherapy. Radiotherapy can also be used, somewhat perversely, as it predisposes to BCC formation, and gives excellent results when used therapeutically, but cannot be used around the eyes or for lesions overlying cartilage, such as pinna or the nose.

What is Moh's method?

It is serial tangential excision of a lesion with frozen section histology. This allows confirmation of complete excision in all planes. It is, however, labour intensive and time consuming, and thus very expensive.

What is the pathology of a squamous cell carcinoma?

The squamous cell carcinoma (SCC) is a very common skin cancer related to chronic sun exposure or certain other carcinogens, such as tar and arsenic. These carcinomas are commonest on the sun-exposed skins of the elderly, and appear as scaly lesions or ulcers (see Figure 6.11). Histologically, keratinocytes show typical malignant disordered growth and cellular atypia. Their behaviour is usually fairly

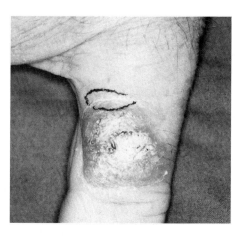

Figure 6.11 The typical scaly appearance of an SCC on a finger.

indolent and metastatic spread unusual. When metastases do occur, they are at a late stage and usually via the lymphatic system. Treatment is by local excision.

What is a Marjolin's ulcer?

The original description was of an SCC developing in a healed burns scar, but the eponym has subsequently been appended to similar malignant transformation in chronic venous or osteomyelitic ulcers.

What is a keratoacanthoma and what is it mistaken for?

It is a benign skin lesion occurring on sun-damaged skin. It grows rapidly for up to 6 months and then regresses. It is highly keratotic, and looks histologically similar to a SCC, which it may be mistaken for. It is self-limiting and of unknown aetiology.

20. DIVERTICULA

What is a diverticulum?

A diverticulum is an abnormal outpouching of a hollow viscus into the surrounding tissues.

What is the difference between true and false diverticula? Give examples

A true diverticulum contains all layers of the wall of the viscus, whereas only some layers are present in a false diverticulum. Diverticula may also be classified according to their aetiology, and be congenital or acquired. Congenital diverticula tend to be true diverticula.

A Meckel's diverticulum is a true diverticulum. It is said to arise in 2 per cent of the population, is 2 inches long and is found 2 feet from the ileocaecal valve. It is a remnant of the vitellointestinal duct and so is congenital. It can be a cause of right iliac fossa pain. The diverticula found in the sigmoid colon are good examples of acquired false diverticula and are presumed to be caused by raised intraluminal pressure causing out-pouchings of mucosa to occur where blood vessels pass between the muscle of the taenia coli.

What are the complications of colonic diverticula?

Colonic diverticula are increasingly common as people age and are estimated to be present in over three-quarters of the population over the age of 75. They have been putatively associated with a Western diet low in fibre, mainly on the observation that they are extremely rare in sub-Saharan Africa. The vast majority remain asymptomatic but, in those that do come to light, there is a variety of possible presentations.

→ *Bleeding.* Irritation of the opening of such a diverticulum is a source of rectal bleeding. This is because the internal opening of the diverticulum is closely related to the vessels that traverse the bowel wall leading to this potential weakness. The blood is often a darkish red in colour and is one of the two common causes of major lower gastrointestinal haemorrhage; the other being angiodysplasia.

→ *Infection.* Diverticulitis is a common cause of admission to the surgical ward with crampy left iliac fossa pain and tenderness associated with a changed bowel habit but rarely bleeding. The patient is pyrexial and often systemically unwell. Treatment is with IV fluids and antibiotics. Surgery is seldom indicated unless further complications occur. In some cases, a chronically thickened inflammatory mass or phlegmon will develop, causing a mass to be palpable in the LIF.

→ *Perforation.* An acutely inflamed diverticulum may perforate. If the body manages to contain it, then a paracolic abscess develops in the LIF. If it is not contained, then the patient presents with peritonitis, often faecal in nature, and requires emergency surgery if fit enough. The operation is usually difficult in the face of extensive contamination of the tissues and gross peritoneal soiling. Many patients end up with a Hartmann's procedure.

→ *Stricture.* Recurrent episodes of diverticulitis may cause an inflammatory stricture in the sigmoid colon that can present clinically as a change of bowel habit or simply as large bowel obstruction, but in either event the differential diagnosis is colonic cancer.

→ *Fistulation.* Perforation of an inflamed diverticulum may present as a colovesical or colovaginal fistula.

A 56-year-old woman presents for the first time with LIF pain, fever and change of bowel habit. How will you manage her?

With a working diagnosis of diverticulitis, treatment is commenced with IV fluids to rehydrate what is often a very dry patient and commence IV antibiotics. Broad-spectrum cover using cefuroxime and metronidazole should be initiated. The patient can have sips of water only until her systemic symptoms are settling and her observations (pulse, temperature) return to normal. The patient normally settles down on such a regime. In a woman of this age, an effort must be made to prove the diagnosis. In the acute stage, most surgeons prefer not to endoscope the patient as there is perceived to be a greater risk of perforation. An ultrasound scan is the recommended first-line investigation to demonstrate the thickened colon and to exclude localized collections. If this does not provide enough information, a CT scan with oral contrast will reveal diverticula, as well as evidence of inflammatory mass or abscess formation. Alternatively, in a simple case that rapidly resolves, outpatient barium enema should be sufficient to prove the diagnosis of diverticular disease, although, because it is so common, it does not prove diverticulitis.

What is a Zencker's diverticulum and describe the relevant anatomy?

Zencker's diverticulum is a pharyngeal pouch. It is an out-pouching of pharyngeal mucosa through a gap between the inferior constrictor and cricopharyngeus, known as Killian's dehiscence. Although the dehiscence is in the midline, 90 per cent of pharyngeal pouches present on the left side. The pouch classically presents with the patient vomiting or regurgitating yesterday's undigested food. Other presentations are halitosis and recurrent aspiration-type pneumonias. Diagnosis is by barium swallow in the first instance, as unwary endoscopy can perforate the pouch; subsequent stapling off and inversion of the pouch may be achieved endoscopically or at open surgery.

21. CELL CHANGES

Define hyperplasia, hypertrophy, metaplasia, dysplasia and neoplasia, and give suitable examples

→ *Hypertrophy* is the response of cells to increased demands by an increase in cell size without replication. An example is the muscle hypertrophy that develops in athletes in response to training in both skeletal muscle and the myocardium of the ventricles.

→ *Hyperplasia* is the response of cells to increased demand by increasing cell numbers. An example is the hyperplasia of bone marrow in individuals living at altitude.

→ *Metaplasia* is the reversible transformation of one type of terminally differentiated cell to another fully differentiated cell. An example is the ciliated respiratory epithelium of smokers turning into a squamous epithelium.

→ *Dysplasia* is increased cell growth in the presence of cellular atypia and altered differentiation. The changes may resolve when the initiating factor is removed. These changes are pre-malignant. Dysplasia in the uterine cervix provides a commonly known example and demonstrates the role of a screening test admirably. Women undergo cervical smear testing in order to identify asymptomatic dysplastic changes, which can be treated before frank malignant transformation occurs.

→ *Neoplasia* means in the literal sense 'new growth', and is defined as an abnormal tissue mass with excessive uncoordinated growth, which persists when the stimulating factor is removed. It may be either benign or malignant; examples are innumerable – any cancer displays neoplasia.

What is Barrett's oesophagus and describe its significance?

Barrett's oesophagus is an intestinal metaplasia of the oesophageal lining. The normal squamous epithelium is replaced by gastric-type columnar epithelium for a variable distance. By definition, the squamocolumnar junction must be greater than 3 cm above the gastro-oesophageal junction to gain the description Barrett's oesophagus. Within the columnar epithelium, areas of genetic instability may develop, probably in response to bile and acid reflux, which lead to dysplasia, and eventually adenocarcinoma. The risk of developing cancer in a Barrett's oesophagus is now thought to be between 30 and 60 times the background risk. Barrett's oesophagus is increasing in incidence and is responsible for the rising number of cases of oesophageal cancer in the Western world. The management of Barrett's oesophagus is controversial, as few surgeons would advocate oesophagectomy for early dysplastic change. The differences between high-grade dysplasia and early cancer can sometimes be very difficult to identify, and severe dysplasia warrants consideration of surgery. Certainly, most surgeons would advocate regular endoscopic surveillance once these changes have been identified, although there are surgeons who take the view that in elderly patients who will never be fit enough to undergo radical resectional surgery, repeated endoscopy is not warranted. They prefer to treat those patients on a symptomatic basis. All patients with Barrett's oesophagus should receive permanent proton pump inhibitor therapy.

What is carcinoma *in situ* and is it necessarily a better diagnosis to have than carcinoma?

A carcinoma *in situ* is an epithelial neoplasm that has all the cellular features of a carcinoma, but has not yet invaded through the epithelial basement membrane. This means that it has not yet reached the potential routes of spread: bloodstream, lymphatics or a serosal surface. Removal of an *in situ* lesion will guarantee a cure from that particular tumour, provided that the resection margins are clear.

For isolated tumours, removal at an *in situ* stage offers the best chance of cure but, for other tumours, it may represent a field change, and is an indicator of high risk for further disease. One example is transitional cell tumours of the bladder, where carcinoma *in situ* has a high risk of transforming to poorly differentiated invasive tumours without becoming exophytic. Because of this, carcinoma *in situ* of the bladder is aggressively treated intravesically and, at any sign of progression, radical treatment is indicated.

Norman Rupert Barrett (1903–79). Born in Adelaide, Australia, he was a British surgeon, educated at Eton and Cambridge. He was a surgeon at St Thomas' and the Brompton Hospitals. He was president of the Society of Thoracic Surgeons of Great Britain and Ireland, and edited the journal Thorax *for 25 years. He was not the first to describe the changes of the oesophagus that bear his name, which was adopted after his article in 1950.*

22. DYSPHAGIA

What is dysphagia and what are the causes?

Dysphagia is described as a difficulty in swallowing; it is not pain on swallowing, which is known as odynophagia. The causes are legion but may be arranged in a sensible order. Whilst there are some congenital causes of dysphagia, such as oesophageal atresia or stenosis, which may coexist with tracheal fistulae, or dysphagia lusoria, where an aberrant vessel, such as the subclavian artery or double aortic arch compresses the oesophagus externally, the vast majority of causes are acquired.

Conditions of the wall
→ *Tumours* – both benign, such as lipoma and leiomyoma, and malignant, adenocarcinoma and squamous cell carcinoma.
→ *Strictures* from gastro-oesophageal reflux disease or ingestion of caustic agents.
→ *Neurological conditions.* These may be infective, such as diphtheria and syphilis, or non-infective conditions like myasthenia gravis, or a brainstem stroke.
→ *Neuromuscular conditions.* Achalasia, a pharyngeal pouch, pseudobulbar palsy or the trypanosomal infection of Chaga's disease are examples.

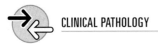
→ *Connective tissue disease*, such as scleroderma, which may be associated with the CREST syndrome.

Intraluminal obstruction

→ Foreign body or food bolus obstruction

→ oesophageal webs of Plummer–Vinson syndrome.

Extrinsic pressure

→ Mediastinal lymph node enlargement

→ increased left atrial size

→ thyroidal compression.

Psychosomatic

→ Globus hystericus.

How would you investigate dysphagia?

The starting point is always a careful history and examination, bearing in mind the diverse list of possible causes. This should then direct the approach to investigation. A full blood count may reveal the microcytic hypochromic anaemia associated with Plummer–Vinson syndrome. First-line imaging for high dysphagia where food sticks in the neck is by a barium swallow to exclude a pharyngeal pouch; for all other cases, upper gastrointestinal endoscopy is the first-line investigation. Video fluoroscopy may be required to give dynamic information in cases such as achalasia or corkscrew oesophagus. Further specialist investigations will be required for specific diseases, such as a Tensilon test for the diagnosis of myasthenia gravis.

Discuss the epidemiology and aetiology of oesophageal cancer

Oesophageal cancer is a disease of the middle-aged and elderly, and is rare before the age of forty. It is 1.5–3 times commoner in men than women. The epidemiology of oesophageal cancer is rapidly changing and, whereas lower-third tumours used to account for only a third of oesophageal tumours, they now account for more than half; only 8 per cent of tumours are in the cervical oesophagus.

Carcinomas are commonly squamous cell tumours, with adenocarcinomas accounting for around 10 per cent of oesophageal tumours worldwide. Adeno-carcinomas are thought to arise out of Barrett's metaplastic epithelium and are increasing in incidence and are now the commoner type in many Western countries. Squamous cell carcinoma has three geographical areas of marked increased incidence: Iran and Russia bordering the Caspian Sea, the Transkei region of South Africa, and the highest incidence of all is in the Henan, Hebi and Shaxi regions of Northern China. There the incidence is over 100 cases per 100 000 population compared to 2–8 per 100 000 in most of Europe.

In these high-incidence areas, dietary factors, such as increased nitrosamines, mould-affected food, trace element deficiency, particularly molybdenum, and deficiencies of vitamins A, C and riboflavin, are thought to be important. Elsewhere common aetiological factors are cigarette smoking and alcohol consumption. Conditions associated with a higher incidence of carcinoma and grouped together as potentially pre-malignant are tylosis, caustic strictures, oesophageal webs, achalasia and Barrett's oesophagus.

Very rarely, the oesophagus may play host to sarcomas or malignant melanoma.

What surgical approaches to resection of an oesophageal carcinoma are used?

Many different approaches have been described. The three commonest are the following.

→ *Ivor Lewis.* An upper midline laparotomy is used to mobilize the stomach followed by a right thoracotomy. It is a good approach for lower- and middle-third tumours. A third incision in the neck was added by McKeown, which allows removal of the cervical oesophagus and an anastomosis out of the chest.
→ *Transhiatal.* As the name might suggest, this approach does not open the chest; the oesophagus is freed by blunt dissection. Popularized by Orringer using a laparotomy incision from below and a cervical incision above to free the upper end, it is a useful approach for upper- or lower-third tumours.
→ *The Sweet approach* utilizes a left thoracotomy or thoracoabdominal incision. It is good for tumours at the cardia, but the heart and aortic arch can make the anastomosis taxing.

23. SALIVARY GLANDS

What does this x-ray (Figure 6.12) show?

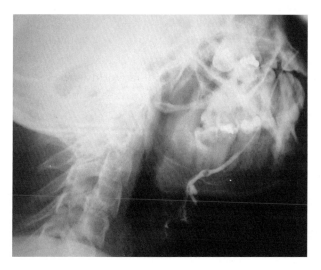

Figure 6.12

This is a submandibular sialogram demonstrating a stone in the submandibular duct.

Discuss salivary stones

Sialolithiasis or salivary duct stone formation is commonest in the submandibular gland and less so in the parotid. This probably reflects the fact that the secretion of the parotid is particularly serous, as opposed to the mucinous submandibular gland secretions, which must flow against gravity, as the duct has an upwards course in the normal upright position. Salivary stones generally have a nidus of organic matter or microbes surrounded by calcium phosphate, although other varieties of stone can be found. They present with pain and gland swelling, particularly at meal times, when the stone is intraductal but may remain asymptomatic, if the stone remains within the gland itself. Infection may supervene in an obstructed gland. Repeated small stones may cause fibrosis of the duct, which may then obstruct in its own right.

How may a submandibular stone be assessed and removed?

On clinical examination, a submandibular duct stone is usually readily palpable on bimanual examination and evident on plain lateral radiography. If the diagnosis is in doubt, sialography will help. Injection of 1.5–2 mm of radio-opaque contrast into the submandibular duct orifice will show a blockage to the flow of saliva; this may be complete or it may outline the stone as a filling defect. If the stone lies in the anterior two-thirds of the duct, it can be excised intraorally. A stay stitch is passed beneath the duct to prevent the stone slipping back out of reach. The mucosa overlying it is incised, the duct mobilized and controlled in a stay stitch, and then opened and the stone removed. The duct is marsupialized, as any attempt to close the duct would lead to stenosis. If the stone lies within the glandular duct system, then excision of the whole gland should be undertaken through a submandibular approach.

What nerves are at particular risk in the operation for removal of a submandibular gland?

The incision is sited 2–3 cm below the mandible to avoid the mandibular branch of the facial nerve that lies close to the gland. The lingual nerve is at risk as it crosses the duct and loops down toward the deep surface of the deep part of the gland, to which it is attached by strands of parasympathetic nerves, which must be divided. The hypoglossal nerve lies behind the gland covered by a thin layer of loose connective tissue that separates it from the deep surface of the gland.

What are the common salivary gland tumours?

The commonest of all salivary tumours is the pleomorphic adenoma, consisting of mixed connective and glandular elements of epithelial origin within a pseudocapsule. It is generally benign but longstanding pleomorphic adenomas can undergo malignant transformation into aggressive squamous cell tumours. Warthin's tumour or adenolymphoma is strongly associated with tobacco smoking and contains lymphoid follicles and cysts, and may fluctuate in size; it generally feels softer than a pleomorphic adenoma and is benign. Oxyphilic adenoma, sometimes referred to as an oncocytoma, is the third of the benign salivary tumours, but accounts for only about 1 per cent of cases and is commoner in women. Malignant salivary tumours are not common, with an incidence of about two per 100 000 and are of a variety of types. Mucoepidermoid tumours are commonest, with adenoid-cystic, acinic cell, adeno- and squamous cell carcinomas all occurring in smaller numbers. The mucoepidermoid and acinic cell tumours exhibit a variety of growth patterns but all, however slow growing and indolent-appearing, retain the ability to metastasize.

A total of 75 per cent of all salivary tumours arise in the parotid, of which 80 per cent are benign and 80 per cent are pleomorphic adenomas. Fifteen per cent of tumours arise in the submandibular gland of which 60 per cent are benign, and 95 per cent are pleomorphic adenomas. Only 10 per cent of salivary tumours arise in the sublingual glands: only 40 per cent are benign but all are pleomorphic adenomas.

What is Frey's syndrome?

Following parotid gland surgery, the salivary secretomotor fibres may regrow to innervate the divided sympathetic nerves to skin of the auriculotemporal area and this gives rise to the phenomenon gustatory sweating. Frey's syndrome occurs in up to 50 per cent of patients undergoing parotidectomy and may not appear until many years after surgery. If problematical and not controlled by topical aluminium preparations, then division of Jacobson's nerve in the auditory canal may help. Patients with Frey's syndrome may also demonstrate thermal salivation!

Luiji Frey (1889–1944). Polish neurologist who described this syndrome in 1923. She was killed by the Nazi regime in 1944.

24. VENOUS ULCERATION

What is an ulcer?

An ulcer is defined as an artificial break in an epithelial surface.

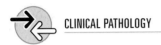

What is the typical appearance of a venous ulcer?

See Figure 6.13. Typically, they are shallow terraced ulcers with varying degrees of granulation tissue and/or infected slough in the base. They appear in the gaiter area of the lower legs, and there is often venous staining and lipodermatosclerosis in the surrounding tissue. They are sensate but not excruciatingly painful. Varicose veins are not invariably associated.

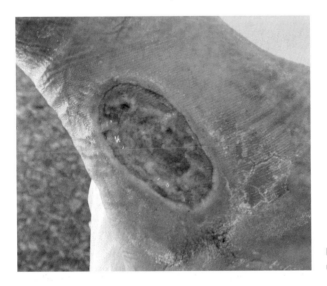

Figure 6.13 A large venous ulcer at the lateral malleolus.

What are the current aetiological theories behind venous ulceration?

There are two proposed theories as to the causation of venous ulceration. Burnand et al. proposed the fibrin cuff theory, which suggests that high pressure in the capillary bed of the ankle skin encourages deposition of macromolecules, such as fibrin and fibrinogen, which form a cuff around the capillaries, preventing egress of oxygen and nutrients into the tissues. This leads to anoxia and susceptibility to tissue damage and slow healing. Coleridge-Smith suggests that high venous pressures cause lymphocytic accumulation within the capillaries, resulting in their blockage, thus causing local tissue hypoxia and sustaining damage. Both sets of events may be demonstrated within the tissues but no clear evidence has accumulated as to which, if either, is the causative pathway.

What is the treatment for venous ulcers?

After careful assessment and confirmation that the patient does not suffer from distal ischaemia, then thorough cleaning of the ulcer, non-adherent dressings and firm compression bandaging are the mainstays of treatment. This is usually in the form of three- or four-layer bandages. This is repeated weekly. Most ulcers heal within 3 months; thereafter the trick is to try to keep them healed and continued use of compression stockings helps. If there are associated varicose veins, either in the long saphenous distribution or calf perforators, then these should be attended to surgically if at all possible, otherwise recurrence or non-healing is likely. In some centres, hyperbaric oxygen therapy is being used experimentally, as are a variety of topical growth-promoting agents, to try to heal these, often recalcitrant, ulcers.

List the differential diagnoses of a lower limb venous ulcer

→ *Ischaemia*. Poor arterial supply is not uncommon in elderly patients and the peripheral pulses should be assessed, using Doppler if necessary. Mixed arteriovenous ulcers are a catch for the unwary.

→ *Malignancy*. Occasionally, a squamous cell tumour will present as a supposed venous ulcer. If suspicious, a punch biopsy from the edge will confirm the diagnosis.

→ *Infective diabetic ulcers*. These are usually obvious, punched out, offensive-smelling deep ulcers in a known diabetic.

→ *Deliberate self-harm*. This is not common but does occur; other skin marks may give a clue to the real diagnosis.

→ *Gummatous ulcers*. These are much less common in the present day. They require appropriate serological testing.

→ *Vasculitic*. Related to rheumatoid arthritis and scleroderma; examination of the whole patient for other stigmata is essential.

→ *Pyoderma gangrenosum*. This condition is of unknown aetiology but gives rise to rapidly growing, necrotic-looking ulcers. Treatment is with steroid therapy. It may be associated with inflammatory bowel disease, myeloma, rheumatoid arthritis or liver disease.

25. ARTHRITIDES

What are the differing clinical features of osteoarthritis and rheumatoid arthritis?

Osteoarthritis gives rise to a joint pain felt on exercise or activity. It gradually increases as the joint is used further and is initially relieved by rest. Weight-bearing joints tend to suffer most. Night pain can become a particular problem and disruption of sleep is one factor influencing the decision for surgery. As reluctance to move the joint increases, this allows other changes to occur, and the joint stiffens and the patient loses movement at that joint; this may progress to fixed deformities. Examination reveals a swollen joint with an effusion and reduced movement, usually with pain and crepitus.

Rheumatoid arthritis is typically polyarticular, affecting the small joints of the hands. The joints are painful, swollen and stiff, which tends to ease off with activity. Disease activity may vary over time and painful inflamed joints may settle down after a few months only to flare up again later. There is often a feeling of systemic malaise and lethargy associated with rheumatoid disease. The joints are swollen and tender with synovial thickening. Gradual progression of the disease leads to joint deformity and instability as ligaments become involved with disease progression.

Which type is shown on this x-ray (Figure 6.14)? What are the common radiological findings of the two?

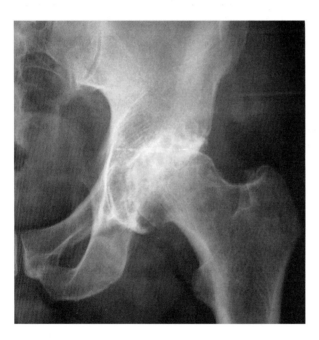

Figure 6.14

This shows osteoarthritis in a left hip joint. Osteoarthritis has four cardinal signs on plain x-ray: osteophyte and new bone formation, loss of joint space, subchondral sclerosis and bone cysts. Rheumatoid arthritis shows narrowing of the joint space and marked osteoporosis with bony erosion. As the disease progresses, bony destruction and damage to capsule and ligaments allows joint disruption to occur and subluxation progresses.

What other types of arthritis impinge on surgical practice?

Virtually any sort of arthritis capable of destroying joints will bring itself to an orthopaedic clinic. The seronegative arthritides, such as those connected with Reiter's syndrome, psoriasis or Crohn's disease, may all present acutely. Ankylosing spondylitis may present to the orthopaedic surgeons but it may impinge on surgical practice in any speciality, since operating on anyone with severe ankylosing spondylitis will present problems.

What are the complications of total joint arthroplasty?

Although joint arthroplasty has revolutionized the treatment of hip and knee arthritis, and changed the lives of thousands of patients, it is not free of complications. As the procedure consists of implantation of a foreign body, the worries regarding infection loom large. The particular problem is that eradication of infection around a prosthesis is notoriously difficult and often requires revisional surgery, which is itself no small undertaking. Loosening of the prosthesis is a further problem, which can be exacerbated by infection. All joint replacements have a finite lifespan before the components wear out and this should be borne in mind when selecting the particular prosthesis for each patient. Specific problems with hip replacements are migration of the acetabular cup, sometimes into the pelvis itself, and of dislocation of the joint, which is said to be more common after a posterior approach. The application of cement to the marrow cavity has its own problems, causing relative cardiovascular instability, so it is essential to inform your anaesthetist when applying cement.

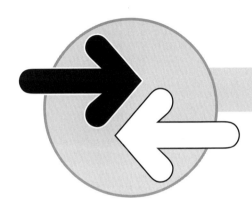

1. BOWEL PREPARATION

How would you prepare a patient for colonoscopy?

The aim of bowel preparation is to purge the colon to allow adequate views of the mucosa of the entire large bowel at colonoscopy. There are several methods of doing this ranging from prolonged starvation allowing natural clearance of the gut, to mechanical cleansing with large volumes of preparatory agent. One such regime popular in the USA is 4 L of 'Kleen-Prep' taken over 4 hours on the day prior to the procedure. Many people find such volumes difficult to ingest and a kinder regimen is two sachets of sodium picosulphate taken 12 hours apart, the latter sachet a minimum of 8 hours prior to the scheduled time of colonoscopy. Both the 'KleenPrep' and the 'Picolax' methods are complemented by restricting the patient's oral intake to clear fluids only for the 24 hours preceding the examination. The patient should be warned that they will suffer diarrhoea for the day and should make efforts to maintain adequate oral hydration.

Preparation of a patient for colonoscopy involves more than clearing the bowel. Informed consent is obtained and, in doing so, the procedure described, explaining the need for pain relief and a hypnotic agent, and also that the examination may feel uncomfortable at times. Complications of colonoscopy, such as perforation, bleeding and the need for emergency surgery should be discussed, and a consent form completed. All patients undergoing colonoscopy should have secure intravenous access sited.

In what instances is extra caution necessary?

Elderly patients, or those who are otherwise at risk of dehydration and electrolyte disturbance from purgative bowel preparation should be admitted to hospital to receive it. They should have a replacement intravenous crystalloid infusion. Patients in whom a stenosing tumour is suspected, which was, for example, impassable at flexible sigmoidoscopy, should have a single sachet of bowel prep, and not receive the other one until it is clear that the patient is able to evacuate their bowels satisfactorily.

In what instances would you definitely not use oral bowel preparation?

Patients with previous allergic or hypersensitivity reactions to bowel preparations should not receive the same type. Any patient undergoing colonoscopy for an obstructing lesion should have a distal enema only and forego oral preparation owing to the increased risk of perforation. Patients undergoing emergency colonoscopy for gastrointestinal haemorrhage will not have time for bowel preparation; in these cases, the intraluminal blood tends to clear the colon and acts as the patient's own purgative.

How do laxatives work?

Laxatives fall into one of the following four main categories.

→ *Osmotic agents.* Agents such as lactulose are composed of complex sugars that are not absorbed by the human gut; consequently, they remain in the lumen and exert a strong osmotic effect, drawing water into the colon and softening the stool. Magnesium hydroxide is another commonly used osmotic agent.

→ *Bulking agents.* These are typified by commercial preparations, such as 'Fybogel', which contain shredded indigestible fibre, ispaghula husks, which form bulky stools that stimulate peristalsis. They should be used in conjunction with an adequate fluid intake to prevent the risk of obstruction. Bulking agents are also indicated for some cases of faecal incontinence as the weakened sphincters can manage to control a bulky stool better.

→ *Stimulants.* A wide variety of agents can cause increased gut motility, the commoner ones being senna and bisacodyl. They are contraindicated in bowel obstruction and long-term usage may result in an atonic colon.

→ *Faecal softeners.* Paraffin is the most well known of this group but its use has waned recently owing to the associated problems of perianal discomfort and the stimulation of granulomatous reactions. It is still part of several 'over-the-counter' laxative preparations.

Before prescribing laxatives for constipation, the patient should be counselled about lifestyle changes that may help, such as increased fluid intake and dietary manipulation to increase natural fibre. A search for any underlying cause or alternative diagnosis should be made before the label of 'just constipation' is made.

2. BLOOD TRANSFUSION

What factors would alert you to an incompatible blood transfusion?

In the conscious patient, an incompatible transfusion presents as a haemolytic transfusion reaction (HTR) with massive intravascular haemolysis of the transfused cells. This may manifest as rigors, lumbar pain, pyrexia and fever, haemoglobinuria, hypotension and renal failure. Activation of the clotting cascade and disseminated intravascular coagulation may occur. It is a life-threatening event.

In the anaesthetized patient, recognition is often more difficult, but persistent hypotension and unexplained oozing from the surgical site may be indicators. If an immediate HTR is suspected, the transfusion should be stopped immediately, and the identification details checked on both the patient and the donor unit. Clerical error remains by far the most common cause of transfusion reaction. The donor unit and a sample from the patient should be sent for immediate compatibility testing. Supportive therapy should be instituted as required for the patient. This may well include inotropes and renal replacement therapy. Intravenous steroids and antihistamines should be considered.

A delayed HTR may occur up to 3 weeks after transfusion, with haemolysis occurring in the sequestered cells in the spleen. Symptoms include fever, rigors and myalgia, accompanied by jaundice. A direct antiglobulin test establishes the diagnosis.

What are the complications of blood transfusion?

Complications of blood transfusion can be related to the mechanics of transfusion or the transfusion itself. Complications due to the mechanism of delivery include cannula site sepsis, haematoma and air embolism.

Complications of the transfusion itself can be described as immediate, early or late.

The only 'common' immediate complication is the major transfusion reaction described above.

Early transfusion reactions include the non-haemolytic transfusion reaction mediated by HLA antigens and granulocyte antibodies; the patient generally displays only a mild pyrexia and headache. There may be a considerable risk of fluid balance problems and circulatory overload when a frail patient receives a large-volume transfusion.

Late complications include disease transmission and immune modulation. Transfusion of donated blood and products exposes the recipients to the risk of infection. UK-donated units are routinely checked for antibodies to HIV 1 and 2, hepatitis B and C, cytomegalovirus and syphilis; however, this is not foolproof, as it is possible to donate infected blood after infection but before seroconversion. The risk of contracting HIV from UK-donated blood is currently estimated at 1 in 2 million transfused units. *Yersinia* species can survive at 4°C and, as such, may be transmissible in donated blood; the ensuing acute bacterial transfusion reaction is spectacular, with the patient rapidly succumbing to a fulminant endotoxic shock.

Other consequences of transfusion include immunosuppression, which has relevance in cancer surgery, and was once used therapeutically in renal transplant surgery when recipients were given pre-operative transfusions to dampen down their immune response to the transplanted organ. Thalassaemia patients who receive multiple transfusions over many years are at risk of iron overload and should be treated with chelating agents such as desferrioxamine.

What are the specific complications of massive blood transfusion?

'Massive transfusion' is defined as replacement of the entire circulating blood volume within 24 hours and presents specific complications. Massive transfusion of cold stored blood risks hypothermia, citrate toxicity, hypocalcaemia from citrate binding and hyperkalaemia from the K^+ that leaches out of the red cells as they are stored. Most of these may be obviated by slower transfusion of warmed blood. Stored blood contains little in the way of platelets or clotting factors, so massive transfusion with red cells alone induces a dilutional coagulopathy as the platelet count falls. Treatment is by infusion of fresh-frozen plasma (FFP) and platelets, if the count is low enough. Massive transfusion is a recognized contributing factor to ARDS.

Describe the ABO and Rh systems

The ABO blood group antigen system is controlled by a pair of allelic genes (H and h) and by three allelic genes A, B and O, of which A and B are dominant. The H-gene codes for enzyme H, which forms the A and B antigen precursors. The A and B genes code for enzymes, which then add specific substances to the H precursor to form A and B antigens. O is amorphic and does not transform H substance and thus is not antigenic.

The combinations of phenotype, genotype, and antigens are shown in Table 7.1.

Table 7.1

Blood group	Genotype	Antigens
O	OO	
A	AA or AO	A
B	BB or BO	B
AB	AB	A and B

The Rhesus (Rh) system is governed by six antigens C, D, E and c, d, e. Individuals will have either the C or c antigen, but not both, and similarly for Dd and Ee. Rhesus positivity is based on the presence of the D antigen, as it is considerably more antigenic than the others. A rhesus transfusion reaction is still possible, therefore, even in someone who is Rh-negative; owing to the presence of the other Rh antigens, these reactions tend to be much less severe.

How do we take and store blood for transfusion?

In the UK, blood donation is voluntary and unpaid. All donors undergo health screening questioning prior to donation, to screen out individuals with behaviours at high risk for HIV or hepatitis virus carriage. Recent malaria is a contraindication to donation, as is recent travel through a malaria-endemic area. A finger-prick blood sample is used to ensure adequate Hb levels. The donor lies recumbent with arm outstretched and blood pressure cuff inflated on the upper arm. After skin cleaning with an alcohol wipe, a suitable vein in the antecubital fossa is needled and 450 ml of fresh blood is collected into a sterile plastic pack containing 63 ml of citrate preservative as well as adenine, phosphate and dextrose.

The removed blood may be stored as whole blood or, more commonly, processed into constituent fractions. It is usual to remove plasma to leave the red cells with a haematocrit of ~70 per cent. Other cellular components derived include leucocyte poor red cells, washed red cells for patients who have had previous anaphylactic transfusion reactions and platelet concentrates. The plasma may then be further fractionated into fresh-frozen plasma (200 ml obtained from 1 donor unit, stored at $-30°C$), cryoprecipitate (20 ml of FFP supernatant containing Factor VII:C, VII:vWF and fibrinogen), clotting factor concentrates (VIII, IX), albumin and immunoglobulins.

3. STERILIZATION

What are the differences between cleaning, disinfecting and sterilization?

Cleaning refers to the process of physical removal of contaminants, but not necessarily to the inactivation of any microbial organism. Disinfection reduces the viable organism count but does not necessarily kill or inactivate all spores, viruses or organisms. Sterilization is the complete eradication of all viable microorganisms including viruses and spores. The term sterilization in this context cannot be applied to living tissue – as it is a tissue damaging process – but only to inanimate objects. Skin is disinfected not sterilized.

What methods of sterilization are there? Give examples of their use

In general terms there are five methods of sterilization.

After cleaning, surgical instruments are generally sterilized in pressurized steam autoclaves, most commonly at 134°C at 30 lb/in^2 for 3 minutes. This is the most efficient method of sterilizing large volumes of equipment but is not suitable for articles such as fibreoptic endoscopes. Dry-heat sterilization (160°C for 2 hours) is used for items such as non-aqueous liquids and ointments. It cannot be used on rubber and plastics, as they would be denatured. It is a relatively inefficient method. Ionizing radiation (γ ray) is used on an industrial basis to sterilize large batches of single-use items, such as swabs and catheters. The last two methods are less commonly employed in the NHS. The first is sterilization with ethylene oxide, a toxic mutagenic agent that is a very effective sterilizing tool, which is used predominantly as an industrial process. Finally, a combination of low-temperature steam and formaldehyde may also be employed, which is useful for articles with integral plastic parts that would be damaged by a high-temperature process. Endoscopes are *disinfected* in a 2 per cent solution of alkaline glutaraldehyde after manual cleaning.

Describe three solutions commonly used for preparing the skin at surgery. What are their relative merits?

→ *Povidone–iodine* – a potent fast-acting bactericidal agent with fungicidal properties, which may be used in aqueous or alcoholic solution. It can, however, cause allergic reactions.
→ *Alcohol* – evaporates leaving a dry surface, but must be allowed time to dry. Alcoholic preparations are flammable and pooling must not be allowed to occur. They can be an irritant to mucous membranes and delicate skin.
→ *Chlorhexidine and cetrimide (Savlon)* – aqueous quaternary ammonium compounds, which can be used for preparation of delicate areas, such as the vagina, anus and perineum. It is bactericidal but not sporicidal. *Pseudomonas* may grow in stored contaminated solutions.

What are the main features to consider when designing an operating theatre suite?

The location is of prime importance as the operating theatres must have easy access to the Accident and Emergency Department, ITU, the X-Ray Department and the surgical wards, and, if practicable, should all be on the same level. The operating theatre complex itself should have three distinct zones.

→ *Outer zone*: this should have a reception office and a patient reception area where pre-operative checks are undertaken. Storage areas for trolleys are located here, and a supply of gowns and overshoes are kept for use by visitors and relatives accompanying patients to theatre.
→ *Clean zone*: a wide clean corridor should give access to the anaesthetic rooms, recovery area, emergency autoclave, staff rooms and storage areas for x-ray equipment.
→ *Theatres*: each theatre should have a laminar airflow system that pipes clean air in through the ceiling ventilation and exits via floor-level swing flaps with

20–40 changes per hour. The normal working temperature is between 19 and 22°C with a humidity between 45 and 55 per cent; both of these may be increased when performing paediatric surgery. There should be an adequate provision of power sockets, piped medical gases and an anaesthetic scavenging system. There should be a 'dirty' corridor, completely separate from the 'clean' one, via which all waste for disposal or cleaning is distributed.

4. CHROMOSOMES

How many chromosomes does an adult cell have? If it had 92 chromosomes, would it be abnormal?

A normal adult cell has 46 chromosomes. If it had 92 chromosomes it would not necessarily be abnormal if it were replicating. During mitosis, each chromosome divides into two so that the daughter cell will have the same number of chromosomes as the parent cell. Thus, a cell viewed during mitosis before the daughter cell has separated will normally have 92 chromosomes.

Describe the terms haploid, aneuploid and diploid

Haploid describes a chromosome complement of a mature gamete (egg or sperm) following reduction division (meiosis). It represents the basic 23 chromosomes.

Aneuploid is an abnormality in the number of chromosomes. There may be more or less than normal. Loss of a chromosome is generally fatal, but additional chromosomes are not necessarily associated with mortality. Diploid refers to a chromosome complement of two copies of each chromosome, i.e. 46, that of a normal adult cell.

What is trisomy? Give examples and describe how it may occur

Trisomy occurs when there is an additional chromosome attached to one of the pairs giving a triple chromosome. The commonest is trisomy 21, Down's syndrome, which occurs in 1 in 700 live births overall. There is a strong association between Down's syndrome and maternal age, with the incidence being 1 in 25 live births to mothers over the age of 45. The trisomy occurs during early meiotic division of the ovum, when, instead of each daughter cell receiving one component of each pair of chromosomes, one cell receives both because chromosomal separation does not occur; this is known as non-disjunction. When, at fertilization, a gamete with 23 chromosomes fuses with one with 24, trisomy occurs, and in Down's syndrome this occurs on chromosome 21. A similar mechanism is responsible for the rarer Edwards' (trisomy 18) and Patau (trisomy 13) syndromes. Klinefelter's syndrome represents a non-disjunction of the sex chromosomes, commonly represented by 47XXY, although there are several variations of genotype within the syndrome.

What is an autosomal dominant condition? Give examples

An autosomal dominant condition is one manifest in both homozygous and heterozygous genotypes. It is exhibited and transmitted by males and females alike, and an index case will usually have at least one affected parent. Examples include familial adenomatous polyposis, neurofibromatosis and Marfan's syndrome.

What is an autosomal recessive condition? Give examples

An autosomal recessive condition only manifests itself in the homozygous genotype; heterozygotes are carriers but are not themselves affected. In general, parents do not exhibit the trait but siblings may well do. Complete penetrance and early onset is usual. Examples include sickle cell disease, cystic fibrosis and phenylketoneuria.

What is the mode of inheritance of a sex-linked disease?

Sex-linked disorders are all carried on the X chromosome with no cases of Y-linked diseases recorded. They can be dominant or recessive, although the X-linked recessive diseases are much more common.

In an X-linked dominant condition such as vitamin D-resistant rickets, females who are heterozygous for the mutant gene, and males with the gene on their X chromosome will manifest the disease. Half the male or female offspring of an affected mother will be affected, whereas all the female progeny of an affected father will be affected.

In X-linked recessive conditions, a male with the mutant gene is always affected, as there is no normal gene on a second X chromosome. In the female, the condition only manifests if homozygous, and so these conditions usually only affect males, while females are carriers. A common example is haemophilia. Half the female offspring of a female carrier will be carriers, and half the male offspring will be affected. For a male with haemophilia, all his female offspring will be carriers, while all his male offspring will be disease free.

John Langdon Down (1828–96). English physician who described the classical appearances of the syndrome in 1866; although it bears his name, it had been described previously by several authors. The genetic aberration was identified by Jérôme Lejeune in 1959.

Harry Fitch Klinefelter Junior (1912–) described the condition in 1942, whilst working under the guidance of Fuller Albright at Harvard, who Klinefelter admits should take credit for naming the syndrome.

Antoine Bernard-Jean Marfan (1858–1942). French paediatrician who described his syndrome in 1896. He published widely on the illnesses of childhood and was elected as an honorary member of the Royal Society of Medicine in London in 1934.

5. GYNAECOMASTIA

What is gynaecomastia?

See Figure 7.1. It is the enlargement of breast tissue in the male of any age. It is benign and the degree of enlargement can vary enormously. It is usually reversible and may be bilateral in up to one in four cases.

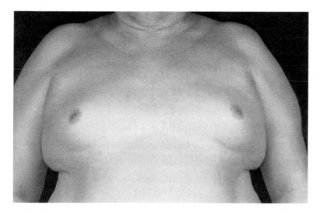

Figure 7.1 An obvious case of bilateral gynaecomastia.

When does it occur and what are the causes?

It typically occurs at three different stages of life. Neonatal gynaecomastia is similar in males and females, and is a result of continued enlargement of the breast bud in the first week or two of life, after which it regresses. Pubertal gynaecomastia is evident in upwards of 30 per cent of pubertal boys if looked for carefully. It is a result of testosterone/oestrogen imbalance and responds to hormone therapy using tamoxifen or danazol in approximately 50 per cent of cases. Adult gynaecomastia, usually in old age, has a legion of causes.

→ Hypogonadism.
→ Neoplasms. They may be β-HCG producers, such as seminoma and teratoma, oestrogen producers, like Leydig or adrenal tumours, or gonadatrophin producers, such as hepatomas, renal cell or gastric carcinomas.

→ Systemic disease, including hepatic failure, renal failure and hyperthyroidism.

→ Drug related – therapeutic hormones, hormone inhibitors (spironolactone, cimetidine and ketoconazole), neurotransmitters affecting prolactin secretion (metoclopromide, methyldopa and tricyclic agents) and cytotoxic agents (busulphan and vincristine).

What is the differential diagnosis?

Gynaecomastia is usually soft and involves the whole gland, and may be bilateral. Unusual, eccentric, hard or ulcerating lesions raise the suspicion of male breast cancer, which should be investigated appropriately with FNAC and mammography.

How would you treat gynaecomastia?

Gynaecomastia unresponsive to other treatments, such as removal of any causative agents or institution of medical therapy, may be treated surgically. Small and moderate-sized swellings may be excised utilizing a circumareolar approach and excising the breast tissue in the manner of a subcutaneous mastectomy, taking care to leave some breast disc behind to avoid an unsightly dint at the site of operation. Large gynaecomastia may require formal reduction pattern surgery. In older patients, the excised tissue should be sent for histology.

What is Poland's syndrome?

This syndrome is characterized by amazia, which is absence of one or both breasts, in conjunction with absence of the sternal portion of the pectoralis major muscle. There is an associated syndactyly. It is commoner in males and occurs in 10 per cent of syndactyly patients. The aetiology is unknown with both sporadic and autosomal dominant inheritance familial patterns seen.

6. ANEURYSMS

Define an aneurysm. Where do they commonly occur?

An aneurysm is a dilatation of a blood vessel over twice its normal diameter; enlargement up to twice the size is referred to as ectatic. Aneurysms may be described as true or false; a true aneurysm contains all the layers of the vessel wall, whereas a false aneurysm does not.

The commonest site for aneurysms to occur is the abdominal aorta and they are found in 2 per cent of the adult population at autopsy. Abdominal aortic aneurysms are often associated with aneurysmal dilatation of the iliac, femoral and popliteal vessels, with popliteal aneurysms (see Figure 7.2) representing the commonest location of peripheral aneurysms and the second commonest site overall. Other intra-abdominal aneurysms are rare, with splenic artery aneurysms being the next commonest after the aorta, with an incidence of less than 1 in 10 000. They are four times more common in women, especially during the child-bearing years and have a 25 per cent chance of rupture, typically during the last trimester. Intracranial 'berry' aneurysms occur at the junctions of the limbs of the Circle of Willis and result from congenital weaknesses at these sites exacerbated by the haemodynamic stresses of the circulation. A carotid artery aneurysm is one of the rarer differentials of lumps in the anterior triangle of the neck.

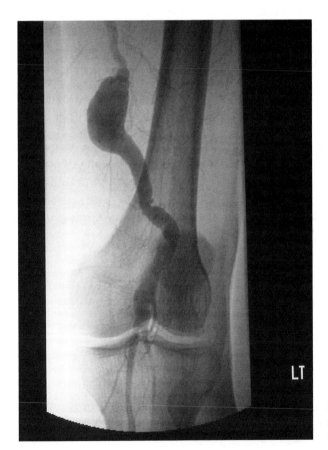

Figure 7.2 Arteriogram demonstrating a large popliteal aneurysm.

In general, how do aneurysms present? Describe the events following a ruptured 'berry' aneurysm

Aneurysms may rupture or leak, thrombose, become a source of emboli, press on adjacent structures or present as a mass noticeable by the patient. Increasingly, they are found as an incidental finding on investigation for other diseases or by screening 'at-risk' populations. Rupture of an intracranial 'berry' aneurysm presents as a subarachnoid haemorrhage. The patient collapses with a sudden onset of the worst headache they've ever had, which is often described as 'like being hit on the head with a hammer'. Examination will reveal meningism and varying degrees of neurological depression, ranging from the near normal through to severe hemiparesis or even coma. Lumbar puncture reveals a uniformly bloodstained CSF and CT scanning will often show subarachnoid blood. Treatment is supportive in the first instance to maintain cerebral perfusion, and prevent vasospasm or rebleeding, both of which will worsen the patient's neurological condition. Patients with no, or relatively little, neurological impairment and no evidence of vasospasm should undergo definitive surgical treatment of their aneurysm within 24 hours to prevent re-bleeding. Patients with greater degrees of impairment are managed expectantly with calcium channel blockers to relieve vasospasm until their condition improves before surgery is contemplated.

Give an aetiological classification for aneurysms

Aneurysms may be congenital or acquired. Atherosclerosis is the leading cause of acquired aneurysms.

→ *Degenerative* – associated with atherosclerosis; most common in the abdominal aorta
→ *Traumatic* – popliteal artery aneurysms in horse riders or, in the case of a false aneurysm, produced by arterial cannulation or other penetrating injury.
→ *Inflammatory* – typically small, whitish, friable AAAs. They rupture at a smaller diameter than would be expected. The surrounding tissue inflammation makes operation difficult.
→ *Mycotic* – these should really be called infective, as they are very rarely of fungal origin. The classical cause was syphilis, giving rise to thoracic aneurysms, but this is now less common. *Salmonella* is now a more common cause.
→ *Connective tissue disorder* – patients with Marfan's syndrome are prone to developing a dissecting aneurysm of the thoracic aorta.

Historically, popliteal artery aneurysms were associated with repeated trauma, typically from prolonged periods of horse riding, and were common in cavalrymen and postal couriers. Surgeons of the eighteenth century either refused to operate on them or ligated them immediately proximal to the aneurysm, risking torrential haemorrhage from the diseased vessel. John Hunter introduced the operation of proximal ligation in 1785, tying off the femoral artery in the subsartorial canal that now bears his name.

7. SUTURES

What criteria would the ideal suture fulfil?

The ideal suture would maintain its tensile strength until its purpose is served. It should elicit minimal tissue reaction and not encourage bacterial ingrowth. It would not be electrolytic, carcinogenic, allergenic or demonstrate a capillary action. It should handle well and knot securely without fraying. In addition, it should be inexpensive and easily sterilized.

Describe how sutures may be classified. Give examples and descriptions of the commonly used sutures

Sutures may be classified as absorbable or non-absorbable. Alternatively, they may be said to be braided or monofilament, natural or synthetic (see Table 7.2). These groupings are not exclusive, as a suture will often be described by several of these criteria. Monocryl™, for example, may be described as a synthetic mono-filament absorbable suture – it handles well with little memory. It will give wound support for 20 days and is absorbed in approximately 90 days.

Describe the needles in common surgical use

See Figure 7.3. Modern needles are virtually all ready-swatched to the suture, i.e. the scrub nurse no longer has to thread the needle each time. One exception to this is the 'aneurysm needle', which is still threaded by hand. Needles may be straight, curved or J-shaped. Straight needles are used for suturing skin wounds, which are easily accessible and are used by hand. Curved needles vary according to the extent of the circle they describe, ranging from ½ to ¾ of the circumference. They are generally manipulated with a needle holder, although there are large 'hand needles' available for abdominal closure, but holding needles by hand is now being actively discouraged to minimize needlestick injuries. Curved needles in their various forms are used throughout surgery. The J needle is used to approximate two tissues that are typically difficult to access deep within a surgical wound. The J needle is commonly used to close the umbilical port site after laparoscopy.

Table 7.2 Sutures

Suture	Type	Description
Catgut	Natural Absorbable	Rapidly hydrolysed. Gives wound support for 7–10 days only. This may be increased by chromic coating. Rarely used nowadays
Polyglactin (Vicryl™)	Synthetic Braided Absorbable	Elicits little tissue reaction; absorbed by hydrolysis between 56 and 70 days, but gives wound support for only 30 days. Vicryl™ Rapide is similar but more rapidly degraded with wound support for only 10 days
Polydioxanone suture (PDS)	Synthetic Monofilament Absorbable	Only slowly hydrolysed (180 days) with good tensile strength for up to 56 days. It is often used as an alternative to nylon for abdominal closure
Silk	Natural Braided Non-absorbable	The original non-absorbable suture, it is used less commonly now as it evokes a marked tissue reaction. It gives active wound support for 1 year but cannot be found in the wound after about 2 years
Polypropyline (Prolene™)	Synthetic Monofilament Non-absorbable	Slides excellently making it the suture of choice for vascular anastomosis, but can be difficult to knot and has a significant memory, making it difficult to handle. Inadvertent crushing will lose 90 per cent of the suture's tensile strength
Nylon (Ethilon™)	Synthetic Monofilament Non-absorbable	Similar handling characteristics to Prolene™ but less memory. It loses approximately 15–20 per cent of its tensile strength per year

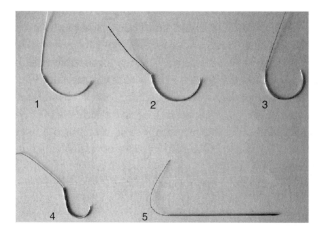

Figure 7.3 Some of the commoner surgical needles in use: 1, ⅜ circle; 2, ½ circle; 3, ⅝ circle; 4, J-shaped; 5, straight.

8. ANALGESIA

What is the analgesic ladder?

It is a stepwise approach to pain control as described by the World Health Organization in which each analgesic is categorized according to potency as mild, moderate or strong. It is an attempt to rationalize analgesic prescribing and suggests that a patient's pain should be treated in a stepwise manner, moving up or down the ladder one step at a time as a patient's pain changes. This principle prevents sudden, irrational changes in analgesia, stops the sequential use of different analgesics of the same potency being used in worsening or uncontrolled pain, and provides a mechanism of reduction in analgesia when pain is improving.

What methods might be used to provide postoperative pain relief?

There is a wide variety of methods of analgesia that may be used alone or in combination for the provision of postoperative pain relief. Some of these techniques are commenced during the operation itself, whilst others are instituted in the postoperative regime. Analgesia may be prescribed on a regular or 'as required' basis.

→ *Oral analgesia.* As soon as the patient is tolerating an oral intake, then this route is appropriate and can be used for all types of analgesics, including opiates.

→ *Epidural anaesthesia.* This generally utilizes local anaesthetic and/or an opiate agent instilled into the epidural space via a catheter inserted prior to surgery; it is usually prescribed and monitored by the anaesthetic/acute pain team. Epidurals can be run as a continuous rate infusion or on a patient-controlled basis.

→ *Patient-controlled analgesia (PCA).* An intravenous cannula is connected to a rate-limited giving set, which in turn is partly controlled by a handset given to the patient. By pressing the handset button, the patient receives a bolus of intravenous analgesic – usually an opiate – on top of a background infusion. The machine is regulated to prevent overdose. A similar method of patient-controlled 'top up' has also been introduced for epidurals.

→ *Local anaesthetic field blocks.* These are most often used for immediate postoperative analgesia as a single block given at the time of the operation, e.g. an ilioinguinal nerve block following an inguinal hernia repair, or infiltration of the wound edges at skin closure. Intercostal nerve blocks are sometimes useful in patients with painful rib fractures to help improve ventilation.

→ *Intramuscular analgesia.* Many opiates are very effective after IM injection and provide pain relief for a reasonable duration.

→ *Per rectum analgesia.* Some agents, such as diclofenac sodium, are particularly effective via this route, particularly in patients who cannot tolerate oral intake.

→ *Transdermal patches.* This route is typically used for chronic pain management as the patches, which usually incorporate an opioid such as fentanyl, are designed as a slow-release mechanism to provide analgesia for up to 72 hours.

What technique may be used in a child who has had a circumcision?

At the time of the procedure, the anaesthetist may employ a caudal block by injecting local anaesthetic into the spinal canal via the sacral foramen. This provides effective means of analgesia for this type of procedure; alternatively, a local anaesthetic penile block may be inserted at the time of the operation. Postoperatively, a non-steroidal anti-inflammatory suppository may be inserted before the patient recovers from anaesthesia and simple oral analgesia taken thereafter.

Compare the use of 'traditional' on demand IM analgesia with PCA

The primary advantages of intramuscular morphine are convenience and safety. At the doses commonly used, there are few side effects, and adequate analgesia is usually maintained for several hours with each injection. The single greatest disadvantage is that the patient must request the analgesia; some patients may be unwilling or unable to do so, and suffer as a result. On a busy ward, there may also be a significant delay between requesting analgesia and its administration. In shocked patients, opioid may accumulate intramuscularly owing to sluggish perfusion, only to be rapidly absorbed when the circulation is restored, leading to unpredictable side effects.

The advantages of an intravenous PCA system are that a more stable blood level of opioid is achieved without the patient having to ask or wait for a nurse to administer it. There is a safety cut out to prevent patients being able to overdose. The disadvantages are that the patient must be able to understand the system and must have the physical ability to press the button required; severely deformed rheumatoid hands can be problematic, as are patients with dementia. This form of analgesia also requires an IV cannula, a pump and a handset to be attached to the patient while they are trying to mobilize postoperatively. Blood opioid levels may fall quickly if no demands are made on the system, so at night the patient may wake up in pain and take longer to achieve a necessary level of analgesia than if they received IM morphine.

9. CONSENT

What are the principles of informed consent?

There are three guiding principles for obtaining informed consent: the person must be competent to give consent, consent must be given voluntarily and it must be an informed decision.

→ *Competent person.* The patient must have the mental power to deal with the matter, based on understanding rather than status. The surgeon must make a judgement as to whether the patient is sufficiently mentally competent to make such a decision. Patients under 16 years may consent, as may patients detained under the Mental Health Act, provided they are competent to do so.

→ *Voluntary consent.* The patient must not feel under constraint or duress, and should be allowed to make their decision freely without coercion.

→ *Informed consent.* The patient must be given sufficient information to allow them to retain, deliberate and make an informed choice about their treatment. Information must given in a form and manner that the individual can understand. They must be told about the proposed treatment, and its potential benefits and commonly occuring risks – usually those occurring in more than 1 in 100 cases. They must be told about any alternative treatments or the risks associated with no treatment. They must also be told about any serious hazards that 'any prudent person would wish to know of' irrespective of how uncommon those hazards might be.

The Department of Health has recently issued new guidelines on the process of informed consent. Those guidelines notwithstanding, the law on consent remains unaltered. As outlined in the DoH guidelines, consent should now be a two-stage procedure. The proposed treatment and anaesthetic should be discussed with the patient and ideally written information provided. At this stage, the patient may sign the consent form. At some later stage before surgery, another health professional should re-discuss the procedure with the patient and ensure that they still wish to go ahead with the procedure as previously outlined. This is then affirmed on the consent form.

Can a child of 15 give valid consent?

Yes, provided he or she is able to understand the procedure, the risks associated with the procedure, and also the risks associated with not undergoing the procedure. However, a child cannot refuse life-saving treatment. For example, if a parent signs a consent form for a procedure on their 15-year-old child, then that consent is valid in law and the child cannot revoke it. Obviously, the practicalities of operating on an unwilling patient raise other medical and ethical issues that would most likely preclude the operation proceeding, but in terms of law, the consent form is valid.

> **In the case of a demented 85-year-old man who requires elective surgery, who should sign his consent form – the wife, the daughter or someone else?**

No one other than the patient themselves can sign a valid consent form. In the event that informed consent is not possible, as in this case, then it is reasonable under common law to act in the patient's best interests. In most cases, it is usual practice for two doctors to document agreement that the procedure is in the patient's best interests and it is usual to gain the assent of the patient's next of kin. This procedure has been formalized in the Department of Health's recent consent guidelines.

> **A man is brought in collapsed with a diagnosis of leaking AAA. He has no relatives with him. Who should give consent and should the operation wait until the form has been signed appropriately?**

No. Again it is reasonable under common law to act in the patient's best interests. This would be to operate immediately, rather than to wait for relatives or for forms to be filled in. In this case, the surgeon should act 'of necessity' and a second opinion is not required.

> **A paranoid schizophrenic is refusing to sign the consent form for a laparotomy to repair her perforated duodenal ulcer. Your house officer suggests sectioning her under the Mental Health Act to force her to have the operation. What is your response?**

Under the Mental Health Act, a patient may be sectioned for psychiatric treatment, but may not be forcibly treated for any other medical condition. As such, sectioning this patient would not allow further treatment of her perforated ulcer. Even in life-threatening illness, **the patient's right to self-determination supersedes the principle of the sanctity of life**. A sensible way to proceed would be to have the patient urgently assessed by a psychiatrist with a view to deciding her mental state and competence. If deemed competent to make decisions regarding her treatment, then the patient's view must be respected and best therapy instituted in the circumstances.

10. LABORATORY METHODS

> **Describe what happens to a pathological specimen from the time you remove it from the patient until you receive the 'path report'**

The specimen is taken from the sterile field and passed out to a theatre assistant and placed in an appropriate transport medium, depending on the nature of the specimen, for transfer to the laboratory. This is most commonly formalin for gross specimens, although some specimens, such as lymph nodes, may be sent fresh. The specimen must be put in a container large enough to allow sufficient formalin to cover the specimen – this is 8–10 times the volume of the specimen. The specimen pot is labelled carefully with patient details, and the nature of the specimen and a request completed by the clinician. This request should contain patient details, clinical scenario and the required tests, including special examinations, such as oestrogen receptor status. The more information provided to the pathologist on the specimen card, the greater the detail provided in the final report.

The specimen is transferred to the laboratory where fixation in formalin continues for at least 24 hours and often longer for large specimens. Once fixed, the specimen is examined macroscopically, including all cavities and lumina, and then 'cut up' into 1 cm sections through the areas of interest. Specific areas of gross pathology are also addressed at this stage, such as lymph node searches.

Each pathological slice then needs to be set in a wax block to allow thin histological slices to be cut. All water in the tissue is replaced by immersion in increasing concentrations of alcohol, before the tissue is finally immersed in a non-polar solvent, such as toluene; this stage taking a further 24 hours. The specimen blocks are then soaked in molten paraffin wax for 5–6 hours before cooling and slicing using a microtome. The wax is then removed from the individual thin slices by the further use of volatile solvents, the slices mounted on glass microscope slides and stained. The staining procedure used will vary depending on both the tissue being examined and the information being sought; however, in general pathology, the initial stain for virtually all tissues is haematoxylin and eosin; specialist stains are then used to elicit specific information and may include immunofluorescence and antibody staining. The slides are then reviewed under the microscope by a trained histopathologist who dictates a report on the appearances.

It is now standard practice for all reports to be double reported by two pathologists after which the report is produced, checked for accuracy and signed before being issued. The report is divided into macroscopic and microscopic sections with a conclusion at the end.

What is Gram staining?

This is a method of rapidly assessing bacteria. A heat-fixed sample on a microscope slide is flooded with crystal violet and then iodine solution stains. Acetone is then used to decolourize the slide, which is then counterstained with dilute carbol fuschin before microscopic examination. Gram-positive bacteria resist decolorization and, therefore, stain blue–black, whilst Gram-negative bacteria stain pink from the carbol fuschin. Differences in Gram staining represent differences in composition of the bacterial cell wall with Gram-negative bacterial walls having an outer membrane permeated by hydrophilic protein transport channels. Gram-positive bacteria include staphylococci and streptococci as well as *Clostridia*, *Mycobacteria* and *Listeria* amongst others. Gram-negative bacteria include *Pseudomonas*, *Haemophilus*, *Campylobacter*, *Neisseria* and *Escherichia* species.

Which three laboratory methods will confirm the presence of pyogenic infection?

The three methods are direct demonstration, culture and serology. Direct demonstration relies on a sample of pus or fluid and cannot be achieved from a swab. Gram staining or other sorts of stain, such as Ziehl–Neelsen and light microscopy, can be helpful in demonstrating pyogenic bacteria, and treatment can begin on this basis. This method is rapid but non-specific, whereas culture is more time-consuming but generally better. Not only will it confirm the diagnosis of pyogenic infection, but will allow bacterial typing and antibiotic sensitivity to be determined. Serology detects antibodies in the blood to the infective organism. It is generally less satisfactory than culture but is useful in diseases where the infecting organism is difficult or impossible to culture, such as Legionnaire's disease or syphilis.

Hans Christian Gram (1853–1938). Firstly, a professor of pharmacology, and then pathology, before becoming Chief of Internal Medicine. He described the appearances of macrocytes in pernicious anaemia and described his staining method in 1884.

11. DIATHERMY

What is diathermy and how does it work?

Diathermy is the passage of high-frequency alternating current (AC) through the body to produce a localized heating effect. It is also known as electrocautery. Low-frequency current up to 50 Hz causes neuromuscular stimulation at amperages of up to 100 mA, but this effect disappears above the 50 kHz threshold. Surgical diathermy operates in the frequency range of 400 kHz to 10 MHz with amperages of approximately 500 mA, which generates a locally concentrated heating effect of up to 1000°C without widespread neuromuscular stimulation.

There are two types of diathermy: bipolar and monopolar. In monopolar diathermy, the current flows from the current generator to the small active electrode held by the surgeon as either forceps or a point, and the tip of the electrode represents a point of high current density where a heating effect occurs.

Current then flows through the patient and exits via the diathermy plate, which is the second electrode. The much greater surface area of the patient electrode ($\geq 70\,cm^2$) ensures that the current density remains low and no heating effect occurs. In a bipolar system, current passes down one limb of the forceps, passes through structures between the tips of the forceps and returns via the other limb. It is safer than the monopolar system in that only tissue between the tips of the forceps is heated, but it cannot be used for tissue cutting and is generally less effective on bulky tissues.

What is the difference between the 'cutting' and 'coag' settings?

In 'cutting' mode, a continuous output is generated, resulting in arcing between the active electrode and the tissue. Cell water is instantly vaporized, leading to tissue destruction, and some coagulation of vessels. In 'coagulation' mode, a pulsed output is generated, resulting in tissue desiccation and sealing of blood vessels with minimal tissue destruction. Some machines have a 'blend' function, which is a mixture of the two mechanisms and allows cutting of tissue with enhanced coagulation.

What are the risks and complications of diathermy?

Not surprisingly, thermal injury is the biggest risk of diathermy. The common causes of diathermy burns are as follows.

→ *Incorrect application of the patient plate.* This results in decreased surface area of contact and subsequent increased current density.
→ *Patient touching earthed metal.* The current bypasses the diathermy plate and reaches a high current density at the point of metallic contact.
→ *Poor technique.* Using monopolar diathermy on pedicled structures results in high current densities and inadvertent tissue injury. Bipolar diathermy is recommended.
→ *Capacitance (inductive) coupling.* This occurs when the electrode is inside an insulator, with a further conductor outside, as used to occur with metal laparoscopic ports.
→ *Direct coupling of instrument to instrument.* This is, of course, used deliberately when picking up a bleeding vessel in forceps and applying monopolar diathermy to the forceps.
→ *Faulty insulation.*
→ *Pooling of alcoholic skin preparation.* This can be ignited by diathermy.
→ *Explosion of bowel gas.* Care should be taken using diathermy on gut.

Diathermy can also interfere with cardiac pacemakers by inducing either complete pacing block or reversion to fixed rate pacing. Modern devices tend to be less susceptible to these effects. Discussion with a cardiologist beforehand will allow prediction of any likely interactions and monopolar diathermy is best avoided, if possible. If monopolar is essential, then the plate should be sited so that the current does not 'cross' the heart and the anaesthetist should have a magnet available to reset the pacemaker, if necessary.

If a patient suffers a diathermy plate burn on the thigh, who is responsible for it?

Although it is usually the Operating Department Practitioner (ODP) who applies the diathermy plate – and is usually the only one who understands the intricacies of the machine – it remains the operating surgeon's responsibility to ensure that the system is safe to use and that the plate is safely attached to the patient.

12. PORTAL HYPERTENSION

Where are the sites of portosystemic anastomosis?

There are four main sites, as listed in Table 7.3.

Table 7.3 Sites of portosystemic anastomosis

Site of anastomosis	Systemic vessels involved	Portal vessels involved
Lower oesophageal plexus	Lower oesophageal veins	Left gastric veins
Periumbilical	Anterior abdominal wall veins	Paraumbilical portal veins
Lower third of rectum	Middle and inferior haemorrhoidal veins	Superior haemorrhoidal vein
Retroperitoneal organs	Retroperitoneal veins	Superior and inferior mesenteric vein tributaries

Which present clinically most often?

The commonest to present clinically are oesophageal varices, which tend to present with haematemesis, which can be of spectacular proportions. Less commonly, major rectal bleeds occur from rectal varices. The emergence of a pattern of engorged veins across the anterior abdominal wall, known as 'caput medusae' is a common accompaniment to portal hypertension but the retroperitoneal anastomoses tend to be symptom-free; they do, however, bleed torrentially if encountered at operation.

What emergency treatments are available for bleeding oesophageal varices?

The initial treatment is resuscitation of the patient: intravenous fluids via two large-bore cannulae, oxygen by Hudson mask, catheterization, urgent cross-matching of blood and simultaneous haematological investigation, including a clotting profile. Any clotting abnormalities should be corrected appropriately.

The mainstay of emergency management of the bleeding varices is endoscopic diagnosis and therapy. This can be by injection sclerotherapy or variceal banding, which is more commonly practised.

Drug treatments are aimed at reducing variceal blood pressure and flow, and are as effective as tamponade. Somatostatin and its analogues, such as octreotide, are commonly used. Vasopressin can be used to reduce portal pressure or its analogues, such as terlipressin, which may have fewer side effects.

In patients who are still bleeding despite the above measures, haemorrhage may be arrested by tamponade, using a specially designed tube, which is passed down the oesophagus and has one or more channels to allow inflation of balloons for tamponade. Various types are available including Sengstaken-Blakemore and Minnesota tubes (see Figure 7.4), which have both gastric and oesophageal balloons and an aspiration channel for each.

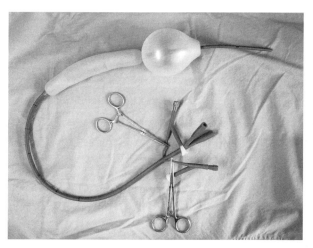

Figure 7.4 A Minnesota tube with both the gastric and oesophageal balloons inflated. Two further aspiration channels can be seen.

Emergency operations are a last resort in variceal haemorrhage and are rarely practised nowadays. The procedures described are lower oesophageal transection or an emergency portosystemic shunting procedure. A newer alternative to surgical shunting is the radiological procedure of transjugular intrahepatic porto-systemic shunting (TIPS). A guidewire introduced through the jugular vein is threaded though the liver and forced into an intrahepatic branch of the portal vein. This track is balloon dilated and held open with a metallic stent, creating a shunt that decompresses the portal system. The decompression itself may actually worsen any encephalopathy and so it should be used with caution. In addition, it is only a temporary solution, as most shunts will thrombose within 1 year.

Does banding varices that have never bled do any good?

There is no evidence to suggest prophylactic treatment is of any benefit.

What is the outlook following a variceal bleed?

The mortality from a first variceal bleed is around 50 per cent. Those that survive have an overall 70 per cent risk of further bleeding and so should be treated aggressively. Repeated endoscopic sclerotherapy or banding of varices should be undertaken until all visible vessels are eradicated and prophylactic atenolol or propranolol should be given, as these have been shown both to reduce mortality from the initial bleed and reduce the risk of rebleeding. Treatment should also aim to improve the underlying portal hypertension and may require hepatic transplantation to achieve this.

13. HUMAN IMMUNODEFICIENCY VIRUS (HIV) INFECTION

Who is at increased risk of acquiring HIV infection?

Human immunodeficiency virus is a highly transmissible retrovirus first suspected in 1981. It is transmitted by sexual contact, blood and tissue products, and *in utero*, and this leads to several well-defined risk groups:

→ homosexual men
→ intravenous drug abusers
→ recipients of blood products, particularly haemophiliacs, prior to 1985
→ residents of endemic areas
→ sexual partners of the preceding groups
→ children of HIV-positive mothers.

Anyone regularly exposed to blood products is at increased risk of HIV infection, which includes health care workers.

How long does it take for seroconversion?

Seroconversion occurs in 85 per cent of cases within 12 weeks of infection. In the remainder it may take as long as 2 years to seroconvert. The 3-month 'seroconversion window' has implications for blood donation, in that it is possible to donate HIV-infected blood before antibody production has commenced, thereby avoiding detection by antibody screening.

What precautions should be taken when operating on a patient who is HIV positive?

Universal precautions should be used routinely for all patients, regardless of HIV or hepatitis status, since the risk of infection is present in all patients. Universal precautions include the wearing of a facemask and impervious gown, with a plastic apron beneath, if heavy contamination is expected. All sharps should be passed between surgeons and scrub nurse using a transit dish. All sharps are disposed of in a self-locking disposable box.

When an operation involves a patient who is known to be HIV positive, then extra precaution should be taken and the theatre staff should be alerted to the 'Category 3' risk, and all clinical specimens should subsequently be labelled as such. Staff in theatre should be kept to a minimum. Surgeons and scrub staff should 'double glove' as the risk of contamination from glove penetration is reduced, and wear a mask with visor or protective eyewear. Protective overshoes are worn. Maximum use of disposable items, including drapes, is recommended and they should be bagged for incineration at the end of the procedure. The use of sharps should be limited, for example, by using diathermy rather than a scalpel to divide tissue. Bodily fluid spills should be cleaned with an appropriate cleaning agent, such as hypochlorite solution.

What surgical conditions are commoner in HIV-positive patients?

Patients who are HIV positive are susceptible to the development of both leukaemia and lymphoma. The surgeon may be called upon to perform excisional lymph node biopsies on these patients to establish the diagnosis. In addition, AIDS-related lymphoma may present in varied extranodal sites, such as perianally, as an intracranial tumour or as an obstructing small bowel tumour. HIV infection is a predisposing cause to the development of fistula-in-ano, anal fissure and perianal sepsis, all of which may present to the general surgeon for management. HIV-salivary gland disease presents much akin to Sjögren's syndrome and sometimes requires superficial parotidectomy to confirm diagnosis.

Aside from risk of infection, are there any other problems arising from operating on HIV-positive individuals?

Many HIV-positive individuals, particularly those in the later stages of the disease, are prone to infection and subsequently are at high risk of developing wound infections after surgery. Healing is often compromised and HIV-positive patients have a higher rate of anastomotic dehiscence than those without the virus. The predisposition to haematological malignancies also interferes with their healing and infection.

Dr Michael Gottlieb described a small group of patients in 1981 who had been treated for Pneumocystis carinii *pneumonia. All were previously fit and healthy, markedly immunodeficient and male homosexuals. He postulated the presence of a new, sexually transmitted, immunosuppresive pathogen. It was a further 2 years before American and French laboratories independently identified the virus to confirm Dr Gottlieb's theory.*

14. LASERS IN SURGERY

What does laser stand for? How do lasers work?

Laser is an acronym that has entered common English usage and represents light amplification of stimulated emission of radiation. It is a device for producing a beam of high-energy electromagnetic radiation. Energy is passed into a lasing medium, usually a gas or crystal, and its constituent electrons release photons of energy as they fall back from an excited to ground state. Amplification occurs by multiple reflection of photons between a pair of mirrors at either end of the lasing cavity, until the laser energy beam eventually escapes the lasing cavity. The laser energy is then channelled into a delivery system, allowing the beam to be produced at the desired site. It is the lasing medium that determines the wavelength of energy emitted.

Which lasers are in common surgical use?

→ CO_2 – an infrared laser that is invisible to the human eye and, therefore, requires a guiding beam. It uses a 'mirror' delivery system. It has very little penetration and is useful in vaporizing surface tissue. Treatment is relatively painless. Healing is rapid, with minimal scarring. It is commonly used in ear, nose and throat surgery for haemostasis and lesion ablation, and in gynaecology for treatment of cervical and vulval pre-cancerous lesions.

→ *NdYAG (neodymium, yttrium, aluminium, garnet).* This is another invisible infrared laser, with penetration of 3–5 mm in tissue. It coagulates larger tissue volumes than a CO_2 laser and leaves an eschar of damaged tissue. It can be used for debulking oesophageal tumours as well as ampullary and rectal cancers. Other indications include control of upper gastrointestinal haemorrhage and ablation of transitional cell carcinomas of the bladder.

→ *Argon*. A blue–green visible laser with little penetration. It is used in ophthalmology for trabeculoplasty and photocoagulation of diabetic retinopathy, and in dermatology for treatment of port wine stains. Both Argon and NdYAG lasers are delivered via fibreoptic cabling.

→ *Ruby*. A visible red laser with superficial effects only. It is used for tattoo removal.

What precautions need to be taken when using lasers?

Each hospital should have a Laser Protection Advisor, and each department a Laser Safety Officer. All persons using the laser should have received adequate training and be named on a designated user list. When in use, a 'laser controlled area' should be established with controlled access and appropriate warning markers. Eye protection is mandatory and should be appropriate to the type and class of laser. The class (1–4) of laser refers to a system reflecting the degree of hazard and power output. Most medical lasers are Class 4. Simple precautions, such as cut-out devices and shrouded foot pedals, should be designed into the machine. The lasing area should be non-reflective.

Is argon beam photocoagulation the same as argon laser? Explain

No, they are different. The argon laser is described above but the argon beam coagulator is a modification of a standard electrocautery circuit. The tip of the electrode emits a stream of inert argon gas that acts as a conducting agent for the current, which can be sprayed on to the tissue without direct contact. It tends to generate only a thin layer of necrotic charred tissue compared to conventional cautery and has the additional advantage that the flow of argon gas will clear away blood from the target site, allowing accurate application of the energy.

15. NUTRITION

How may a patient who is strictly 'nil by mouth' maintain nutritional input?

There are several methods, depending on the circumstances and anticipated duration of restriction of oral input. The ideal is to provide nutrition by the enteral route, which helps to maintain gut mucosal function integrity and decreases bacterial translocation. If the patient is 'nil by mouth' (NBM) to protect an oesophageal anastomosis or following radical maxillofacial surgery, then the enter route may be used by ensuring the food enters the gastrointestinal tract distal to any problem areas. This might be achieved by passage of a nasogastric or nasojejunal tube, although the latter are considerably more difficult to pass. If longer-term enteral nutrition is required, then consideration should be given to the placement of either a gastrostomy or jejunostomy. A gastrostomy can be fashioned operatively at laparotomy or as a percutaneous endoscopic procedure in instances such as long-term feeding in stroke patients. Feeding jejunostomy tubes may also be placed at operation.

If the patient is NBM to rest the gut, then the enteral route is prohibited and feeding will have to be parenteral. In the short term, specially formulated intravenous feeds such as 'Vitrimix' may be used through a standard peripheral cannula, although the high osmolality of the feeds often means a short life span for these lines. Peripherally inserted central lines (PIC lines) are a reasonable compromise allowing peripheral access with central delivery of nutritional mix. Finally, fully-fledged total parenteral nutrition can be given via a central line (Figure 7.5).

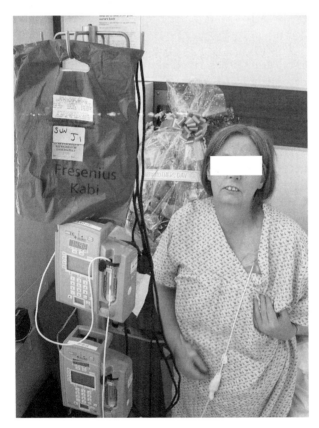

Figure 7.5 Patient receiving TPN. The plastic cover prevents the detrimental effect of prolonged sunlight on the infusion, which is pump controlled and is given in this instance via a Hickman line.

What is the preferred route and why?

If available, the enteral route should be used, as it maintains the integrity of the gut mucosal barrier and reduces bacterial translocation, a primary factor implicated in the pathogenesis of multiorgan dysfunction syndrome and related septic complications. Using this route also obviates the problems of complications associated with central venous access.

What are the complications of TPN?

The complications can broadly be divided into those associated with delivering the TPN and those associated with the metabolism of it.

All those factors that are complications of siting a central line are also the complications of TPN, such as infection, pneumothorax, haemothorax, TPN-thorax, arterial puncture, etc.

TPN gives rise to a wide variety of metabolic disturbances, including hyper- and hypoglycaemia, hyper- and hypokalaemia, hypo- and hypernatraemia, and deranged liver function. This hepatic dysfunction is characterized by intrahepatic cholestasis and fatty infiltration; it is usually self-limiting and resolves after cessation of the TPN.

How many calories and grams of nitrogen should be provided daily?

The requirement for energy and nitrogen in the form of protein varies according to the degree of metabolic stress the patient is under but, in general terms, an adult patient should receive 105–170 kJ/kg per day and 1.3–3.0 g/kg per day of protein. In situations of mild metabolic stress, 1 g of nitrogen should be provided for each 625 kJ of energy provided but, as metabolic stress increases, this ratio falls to 1 g of nitrogen per 420 kJ of energy. A total of 6.25 g of protein provides 1 g of nitrogen.

16. HYPERSENSITIVITY

Describe the four different types of hypersensitivity reaction

See Table 7.4 on page 300.

Discuss latex sensitivity

There are three different types of reactions to natural rubber latex: irritation, contact dermatitis and immediate hypersensitivity. Irritation is classed as a

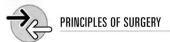

Table 7.4 Types of hypersensitivity reaction

Type	Mechanism	Example
I Anaphylactic	Binding of previously formed antibody on mast cells and basophils on representation of antigen causes degranulation and release of vasoactive amines. IgE-mediated	Anaphylaxis
II Cytotoxic	Antibodies form to normal or damaged cell membrane components, resulting in lysis and phagocytosis of target cell. IgG- and IgM-mediated	Goodpasture's syndrome; transfusion reaction
III Immune complex	Antibodies form to exogenous or non-cellular endogenous antigens. These immune complexes then activate complement and initiate an acute inflammatory response	SLE, some types of acute glomerulo-nephritis
IV Cell-mediated	Activation of sensitized T lymphocytes results in either cytokine release and recruitment of effector cells, such as macrophages or direct T-cell cytotoxicity	Transplant rejection, Mantoux reaction

non-allergic condition. For most people affected, the irritated skin is dry and crusty, and the symptoms resolve when contact with latex ceases. Contact dermatitis represents a type IV delayed hypersensitivity reaction. The affected area becomes dry, crusty and leathery with eruptions of sores and blisters, and typically occurs between 6 and 48 hours post-contact. Repeated latex exposure causes the skin reaction to extend beyond the contact area. A history of atopy, such as dermatitis or asthma, is common in many people with this type of delayed hypersensitivity reaction. Immediate (anaphylactic) hypersensitivity is an example of type I IgE-mediated allergic response caused by circulating antibodies already present at the time of exposure. The cutaneous manifestation of this reaction is a rapid onset urticarial rash extending beyond the area of latex contact. Systemic allergic symptoms include itching eyes, swelling of lips and tongue, breathlessness, dizziness, abdominal pain, nausea, hypotension, shock and, potentially, death in the manner of a true anaphylactic reaction.

Who is at risk of latex allergy?

Latex allergy is still not fully understood, but there is evidence that a history of atopy and a history of latex exposure both increase the likelihood of latex allergy. A history of both appears to be synergistic and confers an even greater risk of allergy than might be expected. People who have regular exposure to latex have an increased risk of allergy and health care workers are a widely affected group. The commonest site of contact is the hands, from latex gloves, which means that surgeons and scrub nurses are two commonly affected groups. All hospitals now provide latex-free gloves for both sterile and non-sterile use.

What precautions should be taken?

A history of latex allergy should be sought in any atopic patient. In known or suspected latex allergy cases, the patient should be put first on the operating list and all procedures undertaken in a latex-free environment. Most anaesthetic departments have a special 'latex-free' trolley for such cases to ensure no equipment that has previously been used with latex is inadvertently used. The patient should have the diagnosis explained to them and advised to carry an 'Alert' bracelet.

17. ONCOGENES

What are oncogenes and proto-oncogenes?

Proto-oncogenes are normal cellular genes that regulate physiological growth and differentiation. If altered or expressed inappropriately, they may give rise to cancer – at this stage, they are referred to as oncogenes and the proteins that result as oncoproteins.

How do oncogenes cause cancer?

Oncogenes and their respective oncoproteins are classified according to their action and mechanism of interference with normal cell-cycle regulation.

→ *Abnormal production of growth factors*. This results in overstimulation of growth and is often coupled with an autocrine loop, as the tumours tend to exhibit receptors for the growth factor. An example is the c-*sis* oncogene causing increased β-chain platelet derived growth factor in astrocytomas.

→ *Abnormal receptors*. Overexpression of growth factor receptors results in inappropriate cellular stimulatory signals and promotion of cell proliferation. This can be seen with c-*erb* B-2, which causes amplification of the epidermal growth factor receptor family in up to 30 per cent of breast cancer.

→ *Abnormal signal transducing proteins*. These transmit stimulatory signals in the absence of physiological stimuli by disablement of the normal intracellular regulatory mechanisms. Thirty per cent of all human tumours contain mutated *ras* genes and the rate is even higher in some tumours, such as colon cancer.

→ *Nuclear proteins.* All subcellular signals ultimately have to be incorporated into nuclear DNA; disruption of the normal nuclear gene transcription in DNA replication is fostered by a wide variety of oncogenes, including c-*myc* in Burkitt's lymphoma.

→ *Cyclin-dependent kinases.* The ultimate step of growth promotion is to stimulate cells to move back into the cell cycle from the resting stage. This is achieved by these kinases and aberrations have been noted in several human cancers, such as cyclin D overexpression in colon and parathyroid tumours.

What is *p53*?

It is a tumour suppressor gene that in healthy cells plays little part in cellular division. If a cell sustains damage to its DNA, through irradiation, for example, then *p53* accumulates in the cell and arrests the cell in G1 phase. Whilst held in G1 phase, the cell has a chance to repair its DNA before continuing to replicate. If the DNA damage is beyond repair, then *p53* forces the cell into apoptosis as programmed cell death will prevent the accumulation of deranged DNA. Aberrations of *p53* function allow increasing amounts of damaged DNA to accumulate, which become entrenched in the dividing cell lines from generation to generation of cell, culminating in tumour formation. Homozygous loss of *p53* is found in virtually all types of human cancers and, in the Li–Fraumeni syndrome, subjects are born with one normal and one mutant *p53* allele, placing them at much higher risk of developing a wide range of cancers.

What is familial adenomatous polyposis? Describe its genetic basis and clinical features

It is a pre-malignant condition that is typified by massive numbers of colonic adenomas at an early age. Left untreated, conversion to malignant colorectal cancer is inevitable before the age of 40 years. It is an autosomal dominant condition with the adenomatous polyposis coli gene on the short arm of chromosome 5. The role of this gene product is not clear, nor is its direct mechanism of tumour formation, but it is believed to regulate cell adhesion molecules, such as E-cadherin. Interruption of these cell adhesion molecules seems to be important in the genesis of colorectal cancer. It accounts for less than 1 per cent of colorectal cancers and has an incidence of 1 in 10 000. As well as colorectal adenomas there are other extracolonic manifestations, including aggressive desmoid disease, duodenal adenomas and periampullary carcinoma. Once identified, genetic and colorectal screening should be instituted for the family concerned. Treatment of choice is elective prophylactic panproctolectomy and ileoanal anastomosis with pouch construction.

After successful colorectal surgery, what is the commonest cause of death in this group?

Approximately 10 per cent of this group will die from duodenal cancers arising from duodenal adenomas and, therefore, after successful colorectal surgery, they should be followed up with regular upper gastrointestinal endoscopy. Any patient who does not undergo proctectomy, such as those treated with colectomy and ileorectal anastomosis, must continue to have the remaining rectal mucosa regularly surveyed to exclude residual adenoma/tumours. All those patients who do have an ileoanal pouch formation should have annual assessment of the anastomotic area, as there is a remaining risk of dysplasia and carcinoma in the remaining transition zone.

Dennis Parsons Burkitt (1911–93). Irish missionary surgeon who described lymphoma of the jaws in African children in 1958; Michael Epstein and Yvonne Barr isolated the implicated virus 6 years later in samples provided by Burkitt. He was a vehement proponent of the benefits of fibre in the diet. He practised throughout his professional life with monocular vision, having lost an eye in a schoolboy fight.

18. MONITORING

How would you monitor a patient under a general anaesthetic?

Monitoring under anaesthesia should ensure that the three components of a balanced anaesthetic – analgesia, hypnosis and paralysis – are progressing correctly, and that the patient's physiological status is as near normal as possible. The monitoring should be a combination of clinical and measured parameters, always remembering to assess the patient, not just the anaesthetic machine.

Pulse is measured continuously and blood pressure regularly, and both may be affected by blood volume changes, analgesic level and drug effects. Oxygen saturation is also measured continuously ensuring that adequate ventilation is occurring. End-tidal CO_2 is continuously measured, which gives a guide to $PaCO_2$, and also warns of any disconnection in the anaesthetic circuit. Muscle relaxation can be assessed by use of a peripheral nerve stimulator, often at the behest of the surgeon. In complex cases, additional monitoring is used, such as arterial lines for continuous invasive blood pressure monitoring, a central line for central venous pressure monitoring, or even a Swan–Ganz catheter to measure left heart filling pressures.

What is end-tidal CO_2 and why is it important?

It is the CO_2 content of the last part of expired air on exhalation, when the CO_2 concentration is at a peak. It is that part of exhaled air that has come from the alveoli, and, as such, gives an approximate guide to the concentration of $PaCO_2$ in the blood. It also functions as an important safety aid, as it demonstrates that the patient is still correctly connected to the ventilator, since end-tidal CO_2 does not rise when the patient is inadvertently disconnected from the anaesthetic circuit.

How would you monitor a patient postoperatively?

The essential monitoring of airway, breathing and circulation in any patient after an anaesthetic should take place in a dedicated recovery area. The airway is kept clear of secretions and the oxygen saturation measured continuously using a pulse oximeter. Blood pressure is measured regularly, or continuously if there is an arterial line in place. Pulse rate is continuously measured by the pulse oximeter. Urine output is monitored hourly, if the patient is catheterized, and any drains and wounds are checked for reactionary bleeding. Temperature is monitored, since hypothermia is a common occurrence during prolonged surgery and the patient should be normothermic before leaving the recovery area. Other monitoring checks take place according to the specifics of the operation and the patient's coexistent medical conditions: diabetics should have blood sugar checked, limb surgery patients should have the limb perfusion checked and neurosurgical patients should have regular GCS recording.

How does pulse oximetry work?

The pulse oximeter is essentially a spectrophotometer. By using visible and infrared light, the ratio of the differences in absorption by oxyhaemoglobin and deoxyhaemoglobin can be calculated. This information is then computed against data obtained experimentally from healthy volunteers and an oxygen saturation calculated. It also resolves the absorption pattern of oxyhaemoglobin found in arterial blood into a pulsatile pattern representative of pulse rate.

Does pulse oximetry detail the adequacy of ventilation?

It does not give any indication of the adequacy of ventilation, as an adequate SaO_2 may be generated by high inspired oxygen concentrations in the face of respiratory failure and carbon dioxide accumulation. In addition, its display lags 20 seconds or so behind real time, so it does not give immediate warning of a catastrophic failure of ventilation.

What are the causes of false readings?

There are several causes and these should always be borne in mind when using a pulse oximeter. Peripheral shutdown, pigmentation, such as deep jaundice and nail varnish, and movement artefact are all causes of false readings. The experimental data against which the machine is calibrated does not extend below O_2 saturations of about 80 per cent, as it was obtained from healthy volunteers; beyond this level the data are extrapolated and an SaO_2 below 70 per cent is inherently unreliable. Pulse oximetry cannot discern between oxy-haemoglobin and carboxyhaemoglobin; thus, in burns cases, the pulse oximeter may markedly overestimate the oxygen saturation.

19. SKIN GRAFTS

Describe the different types of skin grafts

A graft is defined as a tissue or composite of tissues that is transplanted to a new body site independent of its blood supply. The two types commonly used are partial and full thickness grafts, often referred to as split skin grafts (SSG) and Wolfe grafts, respectively. A partial thickness graft takes the surface of the skin, including the epidermis and upper layers of dermis, but leaves the lower dermis and skin adnexa, such as hair follicles and glands intact. This allows regeneration of an epidermal covering at the donor site, primarily derived from the dermal cells surrounding the deep-seated adnexa. Donor-site regeneration usually takes about 10 days. A full-thickness graft takes all layers of the epidermis and dermis, but any underlying subdermal fat that has been inadvertently harvested is trimmed off before grafting at the recipient site. This donor site cannot regener-ate and must be closed as a surgical wound. Because of these differences, partial thickness grafts are thin and hairless and large areas can be harvested, whereas Wolfe grafts tend to be smaller and thicker than SSGs, and contain skin adnexa including hair; they consequently tend to give a better cosmetic match.

Where are the common harvest sites for Wolfe grafts?

As Wolfe graft donor sites must be closed directly as a surgical wound, the com-mon sites are those that will close easily with minimal cosmetic impact. Both the pre- and post-auricular skin can be undermined and closed easily, as can the loose skin above and below the clavicle, particularly in the elderly. The groin and inner arms are further common donor sites, but care must be taken to avoid hair-bearing skin if at all possible.

What sort of tissue bed will not receive a split skin graft?

The obvious consequence of transplanting a graft without its blood supply is that it must be able to acquire a vascular supply rapidly at the recipient site otherwise it will perish. Consequently, avascular surfaces, such as bone without periosteum, tendon, denuded cartilage and irradiated areas will not allow graft 'take'. Areas with movement of the underlying tissue do not take grafts well, as the graft needs to be immobile to allow ingrowth of capillaries; in such instances, steps are taken to immobilize the whole area until the graft has taken securely. Infected surfaces also take SSGs badly, as the increased inflammatory exudate and pus generated tends to float the graft off the recipient bed, which again prevents capillary ingrowth.

What are meshing and fenestration? What are the advantages and disadvantages?

Meshing a split skin graft is a method of increasing the area of the graft by passing it through a special machine that cuts small holes into the graft in a regular pattern, turning the split skin graft into a mesh. Meshing devices can be set to expand the skin graft by a factor of up to six times. Fenestration is a process of perforating the graft by the creation of small holes all over it by hand using a scalpel blade and it creates a porous graft, which allows secretions to pass through.

The only difference between meshing and fenestration is the use of the machine to produce a regular measurable expansion of the graft. The advantages and disadvantages apply more or less equally to both. By creating holes in the graft, it can be used to cover a greater recipient area. It allows tissue exudate to escape from under the graft, thus improving 'take' and it is easier to apply to a complex three-dimensional recipient site, such as an excised pre-tibial laceration. The disadvantages of both of these methods are more scarring and wound contraction, with a less cosmetic final appearance, as the fine mesh pattern remains.

What is the reconstructive ladder when treating wounds?

The reconstructive ladder is the stepwise progression of techniques that can be used to treat an open wound. It escalates from leaving nature to heal itself to complex surgical procedures requiring microvascular anastomoses. The overriding principle of the reconstructive ladder dictates that the simplest approach should be used that will give reliable healing with an optimal cosmetic result. The ladder comprises:

→ healing by secondary intention
→ direct closure with or without undermining or relaxing incisions

→ split skin grafts
→ full thickness skin grafts
→ local flaps – advancement, VY or rotation; these are 'random' flaps utilizing the subdermal plexus of vessels
→ pedicled flaps – here tissue is mobilized on a named vascular supply, which is then inset into the recipient tissue defect, e.g. a pectoralis flap for neck reconstruction
→ free flaps – tissue is isolated on a named vascular supply, which is interrupted and reimplanted at a distant site with microvascular anastomosis of the vessels, e.g. transverse rectus abdominis myocutaneous (TRAM) flap for breast reconstruction.

20. IMAGING

How does ultrasound scanning work, and what are its advantages and disadvantages?

Ultrasound is a medical imaging technique that uses high-frequency sound waves and their echoes to produce an image. The ultrasound machine generates a high-frequency (1–5 MHz) sound wave, which is transmitted to the body via a probe. When the pulse waves reach a boundary between tissues of different characteristics, such as soft tissue and air, some of the energy is reflected and detected by the probe. The remainder of the energy travels further through the body, until it reaches another tissue boundary, where further reflection occurs. The machine analyses the reflected waves in terms of distance to the reflecting boundary, the speed of sound in tissue (1540 m/s) and the time for reflected waves to return to the probe. The machine displays the distances and intensities of the echoes on the screen as a two-dimensional image.

Ultrasonography is safe, quick, cheap and non-invasive. It does not involve ionizing radiation and can be used intraoperatively and endoscopically. Unfortunately, it is highly operator dependent and poor-quality scans make it less useful in obese patients. It gives poorer tissue definition than other modalities and is confounded by overlying gas-filled structures, such as dilated bowel.

How does Doppler ultrasound work and what extra information does it provide?

This is simply ultrasound that employs the Doppler principle. The Doppler effect states that frequency of sound waves reflected from a moving object changes according to the direction and speed of the moving object. The frequency of the

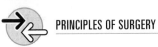

reflected waves is higher if the object is moving towards the probe, and lower if it is moving away from the probe. The magnitude of the frequency shift is dependent on the speed of the target object. Doppler ultrasound uses this principle to assess the speed of a moving target, most commonly intravascular blood, reflecting the ultrasound waves. The information can be represented by an audible signal or by colour-coded flow on the ultrasound machine's screen (duplex scanning). Doppler ultrasound is used mostly to measure the rate of blood flow through the heart and vessels. It can be used to assess arterial supply or venous flow in the investigation of thrombotic disease.

What is a Hounsfield number?

It is a standardized method of representing tissue density on computed tomographic scans. The system of units represents tissue density, reflecting x-ray attenuation, on a scale ranging from −1000 to +1000. Air, by convention, is assigned the value −1000, and water a value of zero. A change of one Hounsfield unit (HU) corresponds to 0.1 per cent of the difference in the attenuation coefficient between water and air.

The use of this standardized scale facilitates the comparison of scans obtained from different CT scanners, and can be used to identify different types of tissue or fluid on a scan; fresh blood has a value of 55HU, for example, whereas a haematoma has a Hounsfield value of 80.

What are the benefits of magnetic resonance imaging over conventional radiology?

Magnetic resonance imaging, previously called nuclear magnetic resonance imaging, generates a three-dimensional image from the energy emitted by hydrogen ions as they realign themselves after being resonated by an array of powerful external magnets. It has many benefits and some disadvantages. MRI scanning does not involve an ionizing radiation dose, which makes it safer than conventional radiology. The data from MRI scanning can be reconstructed in any plane, allowing excellent visualization of abnormalities with high tissue resolution. It is better at delineating between scar tissue, inflammatory tissue and tumour than CT scanning. The MRI can be set to image certain substances selectively, such as certain intravenous contrast agents, allowing MRI angiography. It is the investigation of choice in the assessment of central nervous system tumours and spinal disorders. Although capital outlay costs are high, once established, MRI scanning is relatively cheap. Unfortunately, this cost means that MRI scanning is not as widely available as is desirable. Patients who have metallic implants or fragments may not be suitable for MRI scanning, as it involves lying within an extremely powerful magnetic coil. Many patients find the enclosed tube of the scanner claustrophobic.

List some surgical applications of radionucleotide scanning

→ *Sestamibi scanning* – used to identify parathyroid adenomas. Thallium scanning will outline both thyroid and parathyroid tissue, whereas technetium is only taken up by the thyroid. Subtraction of one from the other images the parathyroid glands.

→ *Red cell scanning* – patients' own red cells are technetium-labelled, re-injected and the patient scanned. It is a method of localizing occult gastrointestinal haemorrhage.

→ *White cell scanning* – labelled white cells are injected into the patient in an attempt to localize foci of sepsis.

→ *Bone scans* – demonstrate metastatic lesions in the skeleton by virtue of their increased vascularity.

→ DTPA (diethylenetriamine penta-acetic acid) and DMSA (dimercapto-succinic acid) scans show the renal pelvis/ureters and the renal cortex function, respectively.

Sir Godfrey Hounsfield (b. 1919). A British engineer and the chief inventor of computed tomographic scanning, which had its first clinical test in 1972. It won him a Nobel Prize in 1979. He had previously led the design team that constructed the first all transistorized computer in UK. He was knighted in 1981.

21. OBESITY

Explain the ways in which the obese patient causes problems to the surgeon

The problems of the obese surgical patient are plentiful. Aside from the technical and anaesthetic problems of operating on the obese, they are at high risk of certain complications and are prone to many coexistent diseases. There are many technical problems encountered when operating on the obese:

→ exposure is limited and the view often obscured by adipose tissue

→ instruments, particularly laparoscopic ones, need to be longer to provide access

→ high pressures are needed for a pneumoperitoneum in laparoscopic work to support the weight of the abdominal wall

→ vessels are less well supported and are more likely to retract causing wound haematomas

→ wounds have increased dead space – collections and infections are commoner

→ the tissues of the abdominal wall are of poor quality and wound dehiscence is commoner.

The anaesthetic problems of obesity are often of even greater importance when considering surgery.

→ Intubation can be extremely difficult in these patients.
→ Higher ventilation pressures are needed.
→ Intravenous access can be problematic.
→ The volume of distribution of drugs is variable owing to variation in distribution in adipose tissue.
→ Respiratory failure owing to hypoventilation consequent on the weight of the thoracic cage. Atelectasis and chest infections are more common postoperatively.
→ Cardiac failure is more common due to increased cardiovascular demands.

The conditions associated with obesity not only increase the frequency with which surgical conditions become apparent but increase the complications associated with subsequent surgery.

→ Diabetes is more common in the obese, increasing wound healing problems and increasing the incidence of vascular disease.
→ Hypertension is more common in obesity and contributes to vascular complications.
→ Obesity is independently associated with increased risk of atherosclerosis, ischaemic heart disease and peripheral vascular disease.
→ DVT and PE in the perioperative period are greater owing to the increased pressure on the calf veins during surgery. This is exacerbated by patient inertia in the postoperative period.
→ Gallstones, gout and osteoarthritis are all more common in the obese. Such patients are poor candidates for surgery for all the above reasons. They are particularly poor candidates for joint arthroplasty because of the excessive wear on the prosthesis.

What is BMI and define the gradations?

BMI stands for body mass index. It is calculated thus:

$$\text{BMI} = \frac{\text{Mass (kg)}}{[\text{Height (m)}]^2}$$

A variety of graduations of BMI have been published and the specifics of them vary slightly. One accepted classification is shown in Table 7.5.

Table 7.5 Graduations of BMI

BMI	Description
<20	Underweight
20–25	Normal
26–30	Grade I obesity – 'overweight'
31–40	Grade II obesity – 'obese'
41–45	Grade III obesity – 'extremely obese'
>45	Morbidly obese

What surgical procedures for treating obesity are in current use? Do they work?

The common surgical procedures are intragastric balloon placement, gastric partitioning and gastric bypass procedures. Jaw wiring is rarely practised these days as it seldom works.

There is evidence that surgery for obesity works but it is heavily dependent on patient selection. The intragastric balloon offers a simple way of assessing whether patients will be able to tolerate and succeed after gastric reduction surgery. A balloon is inserted endoscopically into the stomach and filled with 500 ml of fluid. This limits the gastric capacity. After 3–6 months, however, the stomach adapts, so it is not a permanent solution but, if the patient has maintained some weight loss during this period, then surgery is more likely to have a better outcome.

Gastric partitioning, by vertical banded gastroplasty (Figure 7.6), or more recently by the Swedish laparoscopically placed 'Lap-band', partitions a small reservoir of stomach 30–50 ml in volume in the proximal stomach. The small reservoir prevents large meals being eaten. Gastric bypass procedures involve joining a distal portion of bowel to the stomach, bypassing a portion of proximal

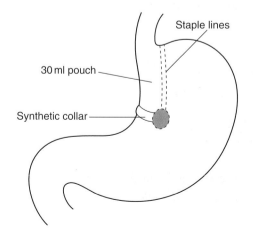

Staple lines

30 ml pouch

Synthetic collar

Figure 7.6 Vertical banded gastroplasty.

bowel. The commonest bypass procedure currently is an anastomosis of the distal small bowel to the proximal stomach as a roux-en-Y procedure, thereby limiting the amount of small bowel absorption that can occur. Given the huge potential for psychological and physical morbidity from these procedures, each patient should be assessed, and treatment options considered, on an individual basis.

Patients can obtain excellent weight loss after these procedures, often to within 30 per cent of ideal weight, but close follow-up is needed to maintain this benefit in most patients.

22. PAEDIATRIC HIPS

What does orthopaedics actually mean?

Orthopaedics is derived from two Greek words; *orthos* meaning 'straight' and *paedion* meaning 'child'. It was originally used to describe the correction of deformities of children, but now denotes the speciality involved in the correction of conditions affecting the locomotor/skeletal system.

Describe the conditions affecting the hips of children and outline your management strategy for each

Four conditions commonly affect childhood hips. They generally occur at different stages of the child's development: congenital dislocation, septic arthritis, Perthes' disease and slipped upper femoral epiphysis.

→ *Congenital dislocation* occurs when the acetabulum is too shallow and the femoral head is allowed to slide off posteriorly. It is suspected by a lack of abduction on Ortolani's test and occurs at a rate of about 1 in 500 live births. The management and subsequent prognosis is related to the age at which it is diagnosed. When diagnosed in the newborn, the hip should be reduced and splinted in flexion and abduction for 3–6 months until ultrasound scanning reveals a congruent acetabular roof and a stable joint. If diagnosis is delayed until between 6 months and 6 years, the hip is reduced by traction on a vertical frame with gradually increasing abduction over 3 weeks with relocation confirmed by scanning. The hips are then held in plaster in at least 90 degrees of flexion and 45 degrees of abduction for 6 weeks before being replaced by a splint. If this fails, then operative reduction is necessary, with or without reconstruction of acetabulum. With late diagnosis, after the age of 6 years, bilateral dislocations are usually not corrected because of the risk of creating asymmetry. Unilateral dislocations are corrected operatively with acetabular reconstruction.

→ *Pyogenic arthritis* in children usually occurs between the ages of 0 and 5 years, and most happen before the infant is 2 years old. Staphylococcal infections are commonest and may arise from a distant septic focus or from an adjacent osteomyelitis. The child is unwell and in pain, although they may be unable to localize the pain. The leg is kept still. Diagnosis is confirmed by aspiration of the joint. Treatment consists of intravenous antibiotics with joint wash out as required.

→ *Perthes' disease* is an avascular necrosis of the femoral head occurring in children usually between the ages of 5 and 10 years. It is more common in boys and the typical patient is a young boy of between 4 and 8 years who presents with a painful limp. Joint movement may be well preserved initially, although abduction is rarely complete. Depending on the stage of the disease, plain radiographs may show nothing at all or increased density of the epiphysis and widened joint space. Treatment initially is the same for all, and consists of bed rest and traction to settle the pain and joint irritability. Thereafter, if the radiological appearances are favourable, no active treatment is needed. If an unfavourable prognosis is expected, then treatment is aimed at 'containing' the femoral head within the acetabulum either by holding the hips abducted in plaster for up to a year or by femoral osteotomy.

→ *Slipped upper femoral epiphysis (SUFE)* is a disorder of teenagers, boys more than girls (Figure 7.7). The very tall and the fat prepubertal boys are most commonly affected, and the onset is sudden in only 30 per cent of cases. If untreated, coxa vara and secondary arthritis are likely to follow. Treatment is surgical and is directed by the degree of slippage. If less than one-third of the width of the epiphysis is displaced, it is fixed where it is with AO screws. If the displacement is between one-third and one-half of the epiphyseal width, then it is fixed in a similar manner, but a later osteotomy may be needed. If severely displaced, surgical correction is needed either by removing a small piece of the femoral neck to allow reduction and pinning or pinning *in situ* coupled with corrective osteotomy. Direct correction of the epiphyseal slip is avoided if possible, as it is likely to result in interruption of the blood supply to the femoral head.

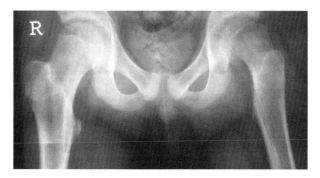

Figure 7.7 A slipped left upper femoral epiphysis.

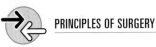

Georg Clemens Perthes (1869–1927). German surgeon who performed many early experiments into the effects of radiation, pioneering the use of radiotherapy for carcinoma of the breast. The condition that bears his name was also described by Jacques Calvé and Arthur Legg, and is sometimes known as Calvé–Legg–Perthes disease or a variation thereof. It was first described by Karl Maydl some 10 years previously.

23. FRACTURES

Classify fractures

In general, all fractures may be classified as open or closed, dependent on whether the overlying skin is intact, or complete or incomplete, according to whether both cortices are involved. Other non-specific methods in common use describe fractures in terms of the displacement, degree of comminution, aetiology (fatigue or pathological) and the pattern produced (oblique, spiral, transverse or impacted). Specific, often eponymous, classifications have developed over time to describe particular fractures, such as the Garden system for intracapsular femoral neck fractures and the Weber lateral malleolar ankle fracture classification.

The AO system for classification of fractures of long bones is a general classification system for fractures. Each long bone has been assigned a number, e.g. humerus – 1, radius and ulna – 2, femur – 3, and a second digit is added to indicate the proximal segment – 1, shaft – 2 or distal segment – 3. The severity is graded A, B or C, with C being the most severe. The further coding is specific to each bone, but consists of a group and subgroup, both assigned a numerical code. Thus, AO 32-A2,1 represents femur (3), mid-shaft (2), least severe fracture (A) oblique fracture (group 2), proximal shaft where medulla is wider (1). It is a complex and unwieldy system to use in clinical practice, but is applicable to all long bones and limits personal interpretation.

What is Gustilo and Anderson's classification?

It is a classification of open fractures, which specifically describes the degree of soft tissue injury.

→ Type I – open fracture with a clean wound less than 1 cm. A low-energy injury.
→ Type II – open fracture with a wound more than 1 cm, not associated with extensive soft tissue damage, avulsions or flaps.
→ Type IIIa – open fracture with adequate coverage of bone despite extensive soft tissue damage; or high-energy trauma irrespective of wound size.

→ Type IIIb – open fracture with extensive soft tissue loss, periosteal stripping and exposure of bone.

→ Type IIIc – open fracture with an associated arterial injury.

There is a high degree of interobserver error with this classification and it tends to concentrate on wound size as opposed to tissue damage; however, it is the system in common clinical use. Note that there is a progression of severity from Type I through to Type IIIb but Type IIIc is essentially a separate category.

How can fractures be immobilized and give appropriate clinical examples?

Fracture immobilization can be by continuous traction, cast splintage, functional bracing, or internal or external fixation.

→ *Continuous traction* is applied along the long axis of a bone to hold a fracture out to length. It can be obtained by using adhesive tape to stick to the skin – skin traction – or more commonly by inserting a distal pin to allow much greater traction force to be applied. It is used, for example, in some spiral femoral fractures with a Steinman or Denham pin through the proximal tibia.

→ *Cast splintage* is the use of plaster of Paris, or newer synthetic substitutes to encase the fracture, completely immobilizing it. It is routinely used for most Colles' fractures.

→ *Functional bracing* is the application of cast segments connected by hinges allowing movement at joints in one plane. It is most commonly used for tibial fractures but, since it is not as rigid as other techniques, is usually used after 3–6 weeks of traction or conventional plaster.

→ *Internal fixation* implies operative reduction of the fracture and the use of pins, screws, plates or nails to fix the reduced fracture in position. Femoral shaft fractures may be fixed by insertion of an intramedullary nail.

→ *External fixation* holds a fracture position by transfixing screws above and below the break attached to an external frame. It is commonly used for open contaminated fractures, typically of the tibia.

24. CHEMOTHERAPY

Describe how the various groups of cytotoxic chemotherapeutic agents work

→ *Alkylating agents* (chlorambucil, cyclophosphamide). These work by the alkyl group combining with intracellular nucleic acids, proteins and cell membranes, damaging DNA linkage, which stops cell division.

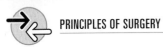

→ *Antimetabolites* (methotrexate, 5-fluorouracil). These compounds are inactive analogues of the compounds required for nucleic acid formation, and are incorporated instead, inactivating the enzyme production pathway.

→ *Vinca alkaloids* (vincristine, vinblastine). These bind to intracellular tubulin inhibiting microtubule formation and arresting mitosis.

→ *Antimitotic antibiotics* (Adriamycin, bleomycin). These work by a number of mechanisms, some intercalate between DNA strands, some impair DNA/RNA synthesis.

What are the principles behind combination therapy?

Clinical resistance to the chemotherapeutic agents can occur and combination chemotherapy reduces this effect. Its underlying principle is to use drugs with different mechanisms of action, allowing a greater cumulative dose of chemotherapeutic drugs with limitation of the side effects of each. It is axiomatic that each drug should be effective as monotherapy against the tumour and have different side-effect profiles.

What are the common complications of chemotherapy?

The complications may be divided into acute and long-term toxicity. Acute toxicity manifests itself in several ways.

→ *Local.* Some cytotoxic agents are extremely damaging to soft tissues if inadvertent extravascular injection should occur. Typical examples are doxorubicin and the vinca alkaloids.

→ *Gastrointestinal.* Nausea and vomiting are common with many agents, including cisplatin, cyclophosphamide and doxorubicin, and are generally due to central stimulation. Dexamethasone, domperidone or 5-hydroxytryptamine antagonists, such as ondansetron, should be given prophylactically before treatment. Methotrexate may cause a mucositis.

→ *Alopecia.* It is often the side effect that worries patients the most and occurs with doxorubicin, cyclophosphamide and etoposide. Patients should be reassured that the hair loss is temporary.

→ *Bone marrow.* This is often the dose-limiting factor when administering cytotoxics and should be checked by a full blood count before each treatment cycle. If granulocyte counts are low, prophylactic antibiotics are indicated and, if very low, granulocyte colony-stimulating factors should be added.

The two main long-term complications are carcinogenesis and gonadal failure. Long-term treatment with agents such as melphalan gives rise to a risk of development of leukaemia. Treatment of Hodgkin's disease is likely to induce complete gonadal failure. Chlorambucil and procarbazine are the agents responsible. Pre-therapy sperm or egg donation is usually recommended.

Describe the use of hormonal therapy in the treatment of prostate cancer

Both breast and prostate cancers are hormone dependent, and control of the disease may be achieved by manipulation of the hormonal milieu. Hormonal therapy in prostate cancer is indicated in those cases where radical therapy is not a sensible step. There is a debate regarding the patient with advanced local disease treated by prostatectomy of whatever sort who is clinically free from metastases, as to when hormone therapy should be instituted. Current evidence suggests that outcome is no worse if hormone treatment is delayed until the appearance of metastases. Those with metastases should receive hormone treatment. The aim of treatment is to suppress androgen production. This may be achieved by bilateral orchidectomy or by chemical castration. Diethylstilboestrol is an effective agent, but has many side effects and is rarely used. Current treatment protocols would begin treatment with a luteinizing hormone-releasing hormone (LHRH) agonist, such as goserelin, given parenterally. The initial testosterone 'flare' from overstimulation may cause worsening of symptoms and should be covered with an anti-androgenic agent, such as cyproterone acetate. LHRH analogues may obtain a good response for months or even years, but eventually all prostate cancers escape hormonal control and attention should turn to effective palliation of symptoms, as second-line therapy is rarely effective.

What is neoadjuvant chemotherapy?

Neoadjuvant chemotherapy is the use of chemotherapy as an initial treatment before surgery. It is commonly used in patients with localized but extensive tumours where local control may be improved by combining two modalities of treatment. This may render an inoperable tumour operable or, in specific circumstances, may allow wide local excision rather than mastectomy for a large primary breast tumour.

25. SURGICAL AUDIT

What is audit?

Audit is defined as 'the systematic, critical analysis of the quality of medical care, including the procedures used for diagnosis and treatment, the use of resources and the resulting outcome and quality of life for the patient'.

Who takes part and how often?

All doctors are required to take part. All the people who are involved in delivering the health care of the particular process being audited should attend the relevant audit meeting. This includes nursing and ancillary staff as well as clinicians.

The Government and Medical Royal Colleges state that audit should be held regularly, and this varies from unit to unit. In some centres, a short weekly meeting is held, whereas in others it is held every 3 months with a session set aside for the meeting.

Is it voluntary?

No. Since 1989, the Department of Health has made it a requirement of every hospital doctor to participate in audit.

What types of audit are there?

The all-encompassing title of audit may be subdivided in several ways. It may be an overall process examining all admissions, investigations, procedures, finances, operations, and morbidity and mortality, or may be topic-based, concentrating on a specific area, such as results of temporal artery biopsy over a 5-year period.

Audit may also be described by the three main elements of health care it looks at, namely; structure, process and outcome. Audit of structure analyses the infrastructure and resources available to provide care, and is not often clinically relevant. Audit of process examines the way in which a patient is treated from start to finish of a clinical episode and might include such things as waiting times, drug prescribing or operative technique. Outcome audit is the sort most familiar to clinicians, and is based on the traditional mortality and morbidity meeting, although other factors may be assessed, such as length of hospital stay and patient satisfaction.

What does 'closing the loop' mean?

Audit is a circular process that runs as follows: an area of concern is identified and a set of ideal standards laid down. This is the level that should be achieved. The relevant data pertaining to that area are collected, examined and a comparison made to the 'ideal' standard. If deficiencies against the standard are identified, corrective measures are instituted into that specific area of practice. After a suitable time, further data are collected and re-examined hopefully to demonstrate an improvement in performance and the attainment of the standards. It is this re-examination after change that is referred to as 'closing the loop'. It is important that audit is a tool for change and improvement rather than merely collection of data, and closing the loop is the means of demonstrating that the audit has been effective. However, it should be noted that audit is an ongoing process and does not end with closing the loop, but is more akin to a spiral, as the new changes are re-audited.

What is clinical governance?

It is defined as 'A system through which the NHS organizations are accountable for continuously improving the quality of their services and safeguarding high standards of care, by creating an environment in which clinical excellence will flourish'. It has been introduced in an attempt to improve the performance of the NHS and is a requirement for all trusts and staff. All NHS trusts must institute effective means of identifying and managing risk, introduce lines of responsibility and have a widespread policy for quality improvement. It is different from audit, although audit is one tool that might be used to demonstrate those improvements that clinical governance requires. It is overseen by the Commission for Health Improvement (CHI), who regularly inspect hospitals to ensure that the relevant standards are being met. For the clinician it involves standard setting, often centrally by the National Institute for Clinical Excellence (NICE), as part of the National Service Frameworks. Professional self-regulation that is transparent should ensure that clinical standards are met, and clinicians should be updated continuously by involvement in continuing professional development (CPD) and lifelong learning. All of this is overviewed by CHI.

Index

Page numbers in **bold type** refer to figures; those in *italics* to tables